Alexa Wright is Reader in Visual Culture at the University of Westminster. She is also a practising visual artist who works with video, sound and interactive digital media.

'Alexa Wright offers an intriguing meditation on the survival of some classical rhetorics of monstrousness in medieval and especially modern visual cultures. Well illustrated and lively, this book will appeal to anyone intrigued by the history of monsters.'

Jeffrey J. Cohen,
Professor of English, George Washington University

'Alexa Wright's thought-provoking new book takes the study of human monstrosity from its earliest manifestation in Pliny's Monstrous Races right up to an analysis of contemporary mass murderers. Using a plethora of illustrations, Wright investigates Foucault's contention that the human monster has vanished from view to be replaced by monstrous character and behaviour to show how iconography still remains crucial to our ability to place and contain those who deeply disturb us. The great strength of Monstrosity lies in the author's deft handling of complex and scholarly images and analysis alongside the expression of her own fascination and puzzlement. The questions "What is truly human?" and even "Who am I?" are never far from the surface.'

Margrit Shildrick,
Professor of Gender and Knowledge Production,
Linköping University, and author of *Embodying the Monster*

'With *Monstrosity*, Alexa Wright offers a provocative and fresh understanding of the monster, the cultural figure that has haunted the human imagination from antiquity to the present. Human monsters, Wright demonstrates, are the unusual and unexpected beings which are on the very edges of the human and onto which we have projected and continue to project our own meanings, fears and fantasies. Alexa Wright's unique contribution to the recent conversation about human monsters comes from her perspective as a photographer. Approaching the human monster from the visual perspective as she does allows Wright to consider the complicated human dilemma about knowing what we see and seeing what we know.'

Rosemarie Garland-Thomson,
Professor of Women's Studies, Emory University

Alexa Wright

Monstrosity

The Human Monster in Visual Culture

I.B. TAURIS
LONDON · NEW YORK

Published in 2013 by I.B.Tauris & Co. Ltd
6 Salem Road, London W2 4BU
175 Fifth Avenue, New York NY 10010
www.ibtauris.com

ISBN: 978 1 78076 335 4 (hbk)
ISBN: 978 1 78076 336 1 (pbk)

A full CIP record for this book is available from the British Library
A full CIP record is available from the Library of Congress

Library of Congress Catalog Card Number: available

Typeset by JCS Publishing Services Ltd, www.jcs-publishing.co.uk
www.bloomsbury.com

Contents

List of Illustrations vii
Acknowledgements x

Introduction 1
1 Monstrous Strangers at the Edge of the World: The Monstrous Races 9
2 Blurring the Boundaries of Nature and Culture: Wild People and Feral Children 27
3 Bodies and the Order of Society: The Greek Ideal, the Monster of Ravenna and Physiognomy 47
4 Monsters in Proximity: Freaks and the Spectacle of Abnormality 79
5 A Monstrous Subject: Representations of Joseph Merrick, the 'Elephant Man' 104
6 Monstrous Images of Evil: Picturing Jack the Ripper and Myra Hindley 125
7 Modern Monsters and the Image of Normality: Ted Bundy and Anders Breivik 145
Afterword 164

Notes 167
Bibliography and Further Reading 193
Index 209

Illustrations

1.1 The Monstrous Races, Arnstein Bible, *c.*1172 (British Library, Harley 2799, f. 243) 8
1.2 Panotii, lintel of Basilique Ste-Madeleine, Vézelay, France, *c.*1125–30 13
1.3 Richard of Haldingham, Mappa Mundi, *c.*1300 (Hereford Cathedral) 22
1.4 Detail from a nineteenth-century facsimile of the Hereford Mappa Mundi, showing Monstrous Races at the edge of the world 23
2.1 Alexander and the Wild Man, painted manuscript illumination, *c.*1420 (© The British Library Board) 36
2.2 Alexander and the Wild Man, painted manuscript illumination, *c.*1410–12 (© Bibliothèque nationale de France) 37
2.3 Jean Bourdichon, 'The Wild Condition', *c.*1500 (© L'École nationale supérieure des beaux arts, Paris) 38
2.4 'What Is It?', poster originally produced in London, *c.*1846 (© The British Library Board) 40
2.5 Oxana Malaya (Courtesy of Animal Planet) 45
3.1 Leonardo da Vinci, 'Vitruvian Man', *c.*1487 (Photo: Luc Viatour) 50
3.2 Gregor Reisch, 'De Astrologia – Astrological Man', 1503 (Wellcome Library, London) 51
3.3 Roman copy of Myron's 'Discobolus' ('Discus Thrower') (© Trustees of the British Museum) 53
3.4 The Monster of Ravenna from a German broadside of 1506 (Bayerische Staatsbibliothek Munich, Einbl. VIII, 18) 55
3.5 Licetus, 'The Monster of Ravenna', 1634 (The Liverpool Medical Institution) 56
3.6 Leonardo da Vinci, 'Five Grotesque Heads', *c.*1480–1510 (Supplied by Royal Collection Trust. © HM Queen Elizabeth II 2012) 63
3.7 Charles Le Brun, 'The Head of an Ox and the Head of an Ox-like Man', *c.*1820 (Wellcome Library, London) 64

3.8 Johann Kaspar Lavater, 'Eight Ways of Looking at Socrates', 1789 66
3.9 Sir Francis Galton, composite portraits, 1883 (UCL Library Services, Special Collections) 69
3.10 Cesare Lombroso, 'Six Criminal Types', 1888 (Wellcome Library, London) 72
3.11 Hugh Welch Diamond, 'Religious Melancholy', *c*.1850–8 (Royal Society of Medicine, London) 76
3.12 Lithograph after Figure 3.11, 1858 (Royal Society of Medicine, London) 77
4.1 'JoJo, the Russian Dog-faced Boy', *c*.1884 (Photo: Charles Eisenmann. Courtesy of Michael Mitchell) 84
4.2 Henry Johnson as 'Zip' with Ashbury Benjamin, the 'Leopard Boy', *c*.1885 (Photo: Charles Eisenmann. Courtesy of Michael Mitchell) 88
4.3 Freak show at the Rutland Fair, Vermont, 1941 (Photo: Jack Délano. Library of Congress, Prints and Photographs Division, FSA-OWI Collection) 91
4.4 Bearded lady, Madame Devere, *c*.1878 (Photo: Charles Eisenmann. Courtesy of Michael Mitchell) 95
4.5 Bearded lady, Madame Devere, with her husband, *c*.1878 (Photo: Charles Eisenmann. Courtesy of Michael Mitchell) 96
4.6 Charles Tripp, calling card, 1885 (Photo: Charles Eisenmann. Courtesy of Michael Mitchell) 98
5.1 Letter written by Joseph Merrick to Leila Maturin, 7 October 1889 (The Record Office for Leicestershire, Leicester and Rutland, ref. DE3644) 106
5.2 Medical photographs of Joseph Merrick, 1886 (Royal London Hospital Archives) 117
5.3 Carte de visite portrait of Joseph Merrick in his 'Sunday-best' suit, *c*.1887 (Royal London Hospital Archives) 119
5.4 Merrick's cap and veil (Royal London Hospital Archives) 121
6.1 Sketches of Jack the Ripper, 20 October 1888 (© Museum of London) 132
6.2 Photo-fit of Jack the Ripper, compiled for police at Scotland Yard in 2006 134
6.3 Widely distributed version of the police mug shot of Myra Hindley, 1965 (Original © Cheshire Police) 138

6.4 Version of the image of Myra Hindley as it appears on the *Daily Telegraph* website 138
6.5 Hindley in prison, *c*.1993 (© The Daily Star. Express Newspapers) 139
6.6 Marcus Harvey, *Myra*, 1995 (Courtesy of the artist) 141
6.7 Police mug shots of Hindley and Brady on the front page of the *Daily Mirror*, 7 May 1966 142
6.8 The photograph of Hindley on the front page of the *Daily Mirror*, 16 November 2002 143
7.1 Some of Ted Bundy's various guises 150
7.2 Anders Behring Breivik, passport photograph 159

Acknowledgements

I owe special thanks to Helen Coxall, without whom this project would never have been realized. Thanks also to David Bate, Alex Warwick, Peter Ride, Stefan Szelkun and others at the University of Westminster who made helpful comments in the early stages of the project. A very big thank you to Clare Waite, whose encouragement and insight helped me to clarify my ideas and reshape later drafts of the chapters, and to Mari Roberts for her incisive editorial suggestions. Thanks to Liza Thomson at I.B.Tauris for believing in this project and for her support as commissioning editor, and to Frances Underhill for helping with image permissions during her internship at I.B.Tauris.

Every effort has been made to contact the copyright holders of images used in this book; if any have been omitted inadvertently, acknowledgement will be made at the earliest opportunity.

In memory of Helen Coxall

Introduction

Some twenty years ago I came across a reproduction of a strangely compelling image entitled 'The Monstrous Races of the World' (Figure 1.1) in a library book. Where did this odd array of people with their faces on their chests, or with hooves or backward-facing feet come from? I was intrigued when, on closer inspection, I saw that one has a dog's head, one has horns and a long, straw-like nose, whilst another seems to be licking the top of its own head with a giant tongue. The awkward but elegant medieval aesthetic of these figures attracted me, but what did they mean? As a visual artist making work about human physicality and the expression of identity, I was particularly interested in the literal way in which these strange creatures embody difference, or 'otherness'. I photocopied the picture and kept returning to it over the next few years. My excursion into the world of human monsters had begun.

It is perhaps significant that the research that has, eventually, culminated in this book began with the Monstrous Races. They seem to provide a good starting point for an investigation into human monstrosity for several reasons, not least because they immediately draw attention to the symbolic power of the human body. Their irregular, transgressive bodies directly and clearly illustrate the main historical purpose of human monsters – that is, to provide a tangible site for exploring the problem of what constitutes acceptable human identity. Whilst the earliest records of the Races date from at least the fifth century BC, they were especially popular during the Middle Ages. Their mixed-up bodies manifest the confusion experienced by early Western travellers as they encountered people with unfamiliar customs and appearances in different parts of the world. It seems that exotic characters such as these were believed by ancient and medieval scholars and lay people alike to actually exist in the uncharted territories at the edges of the geographical world. Europeans believed that here, far from Western civilization, nature was free to create all sorts of strange and magical forms.

As the scope of my research into human monsters began to extend beyond the Monstrous Races I soon realized that the topic of human monstrosity is far reaching and has both political and theoretical implications. The monstrous is of consequence to every branch of learning, from biology, physiology, psychology, sociology and anthropology to criminology and law, history, geography, philosophy and visual culture, as well as many other fields of inquiry. Like its subject matter, this book is eclectic. As a visual artist, my work is not aligned to a particular academic discipline. I have, therefore, freely referenced material from a broad range of different sources in order to formulate this study, which focuses on the *visual* significance of human monsters in particular.

Each chapter of the book is constructed around one or more historical examples, or case studies. Following a trajectory in which they become less and less distinct from 'normal' members of society, the examples are arranged chronologically, starting with the Monstrous Races and ending with the contemporary mass murderer Anders Breivik. But this is not supposed to be a history of monsters. Acknowledging that all histories are plural and subjective, the intention of the book is to analyse the meaning and function of 'real' human monsters in Western visual culture. It investigates the appearance of the monster as a manifestation of that which disturbs the social 'norm', or troubles an existing understanding of what is acceptably human. Michel Foucault uses historical case studies to reconstruct the context and conditions that have given rise to a particular problem, rather than to provide 'historically correct' 'evidence' or proof of past events. In line with his approach, this book aims to offer a context for thinking about the broader social implications of monsters and the monstrous.[1] The examples discussed in the following chapters are intended to build up a picture of the main attributes of all monsters, even if these are expressed differently at different times. Collectively the case studies aim to show how, even though the form that human monstrosity takes changes in line with ideas of self-identity and our shifting social and moral values, the social function of the monster remains constant.

Theoretical Background

Whilst this project draws on ideas from a wide variety of disciplinary contexts, the work of the French philosopher Michel Foucault is key. Foucault's interdisciplinary thinking, his relentless questioning of established structures and his unconventional approach to history are perfectly suited to the study of monsters. The historical transition from morphological to behavioural monstrosity that Foucault outlines in *The Abnormal*, a series of lectures given at the Collège de France in 1974–5, and then again in a 1978 lecture on 'The Dangerous Individual' offers new ways of thinking about 'otherness'. The ideas that he sets out here form the main theoretical foundation for this book.[2] Another key text is 'Monstrosity and the Monstrous', an essay based on a lecture delivered in Brussels in 1962 by the French philosopher and historian of life sciences, Georges Canguilhem.[3] Canguilhem was Foucault's mentor and is said to have profoundly influenced Foucault's thinking.[4] Foucault acknowledges this in his introduction to Canguilhem's *The Normal and the Pathological*, where he writes that Canguilhem 'brought about a significant shift' in the history of science.[5]

As most of the existing literature on monsters confirms, the words 'monster', 'monstrosity' and 'monstrousness' all have their etymological root in the Latin *monstrare*, meaning both to show and also to warn or advise. This original meaning is particularly important in the context of this book because it shows that monstrosity is by definition a visual phenomenon. Although these three words, monstrousness, monstrosity and monster, are generally used as though they were interchangeable, they actually mean different things. This distinction is important because it separates the social and cultural effects of monstrousness from its manifestation. The idea of monstrousness encapsulates the impossible, dreadful, amoral, inhuman, unspeakable and even unthinkable qualities that lie at the periphery of human identity. The monstrous is the inverse or outside of what is acceptably human in any particular social or cultural context.

As the tangible means by which the unspeakable and threatening force of the monstrous is brought into being, monstrosity is both an effect and a cause of monstrousness. According to both Foucault and Canguilhem, up to the end of the eighteenth century monstrosity was understood to be a corporeal irregularity that operated as a manifestation or sign of monstrousness. Canguilhem emphasizes the distinction between monstrosity and the monstrous, whilst at the same time highlighting their interdependence as 'a duality of concepts' which are 'at the service of two forms of normative judgement, the medical and the legal'.[6] Monstrosity is never an intrinsic quality. It is a narrative imposed on certain appearances or behaviours at particular times in specific social contexts.

A monster is the individual object, or subject, in which monstrousness and monstrosity come together. One paradoxical feature of the monstrous/monstrosity/monster triad is that, although monsters and monstrosities act to symbolize or 'realize' monstrousness, what is truly monstrous is that which stands outside the processes of representation or articulation. This book aims to show that once it can be symbolized, monstrousness loses its terrible power.

Foucault and Canguilhem differ in their understanding of the status of monstrosity from the late eighteenth century onwards. Canguilhem argues that corporeal monstrosity, which was once visually identifiable in the distorted bodies of monsters, has been eradicated or rendered 'transparent' by modern science.[7] He maintains that once physical deformity can be understood and controlled by science, the relationship between monstrosity (as an effect of the monstrous) and the monstrous (an infraction of the law that results from monstrosity) breaks down, and the monster disappears. More controversially, he proposes that with the advent of modern scientific explanation all previous forms of monstrousness have been relegated to the realms of myth and imagination.[8]

Foucault builds on the idea that monstrosity was traditionally a physical aberration that points to underlying monstrousness, but he does not insist on a causal relation between the two. In his account, even if by the end of the eighteenth century human monstrosity was no longer manifested in physical deformity, it did not cease to exist. It would become 'something that really will be a monstrosity, that is to say, monstrosity of character'.[9] In this view, modern monstrosity is 'a moral monstrosity . . . a monstrosity of behaviour' which is no longer visual.[10] And yet, as I will argue in the following chapters, the processes of representation and visualization do still play an important part in the attempt to come to terms with what is considered monstrous.

Content of the Chapters

Chapter 1 focuses on the classical Monstrous Races. Whilst from a contemporary perspective it is clear that the majority of these creatures were mythical beings, in the context of this book it is important that they were once commonly believed to be 'real'. For many people the word 'monster' suggests invented and exotic beasts such as the fantastic creatures of children's fiction, or extra-terrestrial beings as in Ridley Scott's *Alien*. But this book is about a different kind of monster. Whilst the term 'real' is complex for many reasons, it is used here to indicate those monsters that are, or have been, understood to have their origins in the world of human experience, rather than in the fictional worlds of novels or films. All monsters are representational constructs, but those that are understood to exist in the 'real world' have a greater impact on the established understanding of what constitutes 'normal' or acceptable human being.

Chapter 2 looks at medieval 'wild people' and feral children in the context of ideas about 'nature' and 'culture', the 'civilized' and the 'uncivilized'. These social outsiders, who live apart from mainstream society, manifest both human and animal features. In the Western, Judeo-Christian tradition, humans have always been thought of as radically separate from other animals thanks to their intellect and possession of a soul. The process of setting us apart from other animals is crucial to the construction of 'normal' human being, which is perhaps why the perceived boundary between humans and animals has always been complex and fraught. One of the most important tasks of the human monster is to draw out some of the confusions that arise at this boundary.

If 'normal' human bodies have acted as a model for interpreting the 'natural' or correct structure of the external world, the unintelligible body of the monster has historically provided an exposition of moral, social or ontological uncertainty.[11] Systems such as astrology and physiognomy can offer a historical context for understanding how monstrousness has been represented in the body of the monster. Chapter 3 examines some of the ways in which the human body, and particularly the face, has been treated as a legible structure from which the order of society or the characteristics of an individual can be determined. The figure of the sixteenth-century Monster of Ravenna is discussed here because it clearly shows how social and political disorder was historically manifested in bodily deformities. The mixed-up body of this strange creature is literally assembled from a collection of parts, each of which transgresses a 'natural' boundary.

Chapter 4 contests Georges Canguilhem's proposal that the scientific explanation of monstrosity, which was elaborated in the nineteenth century, led to 'a reduction of the monstrous'.[12] This chapter looks at freak shows, where the deformed body remained a highly visible signifier of social disorder until at least the end of the nineteenth century. Freak shows in particular demonstrate how deformity and disability have often been confused with monstrosity.[13] In the last part of the chapter, corporeal monstrosity is compared with physical disability to illustrate its relative and contingent nature.

Concentrating on the late nineteenth-century figure of Joseph Merrick, the 'Elephant Man', Chapter 5 investigates the relocation of monstrous significance from the morphology of the body to the character of the individual. In order to examine the apparent effacement of the monstrous effects of Merrick's physical deformities by his socialized character, this chapter follows his progress from freak show exhibit to medical specimen and social subject.

Chapter 6 focuses on the visualization of modern, criminal monstrousness, which threatens to undermine what is established as acceptable human identity when it cannot be visibly situated 'elsewhere', apart from self. The discussion of criminal monstrosity in this chapter is developed through an analysis of the representation of serial killers in the media. Taking the unidentified Victorian figure of 'Jack the Ripper' as an example, the chapter argues that in the modern context the production and public dissemination of visual images represent an attempt to provide a face for the threateningly invisible criminal monster. Later in this chapter the iconic police photograph of the female serial killer Myra Hindley is used to show how the public 'monstering' of images such as this represents an attempt to compensate for the silent refusal of the monster's body to signify. Photographs of 'monsters' are common in the media – recent examples include 'the cellar monster', Josef Fritzl, and the 'Soham monster', Ian Huntley, but their appearance is not particularly unusual, and few are memorable.[14] It is only through widespread publication in association with emotive texts that these pictures become significant. Recognizable visual images such as the iconic photograph of Hindley remain crucial in order to embody monstrousness and situate it in the place of the other, even if the 'monster' depicted looks normal.

Historically, human monsters offer a sense of security by embodying and making visible the threatening and unspeakable monstrousness that is encountered in the world, in society and within the self. Chapter 7 considers the effects of a monstrousness that is not made visible in the morphology of the body, but is brought into being through the actions of individual monsters who show no outward sign of their monstrousness. Modern monsters are social outsiders, and yet the monstrousness they represent cannot be fully contained in what the philosopher

Margrit Shildrick has called 'the place of the other'.[15] The psychopathic American serial killer Ted Bundy, whose veneer of normality was inconsistent with the monstrous acts that he performed, serves as the main example in this chapter. The chapter ends with a discussion of the more recent Norwegian mass murderer Anders Behring Breivik who, like Bundy, looks 'normal' despite his monstrous behaviour.

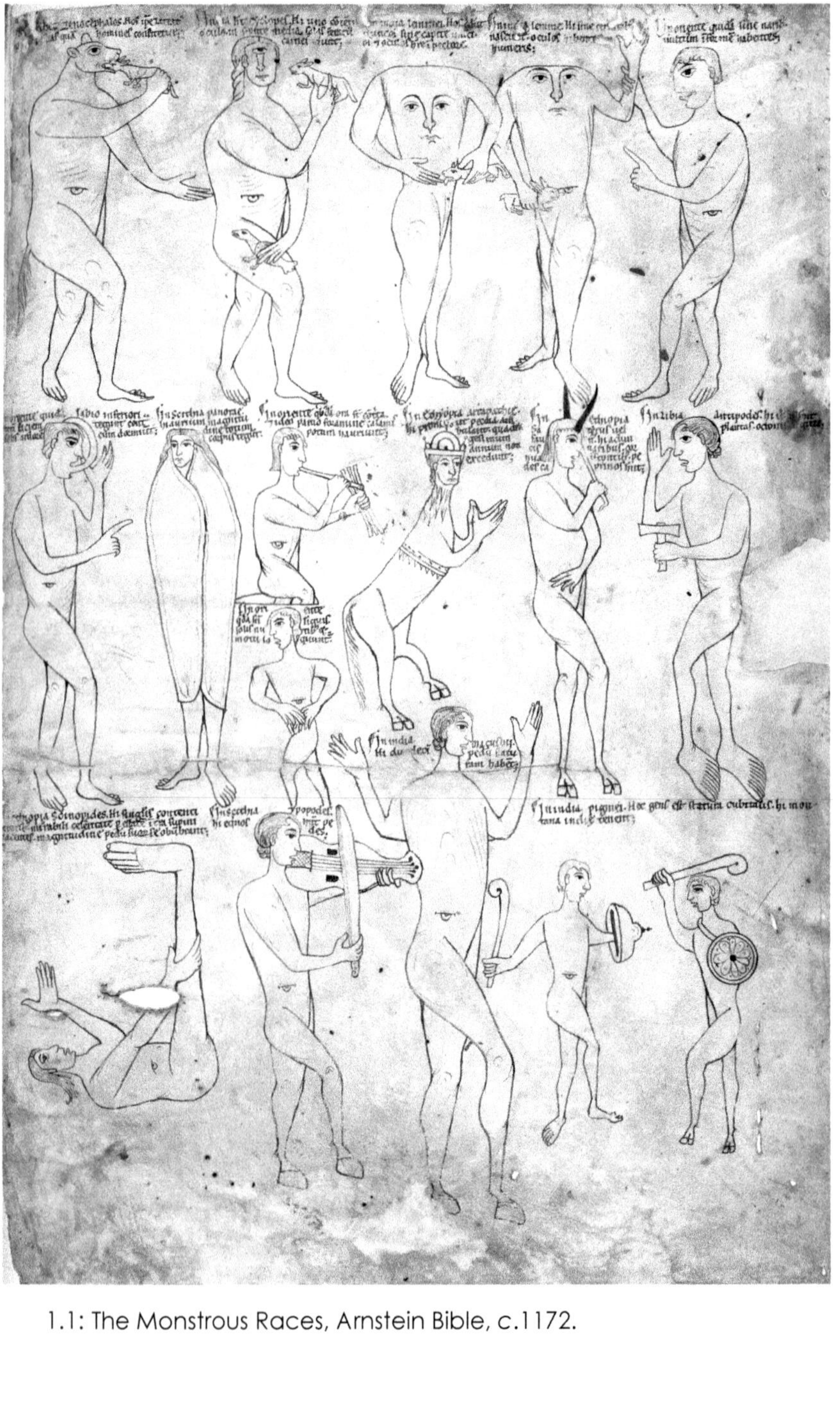

1.1: The Monstrous Races, Arnstein Bible, c.1172.

1 | Monstrous Strangers at the Edge of the World

The Monstrous Races

The Arnstein Bible is a large, heavy book in two volumes.[1] It was hand-written in ink by a German monk, Lunandus of Arnstein, in the late twelfth century. Parts of the text are skilfully illuminated in colour, which suggests that the bible was originally created for public display.[2] But the most interesting and intriguing feature of this ancient book is the collection of sketches on the flyleaves at the back of the second volume. There are several full-page drawings showing cosmographic charts; simple, geometrical world maps; a diagram of related types of human endeavour with philosophy at its head, and, lastly, this pen and ink sketch of the Monstrous Races (Figure 1.1). In these later additions the images and texts are rendered simply and directly, with none of the certainty of the main manuscript. They appear to be private sketchbook drawings or annotations made by someone trying to work out the order of the world during a time of unsettling social and cultural change. Collectively the charts and drawings configured here give a fascinating insight into the late medieval world-view as understood by one anonymous individual. But the most remarkable feature of the bible is the final page of drawings, which is filled with some of the fantastical figures that make up the Monstrous Races. This particular set of drawings may represent one individual's meditation on the order of things, but they also reflect a widespread historical understanding of the body of the human monster as a site for cultural interrogation of the boundaries between nature and culture, human and animal, human and not-human.

The idea of the Monstrous Races is far from unique to this one set of drawings. For a long period, lasting from some time before the fifth century BC until the sixteenth century AD, they were popularly characterized throughout Europe as real creatures that could not be considered fully human because of their remote existence, far from 'civilized' human society. Incorporating human/animal hybrids, exaggerated, misplaced or missing body parts and performing curiously inhuman practices, their mixed-up bodies manifest confusion about what might constitute the boundaries of human society and the limits of acceptable human being.

In the context of this book, the Monstrous Races are especially interesting because they show that, in Western cultures, there is an established history of articulating narratives of self and other visually, in the form of strange bodies and unconventional behaviours. When searching for an interpretation of these oddly configured bodies it is important to bear in mind that, until relatively recently, physical deformity was generally understood to hold negative significance, either for the affected individual or for society as a whole. And yet, like all human monsters, the Races are paradoxical in that they can be read as simultaneously positive and negative, expansive and cautionary, playful and discriminatory – depending on the point of view of the observer.

The apparently whimsical drawings in the back of the Arnstein Bible seem to be infused with a curiosity about the unknown. Whilst each figure is accompanied by a brief annotation in Latin noting its name and geographical origins, they have no visual context. These strange creatures are arranged on the page in what appear to be a series of theatrical vignettes in which they are either performing individually, or interacting with one another. Collectively they seem to point to a sense of wonder at the potential diversity of nature in regions of the world that would have been unfamiliar to most medieval Europeans. Whilst the majority of the figures have human faces, their social status is ambiguous. None of them is clothed, and yet several are holding or using tools, weapons or musical instruments, all of which represent human culture. The top row of figures are all eating or holding smaller animals, which suggests that they have been attributed a primitive nature. The confusion between human and non-human is further emphasized by the fact that many of these quasi-human figures have hooves, and yet some of them are playing music or fighting with weapons. In the centre of the page is a centaur (half human, half horse). The character on the top left has a dog's head and tail. Creatures such as the centaur and the dog-headed cynocephalus, which was believed to communicate by barking rather than speaking, represent a clear transgression of the division between humans and animals which, as we shall see, is one of the most important boundaries defended by human monsters.

In the particular case of the cynocephalus, the animal head on a human body symbolizes a loss of human rationality, suggesting the domination of bestial nature over human culture.[3]

Representing a fundamental breach of the boundary between human and animal, this zoomorphic monstrosity is particularly threatening because it indicates a resistance to human culture. The animal head also indicates a lack of ability to use human language. The use of articulate speech is commonly understood to be the feature that most securely distinguishes civilized humans from beasts, or non-humans.[4] Whilst the cynocephali were reported to bark like dogs, others of the Monstrous Races – such as the Astomi or apple smellers, the straw-drinkers, the snake-eating troglodytes and a race of speechless, gesturing people – were said to lack any kind of speech at all. This in itself would render these particular Races less than human and exclude them from human society in the eyes of medieval scholars, for whom language was a crucial attribute of all socialized peoples.[5]

History of the Monstrous Races

The long and fascinating history of the Monstrous Races is well documented by the art historian Rudolf Wittkower in Chapter 3 of his book, *Allegory and the Migration of Symbols*.[6] Wittkower describes the 'literary transmission' of the Races, from ancient Greek texts, to the Roman naturalist and philosopher Pliny, and then to the encyclopedists of the Middle Ages, charting their gradual decline through the sixteenth and seventeenth centuries. He explains that the confused bodies and strange customs of the Monstrous Races provided a form for anxieties about the limits of human being for a period of perhaps two thousand years, during which time they were discussed and depicted as real, if inaccessible, beings.

Wittkower links the written and verbal history of the Races to a pictorial tradition, claiming that 'we know that pictures of the fabulous races existed in antiquity', although none of these has survived. The earliest remaining images are from the Middle Ages.[7] The strength of public confidence in visual representations of the Monstrous Races during the Middle Ages in particular demonstrates how spoken or written narratives can be 'realized' visually, both in formal religious and academic contexts and, like the Arnstein Bible drawings, within a more popular or personal framework. Although, as Wittkower has shown, the Monstrous Races do have a literary tradition, the available pictures show most clearly how the body of the monster manifests uncertainty. These literal embodiments of difference demonstrate that, by portraying what is understood to be 'other', visual images of human monsters can help to establish and disseminate ideas about what it is to be human within a particular social and cultural context.[8]

The Monstrous Races in Medieval Art and Thought by John Block Friedman provides another detailed account of the Races, again tracing their transmission from antiquity to the Middle Ages and beyond.[9] In addition to a catalogue of all the major types, Friedman offers convincing anthropological explanations for their provenance, which, he writes, were often based on 'errors of perception' on the part of early travellers.[10] He shows how first-hand written or verbal reports brought back by military leaders such as Alexander the Great (fourth century BC) influenced subsequent literary or visual records compiled by people who had never travelled to the regions supposedly inhabited by the creatures they were portraying.

One of the earliest known accounts of the Monstrous Races comes from a treatise on India, published by the royal physician Ctesias of Knidos at around the beginning of the fourth century BC. Ctesias describes a number of marvellous creatures, including Sciopods, who have one giant foot that enables them to hop very fast and is also used to provide shelter from the sun; the Blemmaye, who have no heads but have faces in their chests; and the Panotii, people with enormous ears that they use to cover themselves with when they sleep and which can also be used to fly away from unwanted visitors.[11] These descriptions and the visual images derived from them, such as those shown in Figures 1.1 and 1.2, seem at first glance to be simply naive, charming and playful. However, further research reveals these monsters to be complex, provocative creatures, open to a variety of conflicting interpretations.

According to the nineteenth-century historian J.W. McCrindle, the Races depicted by Ctesias are often misrepresentations of indigenous tribes, particularly those who resisted invasion by Western colonizers.[12] The contemporary art historian Debra Higgs Strickland pursues this idea further, arguing that, in the Middle Ages, representations of the Monstrous Races were crucial to the Christian portrayal of 'godless' non-Christian minorities.[13] But McCrindle also maintains that some of the most influential descriptions of the Races were directly derived from monsters portrayed in two great Indian epic tales and other Brahmanical writings that formed an important part of Indian verbal and literary tradition. For example, the *Mahabharata*

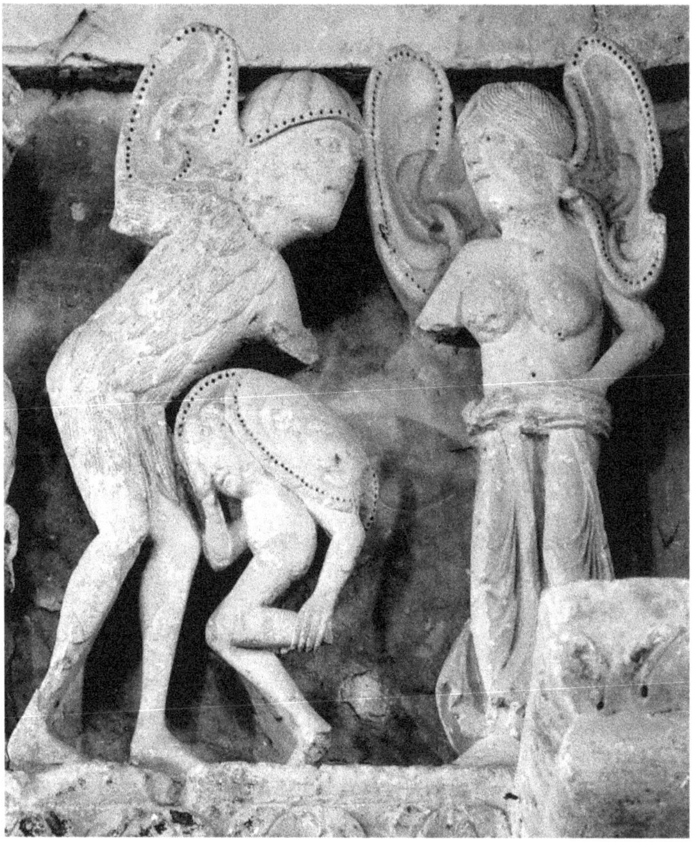

1.2: Panotii, lintel of Basilique Ste-Madeleine, Vézelay, France, c.1125–30.

describes the Karnapravarana, a people who cover themselves with their ears, which clearly served as a model for the Panotii (Figure 1.2).[14] If this is the case, Western travellers must have taken mainstream Indian culture seriously enough to adopt some of its mythology. Wittkower points to the appearance in Arabic illuminated manuscripts of creatures identical to the dog-headed cynocephali.[15] This again suggests that there was some exchange between cultures, ancient Greece being the source of inspiration for both Western and Arabic imagery. So it seems that not everyone whose appearance or culture differed from that of mainstream Western society was labelled a monster. However, the 'East', and especially India, was conceived as a site of potential for wonder and ambiguity for medieval Europeans on account of its distance from their known territories.

The work of the renowned Greek scholars Ctesias and Megasthenes, who was an ambassador to India during the fourth century BC, provided the main source for Western understanding of the culture, history and religion of the East for many years. Their descriptions of the Monstrous Races formed the basis of numerous secondary texts during the course of the next fifteen hundred years, reappearing in influential works by Pliny the Elder, Solinus, Saint Augustine and Isidore of Seville. One of the most significant of these secondary texts is Pliny's encyclopedic *Natural History* (AD 77), which includes an extensive list of the most popular of the Races. Like the earlier Greek accounts, Pliny's descriptions reveal a fascination for the strangeness of 'outsiders' and a sense of awe at what he understands to be the diversity of nature:

> Megasthenes records that on Mount Nulus there are men with their feet reversed and with eight toes on each foot. On many mountains there are men with dogs' heads who are covered with wild beasts' skins; they bark instead of speaking and live by hunting and fowling, for which they use their nails . . . Ctesias . . . writes of a tribe of men called the Sciapods who have only one leg and hop with amazing speed. These people are also called the Umbrella-footed, because when the weather is hot they lie on their backs stretched out on the ground and protect themselves by the shade of their feet . . . further to the east of these are some people without necks and with eyes in their shoulders . . . Among the Nomads of India Megasthenes records a race called Sciritai that has only holes in place of nostrils – like snakes – and has bandy legs. At the extreme boundaries of India, to the East, near the source of the Ganges, he locates the Astomi who have no mouth and whose body is covered in hair. They dress in cotton wool and live only on the air they breathe and the odour they draw in through their nostrils . . . Beyond the Astomi, in the depth of the mountains, so the story goes, live the Trispithami and Pygmies. In height they do not exceed three spans – that is about two and a half feet.[16]

Pliny does not question the truth of the classical texts on which he bases his descriptions, but seems to accept these previous accounts as factual descriptions of actual people. Following the earlier writers, he makes no distinction between clearly mythical characters like the Astomi and real people, such as the Pygmies.

On the one hand the inclusion of Pygmies amongst the Monstrous Races could be taken to indicate that the configuration of many of the Races is based on genuine misperceptions on the part of early travellers, as McCrindle has suggested. This idea is reinforced by Pliny's account of a race he calls the Gymnosophists, who 'remain standing from sunrise to sunset in the burning sun, all the while looking at the sun with a fixed gaze, resting first on one foot and then on the other', which could be a description of Brahmin practising yoga.[17] However, the bodies and customs of the Races could also be read as the emblems of discriminatory and racist beliefs of a xenophobic society, rehearsed without question until travel became more commonplace and people could see the far-off lands they were supposed to inhabit for themselves. We can only speculate on the spirit in which these creatures were originally conceived, but as the examples given so far demonstrate, the Races described by Ctesias clearly do embody many of the perceptual and emotional confusions experienced by early Western travellers. The inhabitants of the 'East' are mythologized in a way that may be considered either charming because of its literal naivety, or disturbing because of its imperialist nature.

Friedman points out that the Greeks, like many closely integrated communities, 'tended to view outsiders as likely to be inferior and untrustworthy'.[18] Whilst the works of classical scholars such as Ctesias and Megasthenes and the writers that followed them demonstrate a fascination with the strangeness of other peoples and places, they do also reveal an intolerance of difference. Friedman maintains that the early accounts of the Monstrous Races are decidedly ethnocentric because the culture, language and physical appearance of the observer are used as the 'norm' by which all other peoples are evaluated.[19] But this is the standard by which all monsters are constructed. Our contemporary understanding of what is monstrous would clearly not include those members of minority cultures who may have provided a source for some of the classical Monstrous Races. And yet the processes by which what is monstrous is identified as 'other', embodied and set apart from self and society, have changed little since the Races held currency.

The Monstrous Races have, understandably, been characterized as precursors to modern racism.[20] From a contemporary perspective this is certainly how they appear when mythical races such as the Blemmaye and cynocephali are grouped together with actual forest-dwelling peoples such as Pygmies. Pliny and other writers seeking subjects for scholarly debate on the limits of human being make no distinction between real and mythical 'others'. These ideas were derived from the ancient Greeks, who imagined themselves to be at the centre of the civilized world, judging all outsiders according to their own culture and customs. Homer, writing some time between the twelfth and seventh centuries BC, is one of the earliest known sources. He describes Pygmies as animals because they were considered too small and too different from Europeans to be men. Although in the contemporary context this seems laughable on the one hand and offensive on the other, it graphically highlights the insecurity and lack of knowledge that engendered the Monstrous Races. For those who first imagined them, much of the terrestrial world must have been an unknown and incomprehensible wilderness. Those distant parts of the globe, where extremes of climate and geography were believed to produce extreme bodies and behaviours, were clearly both intriguing and terrifying to early Europeans.

Whilst the Monstrous Races may be problematic because of the racist connotations that are attached to them, they are nevertheless interesting because, like all monsters, they reflect the cultural values invested in 'otherness'. Because the transgressions they represent are literally displayed on their bodies, the Races provide a clear and straightforward example of the historical function of the human monster as an embodiment of social, moral or ontological disorder. Their hybrid bodies, which combine human and animal, male and female, cultural and natural elements, operate as signifiers of the known and the unknown. They interrogate the boundaries of what constitutes an acceptable human subject on a direct, somatic level. The Monstrous Races demonstrate that, even when it is physically located elsewhere, human monstrosity is a construct that is intimately related to the social and moral values of the observer. By default, then, they also clarify what it means to be a valid member of a particular society. Human monsters are confusing figures lurking on the margins of society. They are strangers, outsiders, law-breakers and, above all, inherently transgressive characters that say more about those who create them than about those that are branded monstrous. In the words of Peter Stallybrass and Allon White, 'what is socially peripheral is so frequently symbolically central.'[21] Individual, social and cultural identities are inseparable from their limits and from the peripheral figures that help to define accepted norms.

Embodying many of the confusing or troubling qualities that must be set apart from self and removed from society, the body of the human monster has historically provided a tangible site for the inscription of transgression. This notion of transgression is interesting because it brings with it the concept of a 'limit' which differentiates one thing or way of being from another. Etymologically, transgression is defined as a violation of the law. It also means crossing over, or going beyond.[22] In the Judeo-Christian tradition transgression is a negative moral term linked, for example, to the biblical account of Adam's 'original sin' in the Garden of Eden. In this context it represents a failure, a fall from grace. For Michel Foucault, however, transgression performs a more interesting and complex role. He proposes that 'a limit could not exist if it were absolutely uncrossable and, reciprocally, transgression would be pointless if it merely crossed a limit composed of illusions and shadows'.[23] In this interpretation, transgression is a creative force that challenges established laws, limits and social structures and compels them to respond to modifications in human understanding, values and belief systems. Transgression is also a political force, in that it disrupts the existing order of bodies and cultures.

As an expression of difference that helps to define the self and the social 'norm' by manifesting what is currently unacceptable, human monstrosity is also closely bound up with ideas of the 'other' and 'otherness'. 'Otherness' literally means 'the state of being different'.[24] But it has come to be integrally related to notions of representation, in which representation of the other is always linked to representation of self. Whilst the self/other relation is accorded different significance in disciplines such as philosophy, psychology, anthropology and cultural politics, the 'other' is never simply a given in any of these contexts. It is never just found or encountered, but is always constructed.[25] Like monstrosity, the 'other' represents what is external to the 'norms' of self and society, but it is also essential to the constitution of the self. The philosopher Richard Kearney points up the paradoxical relation between self and monstrous other: 'in a sense we may say that monsters are our *others* par excellence. Without them we know not what we are. With them we are not what we know.'[26] In other words, the subjective position of the observer is always implicated in the construction of the 'other', whether monstrous or not.

The 'other' and 'otherness' are difficult terms to define because, as the anthropologist Malcolm Crick has written:

> a change in the value of the 'self' invariably alters the image of the 'other' and vice versa; and either change alters the nature of the difference which they constitute and by which they are constituted . . . there can be no final definition of the relation between 'ourselves' and 'others'.[27]

Emmanuel Levinas' philosophical notion of the 'other' as an absolute form of difference that cannot be known or articulated is very close to the concept of the monstrous. Levinas writes that 'the alien being is as it were naturalized as soon as it commits itself within knowledge,' and 'the other, in manifesting itself as a being, loses its alterity'.[28] This 'alien being' is equivalent to the monstrous, which is articulated through the body or behaviour of the monster. When what is monstrous has a visually identifiable, tangible form it can be classified as separate from self and from 'normal' society. Once it has been made known in this way, its terrible power is diffused. What is truly monstrous, therefore, is that which refuses representation and cannot be situated. This form of 'otherness' is profoundly threatening both because it cannot be seen to stand outside, and apart from, the normal subject, and because it undermines existing structures.

On a more practical level, human 'otherness' is traditionally constructed in terms of race, sexuality, gender or physical disability. Culturally and socially, the relationship between self and other is a hierarchical one, based on a need to justify and sustain existing power relations.[29] Racial, sexual or physically deformed 'others' have so often been subordinated to the image of the straight, white, 'rational' and able-bodied European male, which in Western culture has traditionally been the standard by which all 'others' are judged. From this perspective, all that is familiar and similar to the self is considered good, whilst what is other is thought to be strange and evil and must be avoided. In the context of anthropology, for example, Susan Sontag identifies the racial 'other' as a figure of exclusion: 'Europe seeks itself in the exotic . . . among preliterate peoples . . . the "other" is experienced as a harsh purification of "self".'[30]

Within a European tradition that has its roots in ancient Greece, the categorical separation of the European subject from the ethnic 'other' is evidenced in early depictions of the Monstrous Races, whose deformed bodies function as literal, visual representations of cultural otherness. In this case, otherness is aligned with monstrosity, which is the tangible manifestation of what is considered monstrous in any particular context.

Monsters and the Law

However, alterity is not always monstrous. Foucault asserts that, 'there is monstrosity only when the confusion comes up against, overturns or disturbs civil, canon or religious law'.[31] In suggesting that the natural and cultural laws infringed by the monster also determine its existence, he highlights the peculiar nature of the relationship between monsters and the law. The monstrous is powerful because it resists containment by social and natural laws and, in itself, defies language. As an articulation of this terrifying but transformative force, human monstrosity has an impact – which is different at different times – on definitions of what is natural and on the limits of acceptable human identity. It is most interesting when this process occurs in the 'real' world, rather than in the fictional worlds of literature or film. In both being and at the same time representing what is understood to be neither an accepted part of nature nor an accepted part of culture at any given time, the 'real' human monster can act as a powerful and concrete mirror for social and cultural values, whilst at the same time eliciting human empathy.

One example Foucault uses to illustrate his point about monstrosity that overturns the law is that of a pair of conjoined twins, one of which has committed a crime. This act, he says, confounds the law because it is unclear whether one or both of the twins should be executed for the crime.[32] If we understand this to be a 'true' case (as opposed to a fictional one) the potential legal and moral dilemma it raises is simultaneously chilling and fascinating. It is truly monstrous.

In medieval Europe an indication of both human and animal presence in one being represented a direct violation of social and divine laws. In Foucault's words, 'it is because there was a sexual relationship between a man and an animal that a monster appears in which the two kingdoms are mixed. In that respect we are referred to a breach of civil or religious law'.[33] This literal image of the monster as the result of a transgression of the laws prohibiting bestiality, which seem to be more or less ubiquitous in the Judeo-Christian tradition, is highly significant. The monstrous human/animal hybrid both acts as a warning of the consequences of behaviour that contravenes social codes and reinforces the importance of the codes, or laws, that bind a society together. When a clear boundary is established between humans and animals the 'natural', savage, uncivilized characteristics of animals can be set apart from what is human, which is traditionally defined by the possession of culture and of a coherent language, and by the capacity for self-reflection and self-control.[34]

The very existence of laws calling for a clear division between animals and humans indicates a profound anxiety about the potential contamination of human identity by primitive, animal characteristics.[35] The longstanding popularity of the Monstrous Races, which include many human/animal hybrids, suggests that this anxiety has deeply troubled Western cultures for some time. In the sixteenth century the French surgeon Ambroise Paré forcefully described monsters that transgressed the boundary between human and animal as unnatural expressions of evil:

> There are monsters that are born with a form that is half-animal and half-human . . . which are produced by sodomists and atheists who join together . . . with animals, and from this are born several monsters that are hideous and very scandalous to look at or speak about.[36]

In his seminal essay, 'Monstrosity and the Monstrous', Georges Canguilhem explains that, until the late eighteenth century, corporeal monstrosity was generally understood to be the result of a monstrous act such as those described by Paré. It did not happen by chance, but was brought about by 'the license of living beings'. According to Canguilhem, monstrous deformity was read as a sign of a conscious act of defiance, representing a contravention of the laws that segregate particular species, races or types:

> Zoomorphic monstrosity, if one admitted its existence, had to be considered the result of a deliberate attempt at infraction of the order of things, which is one with their perfection; it had to be considered the result of abandoning oneself to the dizzy fascination of the undefined, of chaos . . .[37]

In Canguilhem's view, therefore, someone is culpable – guilty of deliberately bringing about the state of chaos out of which a monster is born by his or her actions. For him, monstrosity is a direct consequence of deviance. But monsters are always paradoxical, simultaneously signifying that something is not right and providing a vehicle for exploring and 'working out' changes to established belief systems. Returning once more to Foucault, we learn that in transgressing the laws of both nature and culture the monster 'combines the impossible and the forbidden'. It is 'a breach of the law that automatically stands outside the law'.[38] He explains this further: 'It could be said that the monster's power and its capacity to create anxiety are due to the fact that it violates the law while leaving it with nothing to say.'[39] Monsters absorb the horror of what is unknown and unregulated by giving form to the unspeakable, and perhaps even unthinkable monstrousness that cannot be contained within existing categories.

In most societies, a sexual act involving humans and animals clearly represents a serious and longstanding violation of the laws of both nature and culture. But in medieval images such as the drawings in the Arnstein Bible (Figure 1.1), even those Monstrous Races whose mixed-up bodies imply that transgressive sexual relations have taken place seem to be depicted as more marvellous than threatening. This is perhaps because, in their geographical location at the very edges of the known world, the Races stood outside the social and symbolic order of Western cultures. Living in a territory beyond the direct experience of most Europeans, they posed little threat to society. Their bodies could be spectacularly reordered without apparent negative consequence because, in the words of the medieval English monk Ranulph Higden: 'at the furthest reaches of the world often occur new marvels and wonders, as though Nature plays with greater freedom secretly at the edges of the world than she does openly and nearer to us in the middle of it'.[40] Confined to this remote and uncharted area, the Monstrous Races locate the transgressions they represent at a safe distance, far from 'civilized' human society.

Monsters and Maps

Medieval maps such as the Hereford Mappa Mundi (Figures 1.3 and 1.4) show a range of monsters in their 'proper' geographical location, at the very edges of the globe. This map, which was drawn on a single sheet of vellum (calf skin), measuring 1.58 x 1.33 metres, dates from the early fourteenth century. Whilst it may be more narrative than utilitarian, the Mappa Mundi functions as an important visual and textual account of medieval cultural values, illustrating the cosmology and theology of the late Middle Ages.[41] Mixing classical agendas with new information provided by more recent commercial travellers, pilgrims and Crusaders, the Hereford map acted as an important and authoritative source for medieval scholars.

According to this map, Jerusalem is located at centre of the (Christian) world and monstrous 'others' are arranged around the edges, beyond the Nile.[42] The monsters depicted include real and imaginary exotic beasts, such as an elephant (with a castle on its back), a manticore (a legendary creature similar to the Egyptian

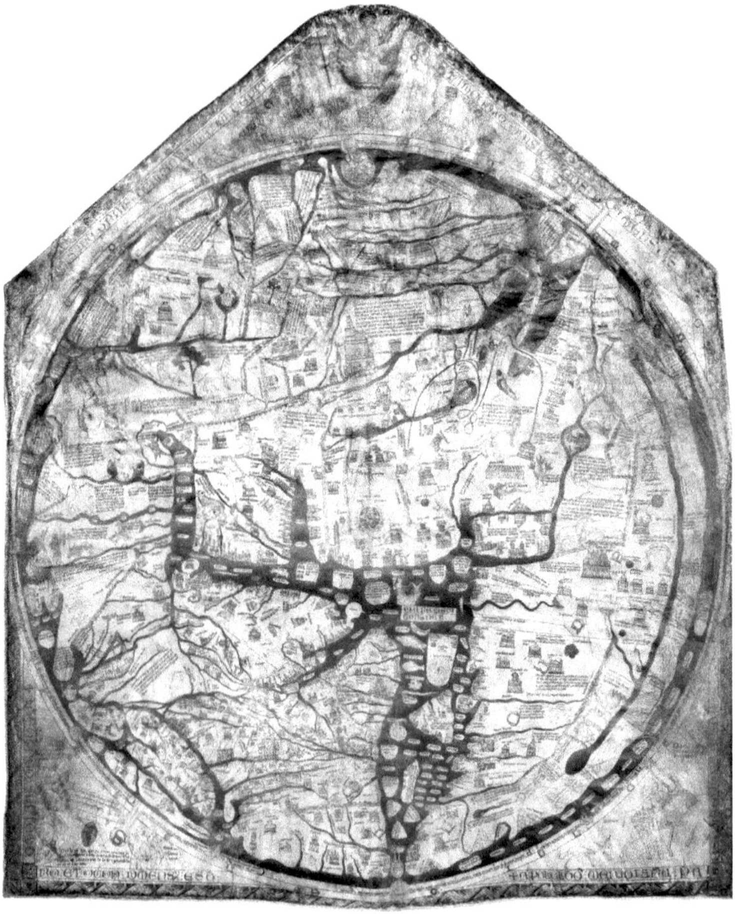

1.3: Richard of Haldingham, Mappa Mundi, c.1300.

sphinx), a parrot, a camel, a unicorn and a dragon as well as many of the Monstrous Races. This grouping of human and animal, fantastical and 'real' creatures seems to suggest an openness to the range of possibilities that may exist in the undefined territory

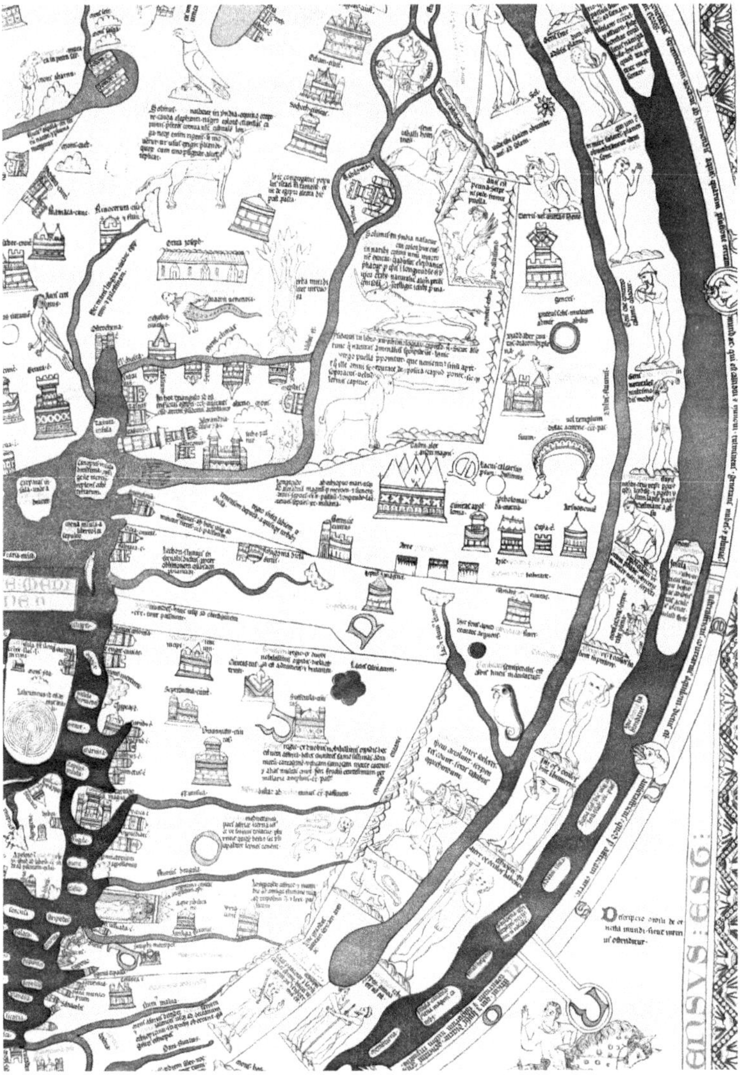

1.4: Detail from a nineteenth-century facsimile of the Hereford Mappa Mundi, showing Monstrous Races at the edge of the world.

beyond the concrete world of immediate experience. However, Friedman paints a rather less benign picture of the presence of the Races at the edges of the map:

> In the antipodal space defined by the edge of what separated us from them, and ringed by the river of Ocean believed to circle the very edges of the earth, is a cultural other, a sciopode or shadow-footed man, whose single great foot protects him from the heat of the sun . . . His physical form defines the oddness beyond the border, for he is half like us and half like them. This map encloses the cultural other and renders him a harmless anecdotal representation . . .[43]

From a contemporary perspective we can only speculate about the true spirit in which the Races were conceived. Perhaps the symbolic other that is being exiled is not so explicitly racial; maybe it is simply difference per se that is anthropomorphized in the bodies of the Monstrous Races.

What is clear is that, even though very few people could claim to have seen any of them 'in the flesh', the Monstrous Races played an important role in the order of the world for classical and medieval scholars and lay people alike. Living at the extremities of the known world, the Races could inhabit the realms of the imaginary and the mythical and yet still be considered entirely 'real'. This is perhaps because, in medieval culture, figures of the imagination and of myth were not differentiated from everyday reality in the way that they are today.[44] The historians of science Katherine Park and Lorraine Daston offer an explanation for this: 'medieval readers and writers shared an approach to truth more complicated and multivalent than the post-seventeenth-century obsession with the literal fact . . . For them, truth could exist on various levels, both literal and figurative.'[45] In the twenty-first century we are led to believe that modern science enables us to separate 'myth' from 'reality', which makes it difficult to understand how people could ever have 'believed in' the Monstrous Races. However, these ancient creatures are not so different to the more modern human monsters introduced in later chapters of this book. They are all, to some degree, mythical figures, constructed in order to help sort out what is acceptably human from what is unacceptably 'other'.

Myth

The term 'myth' is often used to indicate what is imaginary or fictitious. It is associated with something that is not 'real'. In the sense it is used here, a myth is a narrative that assigns meaning to a particular body or action. Roland Barthes has explained that myth is 'a system of communication, a message . . . a type of speech, everything can be myth provided it is conveyed by a discourse'.[46] So mythical human monsters are not necessarily 'unreal'. They are figures around which narratives have been constructed in order to help explain a newly experienced aspect of, or idea about, human being. As mythical figures, the Monstrous Races are imaginative (as opposed to imaginary) creatures that combine elements of observed material reality with signifying features in order to explain something. Barthes goes on to argue that 'myth does not deny things . . . its function is to talk about them . . . it purifies them, makes them innocent, gives them a natural and eternal justification . . . a clarity which is not that of an explanation, but that of a statement of fact'.[47] In this interpretation, a mythical creature is the embodiment of an idea. In giving physical and visual form to a particular belief, the mythical monster can fix it in place and render it 'real'. Whilst Barthes has claimed that 'there is no fixity in mythical concepts – they can come into being, alter, disintegrate, disappear completely', mythical concepts can have lasting effects.[48] This is evidenced by the longevity of the Monstrous Races, whose existence was debated and often defended by scholars throughout the Middle Ages and beyond.[49]

Barthes makes another remark about myth that is particularly interesting in the context of this book. He writes, 'myth is not defined by the object of its message, but by the way in which it utters this message'.[50] Here he draws attention to the constructed nature of myth and to how that narrative can change the way in which an existing object is perceived. In relation to creatures such as those that make up the Monstrous Races, myth can assign meaning to that which is otherwise unintelligible or, in the case of modern monsters, it can assign particular significance to an ordinary-looking face or body. Barthes characterizes myth as a form of representation that is informed by history.[51] For him, the signifier of myth 'presents itself in an ambiguous way: it is at the same time meaning and form' – this is precisely the place of the human monster.[52]

By the beginning of the sixteenth century, the idea of monsters as symbolic 'moral prodigies' was becoming popular in Western culture. Creatures like the Monster of Ravenna (discussed in Chapter 3) appeared, signifying the presence of moral or social unrest within Western society. And yet the strange and distant figures of the Monstrous Races described by early Greek travellers also continued to function as emblems of human difference up until at least the end of the sixteenth century. Wittkower attributes this longevity to the fact that well-educated travellers, who knew the classics and understood natural science, would have seen the Races marked on their maps and would have heard about them from childhood.[53] Even when geographical knowledge became widespread, therefore, travellers found these monsters in the East simply because they believed they would.[54]

The representational function of the Monstrous Races as corporeal signifiers of difference can perhaps be seen in the context of a classical world-view in which the 'normal' human body acted as a model for the universe and social values were directly embodied in the human image. The importance of the 'proper' body as an expression of acceptable human identity is illustrated in a comment made by the medieval teacher, papal adviser and authority on Roman law Baldo degli Ubaldi, who wrote: 'that which does not have the body of a man is presumed not to have the soul of a man . . . since form gives essence to a thing, that which does not have the form of a man is not a man'.[55] In Chapter 3, which focuses on the significance of the body, the idea that human monstrosity represents that which is disproportionate or out of place is examined in the light of a historically widespread belief that a person's character and moral status is mirrored in his or her physical characteristics. This belief, which offers a background to understanding the configuration of the Monstrous Races, is perhaps another factor that contributed to the longevity of belief in their existence.

No matter where the Monstrous Races appeared, they were always geographically distant from their observers. As remote social outsiders, they could pose little threat to established social laws, or to the identity of individuals living within society. Because of their historical and geographical distance the Monstrous Races provide a relatively uncomplicated visual introduction to the study of monsters, whilst touching on several key themes that will be explored further in the following chapters. The next chapter takes up the theme of the monster as outsider and, focusing on the figures of the medieval wild man and the feral child, further explores the contested but fiercely defended boundary between humans and animals.

2 | Blurring the Boundaries of Nature and Culture

Wild People and Feral Children

Throughout the Middle Ages wild men or 'wodewose' (men of the woods) were believed to dwell at the outer edges of the Western world. Favouring liminal or boundary zones, where one state of existence gave way to another, they inhabited the largely unexplored forests and mountains that surrounded European towns and cities. These primitive social outsiders combined human and animal, natural and unnatural attributes, but they were not strictly monsters. Nor were they fully human. Acting as a projection of social anxieties and fears, they embodied complex and shifting perceptions of the relationships between nature and culture, humans and animals, self and other.

By the late sixteenth century these medieval 'men of the woods' were no longer taken very seriously, yet accounts of children living within nature, independent from human society, and either alone or with animals have continued to haunt our collective imagination. Occupying an uncertain place between myth and reality, human and not-quite human, feral children are social outsiders who, like wild people, are thought to exhibit animal characteristics, manifesting both civilized and wild traits. Portrayed as innocent victims of circumstance, these wild children are often presented as objects of pity or fascination, evoking fantasies of rescue and redemption on the one hand and fear and suspicion on the other. Whilst in reality a child described as feral is most likely to be a product of social neglect, wild children are usually characterized as coming from 'an elsewhere', as Michael Newton put it in his book *Savage Girls and Wild Boys*.[1] Organically they are part of 'us', and yet we cannot quite reach them.

Like human monsters, stories of wild folk offer a way of exploring and coming to terms with what might and might not be considered acceptably human in any given context. Monsters, wild people and feral children are all outsiders who never fully conform to our definition of what it is to be human. Within Western culture, the idea of the outsider has a long history that can be traced back to a classical Greek understanding of social hierarchy. For example, in *Politics*, which forms part of his treatise on political philosophy, Aristotle (384–322 BC) describes the *polis*, meaning either the community or the state, within which an individual can live to his full potential.[2] According to classical Greek thought, only the (male) citizen living within the *polis* and subject to its laws could be considered fully human. Along with women, all others were thought to be inferior. Whilst Aristotle wrote that 'in many states the law goes to the lengths of admitting aliens', this was only in extreme cases when 'there is a dearth of legitimate citizens'.[3] Along with those classes who could not, or would not fit into 'civilized' society, most outsiders were regarded as primitive and brutal. They were, perhaps, precursors to the medieval wild man. This ancient insistence on the importance of the law as a force for containing and ordering what is acceptably human continues to inform the way in which criminal or anti-social figures are portrayed today. For example, those who stand outside the law are often described in the popular media as 'animals' or 'brutes', a characterization that casts them in a similar role to the medieval wild man.

In one way or another, wild men, feral children and monsters all embody the loss of order and meaning that may be inherent in a return to a state of nature. And yet, whilst each of these figures provides a locus for sorting out the confusions that arise at the boundary between humans and animals, there are some crucial differences in the manner in which monsters and wild folk are perceived. Even though wild men and women and feral children all directly embody some of the 'uncivilized', brutal and 'natural' characteristics that are to be excluded from civilized society, they have never been seen as portentous in the way that pre-modern monsters were. As we saw in Chapter 1, the presence of a monster usually indicates that there has been a serious and symbolically significant transgression of the laws of both nature and culture. Human monsters, particularly those that possess animal characteristics, are, therefore, highly charged, inherently symbolic creatures.

In his lecture on the abnormal of 22 January 1975, Michel Foucault draws out the paradoxical relationship between nature and the monstrous: 'the monstrous is, so to speak, the spontaneous form, the brutal form, but, as a consequence, the natural form of the unnatural'.[4] Here he presents the monster as a conundrum that characterizes 'the natural' as a construct that mirrors the equally constructed idea of 'the unnatural'. As an embodiment of social and moral confusion, human monsters represent disorder and uncertainty, perverting any simple correlation between the natural and nature, or culture and the unnatural. Wild people and feral children also trouble the boundaries between nature and culture, humans and animals, but in a more straightforward way. The meanings attributed to them are more secular and localized.

Nature and Culture

Nature and human culture are perhaps the most enduringly problematic and unstable of all of the ideas that inform the construction of 'normal' human being, and consequently of 'outsiders' such as monsters and wild folk. In fact, as the cultural critic Raymond Williams has remarked, 'nature' is perhaps the most complex word in the English language.[5] It therefore seems important to identify some of its meanings here, especially as the need for boundary figures such as wild men, feral children and monsters arises out of a basic desire to sort out what is natural or unnatural at any given time. Closely aligned with social and cultural values and beliefs, the idea of nature takes on very different meanings in different contexts. In some cases it denotes a harmful and threatening force, something that must be controlled and tamed, whilst in others it represents a benign and inherently good state that should be preserved and nurtured. As the philosopher Kate Soper has written, the idea of nature 'may be viewed as a register of changing conceptions as to who qualifies, and why, for full membership of the human community'.[6]

Amongst the many possible interpretations of the word 'nature' Soper has identified three distinct concepts that form the basis for our modern understanding. The first of these is the metaphysical concept, which describes nature as that which is other to humanity:

> In its commonest and most fundamental sense, the term 'nature' refers to everything which is not human and distinguished from the work of humanity. Thus nature is opposed to culture, to history, to convention, to what is artificially worked or produced, in short, to everything which is defining the order of humanity.[7]

Even though ideas about what constitutes 'nature' and the 'natural' world are constantly changing in the light of shifting ideas about what we are as humans, Soper has proposed that this formal distinction acts as a foundation for all other readings of the terms 'nature' and 'culture'.[8] And yet, even if we think of nature as absolutely other to culture, comprising all that is not human, humanity is paradoxically also seen as a constituent part of it. In this case, nature is conceived of as both 'that which we are not and that which we are within'.[9] Within this 'realist' conception, we are subject to the laws of nature, and can neither escape nor destroy its effects on the material world.[10] But we are still different to the rest of nature in that we are able to exert conscious control over it. Thirdly, Soper identifies a 'lay' or 'surface' concept of nature which comprises the ordinary, observable features of the world, such as rural landscape, wilderness or countryside.

These three ideas have a variety of meanings, and take on different values at different times according to modifications in our individual and social beliefs and principles. In summary, nature is, on the one hand, thought to be a wild, unruly and unpredictable state that precedes human intervention and to which the world will revert if it is not tamed and suppressed by human culture. According to this way of thinking, it is a disturbing, disruptive and counterproductive force. On the other hand, nature is characterized as an inherently creative energy that animates and motivates the world. In this case, the natural world is understood to be a beautiful and vulnerable place that must be protected and preserved from the destructive influence of human culture. These contradictory interpretations are often coincident and are therefore difficult to tease apart, especially when we consider the traditional understanding of nature as that which is opposed to culture.

If nature is the world of things that exist outside human control and is ultimately 'the idea through which we conceptualise what is "other" to ourselves', the word 'culture' is normally used to describe purposeful human activities and processes.[11] Closely linked to human identity, the concept of culture may be applied to scholarly, spiritual and aesthetic development, a particular way of life or the products and practices of intellectual and creative activity.[12] Culture is another very complex idea; indeed, Raymond Williams devotes almost five pages of his book *Keywords* to an explanation of its etymology.[13] He shows how its various representational and practical meanings are, like those of nature, multifaceted and overlapping.

Although it has always referred to some form of human endeavour or human development, the use of the word 'culture' to indicate the practices and products of intellectual, spiritual and aesthetic development is relatively recent.[14] Williams describes anything that sets people apart from nature or enables us to have control over aspects of the natural world as a cultural process. Civilization, or advanced social development, is the ultimate example of this. According to Williams, this is 'an achieved condition of refinement and order', a normative quality that can be lost as well as gained.[15] Rooted in ideas of social order, the word 'civilization' indicates a conscious or culturally contrived contrast to a wild or savage state of nature. In different ways at different times, wild men and women, feral children and human monsters all interrogate and even subvert the categories and processes described by the terms 'nature', 'culture' and 'civilization'.

Structures of Classification

Throughout the history of Western culture, the ability to set humans apart from other animals has, in one way or another, always been crucial to the idea of 'man' as a civilized being. Although the relationship between humans and animals is understood differently at different times, attempts to make a categorical division between the two can be traced back to the classical age. In the fourth century BC, for example, Aristotle argued for the existence of a divinely inspired universal hierarchy, where all of nature was fitted into a pre-ordained plan. At the head of this single, 'natural' scale was a perfect and unchanging being. Below this was 'man', followed by the animals, each positioned according to the degree of perfection of its soul.[16] Based on Aristotle's propositions, the idea of a *Scala naturae*, or 'Great Chain of Being' was given more concrete form during the Middle Ages, when it was accepted without question by most philosophers and scientists. The Great Chain was depicted as a vertical structure with God at the top, followed by the angels, humans and then animals, with plants and minerals at the lower end. In accordance with this plan was the belief that all things have a particular place and function in the universe. Therefore, to depart from one's proper place, or to transgress a categorical boundary would be to betray one's nature.

To act against human nature by not ensuring that reason ruled the emotions indicated a descent to the level of the beasts. This was a much-derided position that, from the early Middle Ages until the sixteenth century, was symbolized by the figure of the wild man.

The basic premise of the Great Chain of Being, which dictated that species were fixed and could never evolve, seems to have been widely accepted until the eighteenth century, when there was a surge of interest in classification and in sorting out what could and could not be classed as human. One of the most influential scientific figures of the eighteenth century, the Swedish naturalist Carolus Linnaeus (1707–78), sought to build on the historical concept of the divine order of things by classifying all the products of the natural world according to their intrinsic physical characteristics. In the tenth version of his encyclopedic *Natural History* (1758), Linnaeus categorizes humans as *Homo sapiens*, further breaking down humankind into sub-genres: *Europaeus*, *Asiaticus*, *Americanus*, *Afer*, *ferus* and *monstrous*.[17] Like *Homo monstrous*, the sub-category *Homo ferus* lies between humans and animals. This class of being, which is by nature 'four footed, mute and hairy', was the source of the name, and perhaps also the modern idea, of the feral child.[18]

By the late eighteenth century, travel had become more widespread, enabling the discovery of new species of animals and plants and a greater awareness of cultures in other parts of the world. This new knowledge started to undermine the fixed conception of the universe that Linnaeus and other taxonomists had initially attempted to accommodate in their classifications. This lead to new speculation about 'man's' place in the world.[19] Thinkers such as Jean-Jacques Rousseau (1712–78) and the French naturalist Georges-Louis Leclerc, Comte de Buffon (1707–88), started to question the structure of the hierarchical Chain of Being passed down from Aristotle. Assuming that human beings were originally solitary creatures living an unfettered, nomadic existence, Rousseau located 'man' amongst the other animals:

> if we consider [man] . . . just as he must have issued from the hands of nature, we behold in him an animal weaker than some, and less agile than others; but, all in all, the most advantageously organized of all.[20]

In his *Histoire naturelle* (1766) the Comte de Buffon also proposed that human beings and apes share a common ancestry.[21] This interest in tracing the origins of humankind seems to have been primarily the result of an attempt to form a new understanding of the 'true' nature of humanity. At this time, however, the suggestion that humans and animals have a shared ancestry was not taken very seriously. This is perhaps unsurprising, as Rousseau's image of early man coincides almost exactly with the medieval wild man character who had traditionally represented all that stood outside 'civilized' human society.

The term 'savage', meaning 'uncivilized', first appeared in English in the late Middle Ages, although notions of wildness and savagery were used by Europeans to distance themselves from peoples of other 'uncivilized' cultures long before that.[22] In the eighteenth and nineteenth centuries the perceived connections between racial 'otherness' and ideas of wildness or 'savagery' became more explicit. Linnaeus and other eighteenth-century scientists such as the French naturalist and zoologist Georges Cuvier (1769–1832) believed that there were many different human races, with separate origins. The most distinct of these, Cuvier asserts, are 'the Caucasian, or white, the Mongolian, or yellow and the Ethiopian, or negro'.[23] Almost like different species, these races were divided according to geographic location and skin colour, each with distinct and value-laden attributes. Caucasians 'with oval face, straight hair and nose' – the group to which Cuvier assigned himself – were those to whom he believed 'the most highly civilized nations, and those which have generally held all others in subjection, are indebted for their origin'.[24] Cuvier believed that whilst members of the 'Mongolian race' had established great empires, their civilization remained static. By contrast,

> The Negro race . . . is marked by black complexion, crisped or woolly hair, compressed cranium and a flat nose. The projection of the lower parts of the face, and the thick lips, evidently approximate it to the monkey tribe: the hordes of which it consists have always remained in the most complete state of barbarism.[25]

Here Cuvier establishes the idea of the 'Ethiopian, or negro' race as a kind of monstrous species, or ethnic wild man, between human and animal.

By the mid-nineteenth century there was further serious, if deeply flawed, scientific discussion concerning the relationship between 'man' and other primates. The idea of a racial hierarchy became strongly entrenched in Western thought. Evidence of the connection between humans and animals was gathered and published in works such as Charles Darwin's *On the Origin of*

Species (1859) and *The Descent of Man* (1871), Thomas Huxley's *Evidence as to Man's Place in Nature* (1863) and Charles Lyall's *Geological Evidences of the Antiquity of Man* (1863).[26] Much of the final chapter of Lyall's book is devoted to a thorough review of previous ideas about the origins of 'man', followed by evidence in support of his contentious argument that 'if man was made in the image of God he was also made in the image of an ape'.[27] Huxley also provides lengthy biological and physiological evidence for a connection between 'man' and other animals. Comparing 'man' to the gorilla, he too concludes that 'the structural differences which separate Man from the Gorilla and the Chimpanzee are not so great as those which separate the Gorilla from the other apes'.[28] Again, both men make it clear that it is the 'lower' (non-European) races they consider to be closely related to other primates, not the more 'civilized' Europeans. In this context it seems that the concept of race was used as another device to distance 'civilized' men (as these scientists perceived themselves to be) from brute nature, whilst at the same time acknowledging the evident connections between humans and animals. For those who believed that mythology had been replaced by scientific 'reason', the categorically separate racial groups imagined by Cuvier offered a means of symbolizing ontological uncertainty. These visibly different racial 'others' gave tangible form to the fears experienced by 'ordinary' members of Western society about the potential links between mankind and other animals. The hierarchical notion of 'race' was perhaps also an attempt to protect the perceived sovereignty of the white Western man.

Wild Men

Against the background of this longstanding preoccupation with dividing nature from culture, human from animal and 'civilized' self from savage 'other', stands the figure of the wild man. Although the wild man as such first appeared in the Middle Ages, his antecedents can be traced back to the biblical king Nebuchadnezzar, who was rendered insane and forced to live like a wild animal for seven years as punishment for his excessive pride. Connections have also been made with Enkidu, the central character in one of the earliest known literary works, 'The Epic of Gilgamesh' (*c.*2000 BC). Enkidu lived in the wild and was raised by animals until he was seduced into human society and taught human ways. Some of the half-human, half-animal creatures amongst the classical Monstrous Races, such as the dog-headed cynocephalus, whose animal head points to a lack of reason, might also be seen as precursors to the medieval wild man.

Whilst the Monstrous Races appeared in distant regions of the globe, wild people were said to live closer to home, in the woods or mountains of central Europe. These lands were not far from civilized society, but were nevertheless considered too harsh or remote for 'normal' human habitation.[29] Avoiding human contact, wild people remained just out of sight and could, therefore, pursue a lawless existence beyond the strict and hierarchical jurisdiction of the Church and State. In the Middle Ages stories of wild men offered a means of both reinforcing and negotiating accepted social attitudes towards nature and the uncivilized 'animal' aspects of human being.

Writing in the 1950s, Richard Bernheimer begins the first chapter of his book, *Wild Men in the Middle Ages*, by emphatically stating:

> wild men are imaginary creatures . . . [the wild man is] a literary and artistic figure whose imaginary character is proved by its appearance: it is a hairy man curiously compounded of human and animal traits, without, however, sinking to the level of an ape.[30]

Timothy Husband also consigns the wild man entirely to fiction, introducing him as a 'purely mythic creature'.[31] But this does not seem to tell the whole story. It seems that these mythical creatures are modelled on actual social outcasts, such as tramps and disenfranchised peasants, the mentally ill, racial 'others', or simply those who do not 'fit in'. An interesting tension exists, therefore, between the constructed idea of the wild person – which arises from a particular social or cultural need to externalize certain unacceptable characteristics, and the 'real' individuals attributed with these mythical qualities.

In his essay 'The Forms of Wildness' Hayden White makes the point that 'the idea of wildness does not so much designate a particular state of being, but rather an attitude towards a particular, troubling, aspect of existence'.[32] In this understanding it is not the veracity of the story of the wild person that is at issue, but rather the meanings that are attributed to him or her. In other words, as an embodiment of the idea of wildness, wild men and women function like monsters in that they reveal the values and uncertainties of those that create them. The changing implications of a life unconfined by the strictures of Western 'civilization' are directly reflected in the character of the wild man, who shifts between a state of brutal unreason and savagery, and one of natural harmony and enlightenment.

Until the late Middle Ages, wild men were generally portrayed as barbaric and enslaved to nature. In most visual representations they are shown unclothed, covered in hair and of immense strength, usually carrying a large wooden club or stick. Living in the wilderness, this 'natural man' was thought to have regressed to a primitive, bestial state, without language or spirituality. Devoid of reason, he was considered sub-human. According to medieval writers, this lowly state of being was brought about by 'degeneration caused by extraneous circumstances', such as 'loss of mind, 'upbringing among beasts' or 'outrageous hardships'.[33] The existence of the wild man, therefore, acted as a warning of what could happen to anyone who did not conform to the strict social, moral or religious rules of society.[34]

An early fifteenth-century French painting of Alexander the Great (Figure 2.1) shows an army of clothed warriors rescuing a naked woman from the clutches of a hairy savage at night. In this somewhat chaotic image, the wild man is shown to be a dangerous character. He is a barbaric, perverse and lascivious creature, driven by desire and instinct. A symbol of unruly passions, he is the antithesis of the civilized figures of

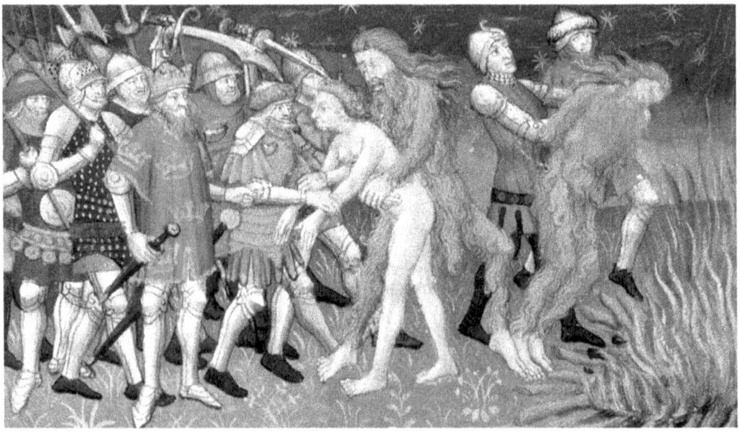

2.1: Alexander and the Wild Man, painted manuscript illumination from 'Le Livre et le vraye hystoire du bon roy Alixandre', c.1420.

Alexander and his knights. The nature he inhabits is a difficult, frightening and uncontrollable place. Whilst on one hand this unruly character stood for all that should be avoided by 'civilized' people, he must also have appeared to be an attractive and liberating figure for those oppressed by the strict regimes of Church and State.[35] In fact, from the late fourteenth century onwards, wild men were more likely to be seen as characters freed from social constraints, who consequently provoked envy and admiration, than objects of fear and loathing. As attitudes to nature changed, so the wild man became a romantic token of a lost age of innocence and, as the historian Timothy Husband has shown, 'a symbol of all that man should strive to achieve'.[36] Another, rather more serene picture, also painted in France in the early fifteenth century (Figure 2.2) supports this interpretation. It shows a seemingly peaceful encounter between Alexander and a much more respectable-looking hairy man. In this romanticized image, the sky is blue, the natural landscape is idealized and the upright wild man is represented as a 'noble savage', standing for all that is innocent and good in human nature. Although these two paintings were created at around the same time, they clearly illustrate a change of attitude towards the natural world. But this was neither straightforward nor complete. In the words of sociologists Paul Hirst and Penny

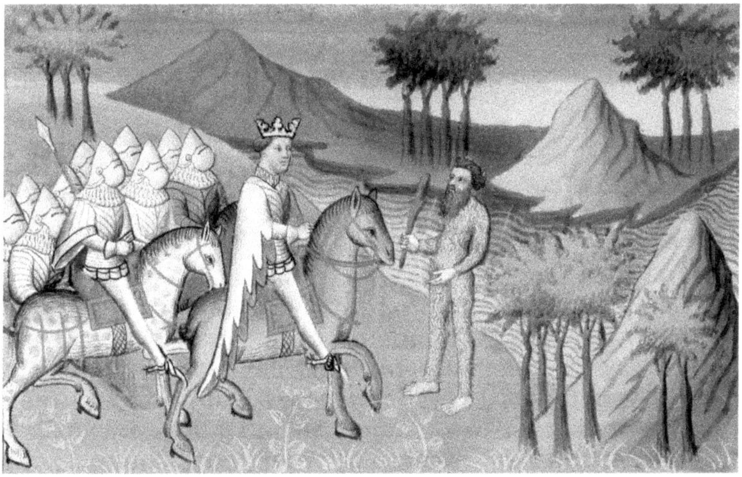

2.2: Alexander and the Wild Man, painted manuscript illumination from Fleur des histoires d'Orient: le livre des merveilles, c.1410–12.

Woolley, the transformation from 'savage' to 'noble savage' could be seen to represent 'one unstable complex of images which present both the fear of and the desire for a transgression of the limits of culture'.[37]

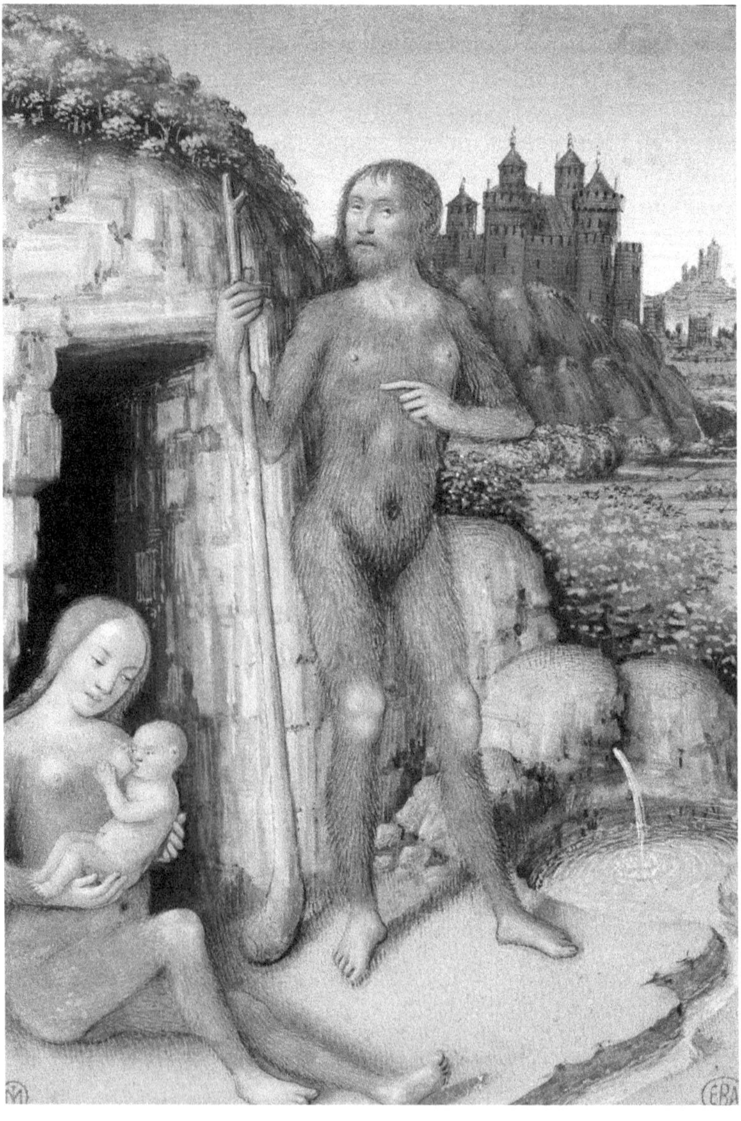

2.3: Jean Bourdichon, 'The Wild Condition', from 'The Four Conditions of Society', no. 32, c.1500.

If, as Hayden White has argued, the wild man represents 'a projection of repressed desires and anxieties' regarding the relationships between society and nature, humans and animals, the much less common wild woman (Figure 2.3) seems to be a symbol of more specifically sexual, or gender-related, anxieties.[38] Like her male counterpart, the wild woman is depicted as either abhorrent or seductive, acting as an incarnation of anxiety on one hand and of desire on the other. Embodying either a negative or positive female stereotype, the wild woman is sometimes portrayed as a dangerous, ugly and hairy seductress, or alternatively as a passive and dependent wife and mother living an idyllic rural life with her wild man husband and children.[39] Whilst there are fewer available images of wild women than wild men, art historian Richard Bernheimer has argued that 'her presence is recorded in areas which either never possessed any wild man mythology or have allowed it to fade out'.[40] According to Bernheimer, the nature of the wild woman was particularly diversified because of the variety of her habitat, which extended from forests and mountains to plains. Wild women living in the mountains were supposed to be giant ogres, enormously strong, appallingly ugly and prone to eat human children. In this abhorrent incarnation, their bodies were bristly all over, their hair wild and full of lichen, and their breasts so long that they dragged on the ground. By contrast, wild women who lived in the milder landscape of the plains were reportedly smaller, gentler and more retiring. They were hairy and clad in moss, with wrinkly faces, but long silken hair.[41] These images seem to suggest that the main role of the wild woman was either to reinforce 'man's' sexual dominance, or to embody a fear of his own sexual nature. The most persistent trait of any lone wild woman was an obsessive craving for the love of ordinary men, which was often achieved by using disguise and deception.

A Nineteenth-Century Wild Man

During the later Middle Ages the European forests inhabited by wild men and women were greatly depleted.[42] These quasi-monstrous creatures also faded from view and images of wild folk became scarce after the early sixteenth century. In the mid-nineteenth century, however, new fears of boundary confusion provoked by the revolutionary ideas proposed by Darwin, Huxley and their colleagues gave rise to another kind of wild man figure in the mid-nineteenth century. This theatrical creature, instructively named the 'What Is It?' first appeared live on stage in 1860. Manifesting a surge of anxiety concerning the boundary between humans and animals on the one hand, and a widespread fear of racial diversity on the other, this hybrid being was supposed to represent the 'missing link' between animal and human. In a poster advertising the 'What Is It?' (Figure 2.4) the problem of the relationship between wild nature and civilized culture is graphically illustrated. A large, ape-like being is depicted, clutching the trademark wooden staff of the wild man, whilst in the background is a table set for tea, a comforting symbol of refined English culture. According to the narrative on the poster, the 'What Is It?',

> can do anything which man or animal can do, except speak, read or write. It leaps, climbs, runs etc. with the agility of a monkey; it lays the cloth and sets a table with the *sang froid* of

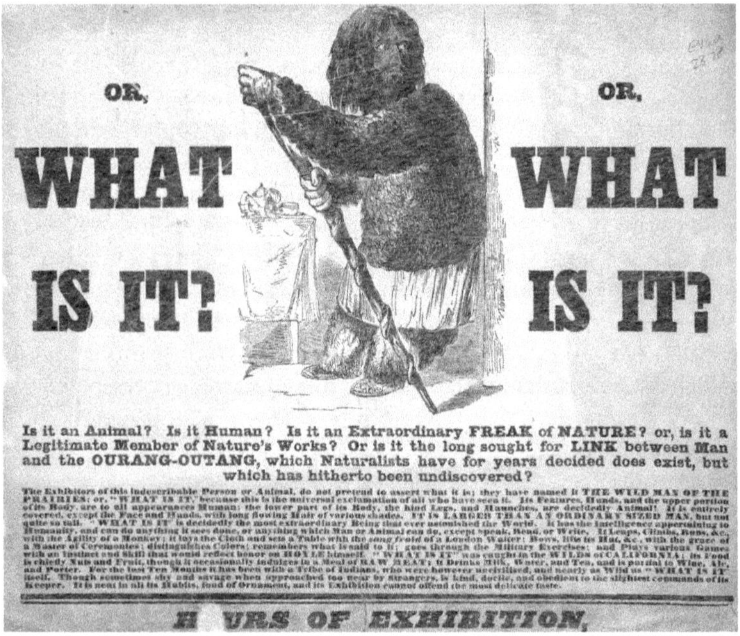
OR,
WHAT
IS IT?
OR,
WHAT
IS IT?
Is it an Animal? Is it Human? Is it an Extraordinary FREAK of NATURE? or, is it a Legitimate Member of Nature's Works? Or is it the long sought for LINK between Man and the OURANG-OUTANG, which Naturalists have for years decided does exist, but which has hitherto been undiscovered?
H URS OF EXHIBITION,

2.4: 'What Is It?', poster originally produced in London, c.1846.

> a London waiter . . . it was caught in the wilds of California . . . living with a tribe of Indians, who were however uncivilized and nearly as wild as 'What Is It?'

Whether or not audiences actually believed any of the rhetoric that surrounded the 'What Is It?', this primitive but refined character proved a highly popular figure on the freak show stage during the latter half of the nineteenth century.[43] Perhaps this was because it enabled ordinary people to speculate about the new scientific ideas put forward by Darwin and his colleagues.[44]

Feral Children

Another more intriguing, complex and subtle character that continues to inhabit the boundary between humans and animals is the feral child, otherwise known as the wild child, or wolf child. The origins of this enigmatic figure may be traced back to ancient myths such as that of Romulus and Remus, the abandoned twins suckled by a wolf, who, according to legend, founded the city of Rome. Whilst it is impossible to know whether mythical characters such as these were based on any actual events, since antiquity there have been many reports of children who have survived for long periods of time outside society with no experience of human care and no exposure to human language. In his book *Wolf Children*, the French writer Lucien Malson lists fifty-three known cases, dating from the mid-fourteenth century to the mid-twentieth century. Other sources suggest that there may be in excess of a hundred recorded cases, and the list is growing.[45]

One of the most thoroughly documented historical wild child stories is that of Victor, the 'Wild Boy of Aveyron', who was first seen in France in 1797. After eluding capture for three years, Victor was eventually taken to Paris in 1800, where Georges Cuvier and a doctor of psychiatry, Philippe Pinel, dismissed him as a 'congenital idiot'. But a junior doctor, Jean Marc Gaspard Itard, thought differently. Itard worked with Victor intensively over a five-year period to try to socialize him. His detailed account tells of a boy who was captured at the age of about eleven or twelve after subsisting for several years on roots and berries in woodland in the Aveyron region of France.[46] In line with the long-held cultural belief that human life can only be realized within society, Itard developed a personalized programme of treatment and education for Victor, aiming 'to attach him to social life, by rendering it more pleasant to him than that which he was then leading'.[47] Itard's project was, however, only partially successful as Victor's behaviour apparently remained wild and uncontrollable, and he never learned to speak.

In her recent study of feral children, historian Adriana Benzaquén sorts wild children into three different categories.[48] The first of these is the confined child who, like thirteen-year-old 'Genie', who was discovered naked and harnessed to a chair in a bare room in a California suburb in 1970, is in an abusive situation, deprived of a normal life by his or her parents.[49] Second is the 'free' wild child who, without a name and of unknown origin, lives entirely 'in the wild'. This type, which is clearly the most romanticized of all, is understood to be extremely rare. Benzaquén names only one example: the so-called Gazelle Boy of the Sahara, who was reportedly observed by the artist and explorer Jean-Claude Auger (alias Armen) throughout the 1960s. However, the fact that Auger apparently made no attempt to capture or even communicate with the 'Gazelle Boy' makes even this example seem highly implausible.[50] Benzaquén describes her third 'type' as the 'most inhuman and brutalized form of the wild child', the 'wolf child', who is brought up by animals.

Perhaps the only reliably documented modern example of this type of feral child is John Ssebunya, the 'Ugandan Monkey Boy'. Ssebunya was born in a small village during the Ugandan civil war of the 1980s. Since a villager discovered him living a feral existence in the forest in 1992, John's story has been widely reported in the international media. He has been the subject of numerous documentaries, and on 23 April 2007 appeared on the Dutch talk Show *Jensen!*, along with his adoptive parents, Paul and Molly Wasswa.[51] Speaking in Swahili, with his parents translating, Ssebunya recalls that, at a very young age, he fled to the forest after his mother was killed. There he formed a friendship with a troupe of vervet monkeys, which he relied on for food and comfort for a period of two to three years. Stating that he was able to communicate with the monkeys, Ssebunya briefly performs an imitation of their behaviour in front of a laughing talk show audience. But, when asked by Robert Jensen whether he still climbs trees, he replies with dignity and a hint of irony that, as an adult, he is now too old for this. Ssebunya speaks with a pronounced stutter, which, along with his slightly awkward gait, is one of the few remaining traces of his feral existence. Like other 'feral' children he is fascinating to watch, perhaps because his presence is a tangible reminder of the fragility of the boundary between savage nature and civilized culture.

The first episode of a three-part documentary series on feral children, made in 2011 for the Sky TV channel Animal Planet by anthropologist Mary-Ann Ochota, recalls the uncontrollable, animal state in which John was found.[52] Filthy and severely malnourished, with long, curved fingernails and calloused knees, he was apparently unable to walk upright. Terrified of humans and incapable of human language, he would scream, cry, scratch and bite, using gestures similar to those used by the monkeys. He was also reportedly covered in hair, although an early photograph shows no indication of this. Villagers recall that many people came to see this oddity, wanting to kill 'it' because they thought 'it' was an evil spirit. In the documentary, a teacher at the school John later attended states that, after three years living in the forest, 'this [John] was totally different, it was too much'.

Stories of children who, like 'Genie', have been forcibly isolated from human society are certainly compelling, but those who, like John Ssebunya, have survived 'in the wild' are most interesting because of what they represent. As Benzaquén points out, 'the confined child presents us with no mystery because her or his confined life is one of maximum control and immobility'.[53] His or her condition is a direct and tangible consequence of abuse. On the other hand, the image of the 'wild child' living in a state of nature gives form to the fantasy of escape from the routine of human life and freedom from social control. In this incarnation, the wild child personifies Rousseau's idea of an essential humanity. Yet this figure of the free, natural child also provokes a sense of unease. As Hirst and Woolley have argued, 'a genuinely feral existence on the part of a human child threatens . . . both the divide between man and nature and the place of culture as definitive of the human as against the animal'.[54] Although extremely rare, documented cases such as that of John Ssebunya act as reminders that if children really can be brought up by animals, adopt animal qualities and survive without the influence of human culture, the boundary between humans and animals may be more porous than we would like to believe.

Children who have survived outside human society may be seen as valuable objects of scientific knowledge, but the details of their lives are always interwoven with mythic, literary and moral narratives in a way that keeps us uncertain as to what might be true about them. Wild children continue to fascinate us because, like human monsters, they challenge the definition of what it is to be human. But it is perhaps the uncertain interplay between the 'real' and the 'constructed' aspects of their stories that most intensely provokes our curiosity. One particularly intriguing and contentious wild-child story is that of a Ukrainian girl, Oxana Malaya, who was born into a remote farming community in 1983. Since her story first came to the attention of the international media in the early 2000s, it has been widely reported that from an early age Malaya was left outside in the yard by her alcoholic parents, who were apparently too drunk to care for her. During an interview with British child psychologist and expert on feral children Lyn Fry in 2006, Malaya herself stated that, at the age of three, she had reasoned that 'mum had too many children and there weren't enough beds, so one night I called to the dog and started living with her'.[55]

Malaya's story was initially made public by the Ukrainian tabloids, which published claims that she was kept chained up in the yard of her family home, where she survived by suckling the farm dogs and eating raw meat. An enormously popular television documentary, *Mindshock*, first shown in the UK on Channel 4 in 2006, states that she continued to live with the farmyard dogs until the age of eight, when a neighbour eventually reported her condition to the authorities and she was sent to a children's home.[56] The documentary includes some archive footage that shows her perform a re-enactment of the animal behaviour she is said to have exhibited when living as a feral child. As she barks and growls at the camera, walks on all fours, laps water from a tap and shakes herself, her mannerisms are certainly more dog-like than human.

Mary-Ann Ochota disputes the story that Malaya grew up with dogs. In a radio interview she has said,

> When we arrived [in Ukraine to film the second episode of the Animal Planet series] I discovered that [Oxana] was taken into care at the age of eighteen months, and she had grown up in state Soviet orphanages, so suddenly you think . . . 'is this all a massive hoax?' Someone is making money, perhaps, out of peddling this story about a dog girl who barks and howls and crawls around on all fours.[57]

In this new documentary, the archive footage of Malaya performing dog-like behaviour is used to demonstrate how she began to imitate the dogs as an escape from the trauma of living in the Soviet orphanage.[58] According to Ochota, the dogs offered physical comfort and an emotional connection that was missing in Malaya's experience of human relationships. Whether at her home or in the orphanage, it is clear that Malaya was sufficiently neglected by humans to develop a special relationship with dogs. Anna Chalaya, director of the Baraboy Clinic, where Malaya now lives as an adult, has commented that 'she didn't think it was necessary to speak at all . . . she used to show her tongue when she saw water, and she used to eat with her tongue and not her hands'. When she was stressed Malaya would apparently 'go outside into nature . . . and bark'.[59] Malaya herself has described the way that she would converse with the dogs like this: 'they would bark. I would repeat it. That was our way of communicating'.[60]

Whilst Malaya is unable to read or write and, as a young adult, was deemed by Fry to have a mental age of five to six years, it remains unclear whether or not her learning difficulties were

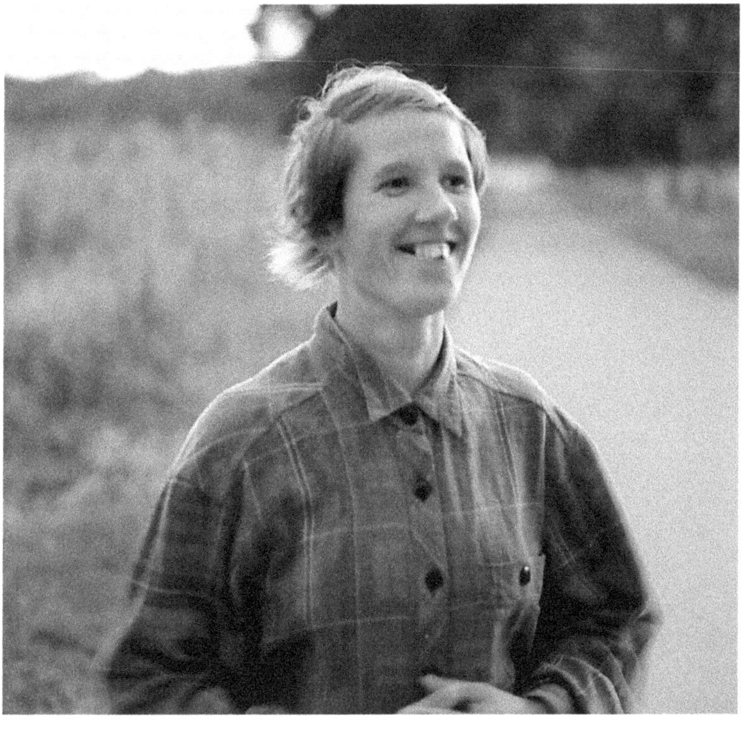

2.5: Oxana Malaya.

compounded by spending many of her developmental years in the company of dogs. More recently, she has certainly been able to live a relatively normal life at the clinic in Odessa, where she shares a bedroom with five other women, takes care of herself and regularly works in the dairy. Whatever the correct details of her life, Malaya's 'true' story is one of neglect and abuse, her dog-like behaviour the manifestation of a desperate desire to belong somewhere within what Edward Dudley and Maximillian Novak have termed a 'socially provided world' in their book *The Wild Man Within*.[61]

Nevertheless, in the popular imagination Malaya remains both an object of fascination and an outsider figure. For example, an article in the *Telegraph* newspaper from 2006 reported that, whilst she has had boyfriends, at least one was 'scared off' by her show of canine behaviour because 'to be confronted with what she was . . . put him off'.[62] Emphasizing the irreconcilable differences between a creature like Malaya and a 'normal' child, and at the same time drawing on our sympathy, the article concludes with the comment that: 'although the amelioration of her terrible history has gone a long way, it can probably go no further'.[63] Behind these words is the suggestion that, as a child who has transgressed the boundary between humans and animals, Malaya is ultimately irredeemable. Perhaps she is dismissed because, on a symbolic level, the existence of a child who identifies as much with animals as with humans remains a threat to our understanding of what it is to be human.

3 | Bodies and the Order of Society

The Greek Ideal, the Monster of Ravenna and Physiognomy

> The body . . . is a powerful symbolic form, a surface on which the central rules, hierarchies, and even metaphysical commitments of a culture are inscribed and thus reinforced.[1]

There are many ways in which human society depends on the signifying function of the human body. Most obviously, the visual signals conveyed by the structure and dynamic features of the body, and the face in particular, form a basic element of human communication. But ancient systems such as astrology and physiognomy also treat the body and face as codified structures that can be visibly related to the cosmos, to the order of society as a whole or to the character of a particular individual. Within these systems the human body functions as a collection of visual images that correspond to general beliefs about the order of the world, or to particular ideas about human character. Whilst neither astrology nor physiognomy is taken very seriously in contemporary academic or scientific contexts, the belief that a person's face can reveal his or her 'true' character is certainly still current within popular culture. Modern portraiture relies on what the art historian Martin Kemp has called the 'physiognomic imperative', and photographic snapshots and 'mug shots' of celebrities or criminals published in the media are generally expected to reveal correspondingly positive or negative characteristics.[2]

According to the anthropologist Mary Douglas, the representational function of the body is crucial, and inevitable. It is perhaps because, as Douglas suggests, the human body offers 'the most readily available image of a system' that it is always treated as an image of society.[3] Most importantly, Douglas asserts that, 'there can be no natural way of considering the body that does not involve at the same time a social dimension'.[4] She describes a continual exchange of meanings between body and society, within which the physical experience of the body is modified by society, which in turn is represented by the body.[5] This reciprocal dynamic between body and society is crucial to the construction of meaning in deviant or monstrous bodies.

With the intention of establishing a historical and cultural context for understanding monstrosity as a visual phenomenon, the chapter takes up the idea of the body as a legible surface, focusing on the practices of astrology and physiognomy. The strangely mixed-up figure of the sixteenth-century Monster of Ravenna is introduced here as an extreme example of the way in which the body of the monster can act as a visual image of social and political disorder.

Within a world-view that understands the 'normal' human body as an ideal physical and symbolic expression of certainty and order in society, the body of the monster has historically represented that which is disproportionate, or out of place. In fact, all the strange, uncertain and often monstrous bodies discussed in the previous two chapters owe their symbolic power, and perhaps even their existence, to the traditional understanding of the 'normal' human body as a legible and significant structure. As a counterpart to the rational order of the 'normal' body, the deformed body of the monster visibly manifests troubling boundary confusions in the form of excess, deficit or bizarre and illegal combinations. In the third of his lectures on the abnormal, given on 22 January 1975, Michel Foucault explains that,

> From the middle ages to the eighteenth century . . . the monster is essentially a mixture. It is a mixture of two kingdoms, the animal and the human: the man with the head of an ox, the man with birds feet – monsters. It is the blending, the mixture of two species: the pig with a sheep's head is a monster. It is the mixture of two individuals, the one who has two heads and one body, or two bodies and one head is a monster. It is the mixture of two sexes: the one who is both male and female is a monster. It is a mixture of life and death: the foetus born with a morphology such that it cannot live, but which however manages to live for a few minutes or days, is a monster. Finally, it is a mixture of forms: the person who has no arms or legs, like a snake, is a monster. Consequently, the transgression of natural limits, the transgression of classifications, of the table, transgression of the law as a table: this is the real question of monstrosity.[6]

Foucault describes the monster as an 'anti-cosmological being' that contradicts the natural order of the universe.[7] The various examples he gives in the passage quoted above illustrate how monsters are, by nature, unclassifiable creatures, their mixed-up bodies displaying all kinds of morphological abnormalities. The human monster is essentially a kind of 'nondescript' that resists containment by any legal, scientific, natural or cultural system. The grotesque distortions of its formation simultaneously create and signify the presence of structural disorder in the world around it.

The 'Normal' Body

There is much historical evidence that the 'normal' human body has been used as an important model for interpreting the 'natural' or correct structure of the external world for millennia. As early as the fourth century BC, for example, Plato set out the idea of the human body as a microcosm that 'can stand as a conceptual framework for all that follows'.[8] According to the American scholar Leonard Barkan, this cosmological view of man characterized the study of natural philosophy until at least the sixteenth century. It informed the work of artists such as Leonardo da Vinci, whose 'Vitruvian Man' drawing (*c.*1492) (Figure 3.1) offers a literal illustration of earlier ideas about the structure of the world. The Roman architect and writer Vitruvius (*c.*70–25 BC) believed that the configuration of all natural forms, including the human body, was based on universal laws of proportion and symmetry. By showing that the 'ideal' body fitted precisely into both a circle and a square, Vitruvius aimed to demonstrate that there was a link between natural proportions, perfect geometric forms and the ideal human body. These beliefs, which were taken up by da Vinci, formed the basis of the Renaissance understanding of proportion.

Barkan has noted that, 'for Western civilization to study man was to study the cosmos, and to know the cosmos was to know oneself'.[9] He points to the 'crucial and central' position of the body within the ancient tradition of astrology, which relies on a pictorial correlation between the human image and the cosmos.[10] The zodiacal system divides the human body into sections according to the relative positions of the moon, planets and stars, proposing a literal correspondence between character traits, the body and the universe. Within this system, the human figure in general functions as a legible image of the cosmos, whilst the configuration of each individual body is determined

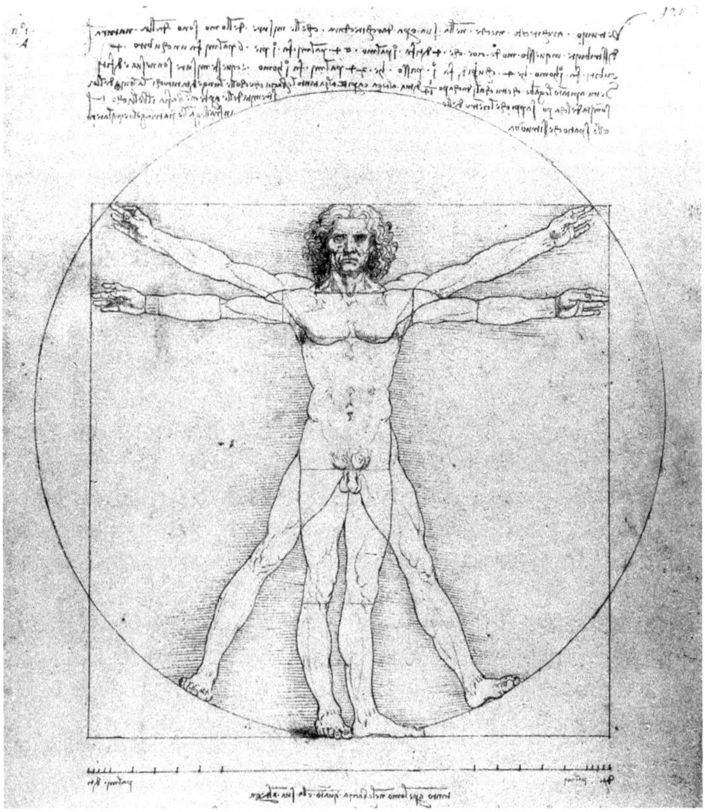

3.1: Leonardo da Vinci, 'Vitruvian Man', c.1487.

by a particular arrangement of the planets. Images such as the picture of astrological man (Figure 3.2) show how the planets are supposed to influence individual parts of the body.

According to ancient astrologers, it is the zodiacal signs present at the birth of an individual that govern the formation of his or her anatomical features, and changes in the configuration of the planets are thought to determine the dynamic state of the body.[11] This belief system, in which 'man' is seen as the centre of the world and the 'normal' human body functions as a model for a well-ordered world, offers a clear context for the idea of the deformed body of the monster as a negative indicator. From this point of view, human monstrosity is thought to be caused by negative forces in the external world that leave their mark on the structure of an individual human body.[12] The bodily

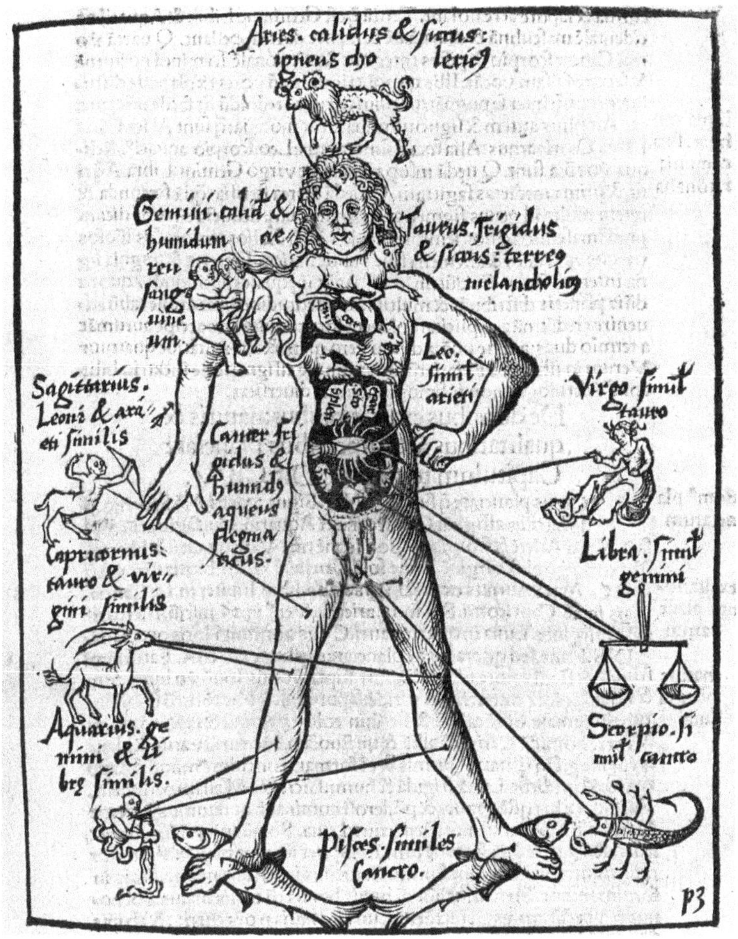

3.2: Gregor Reisch, 'De Astrologia – Astrological Man', *Margarita philosophica*, 1503, woodcut.

appearance of the monster provides an obvious visual indication that something is wrong.

The Greek Ideal

In direct contrast to the deviant body of the pre-modern monster, the idealized figure of the classical Greek athlete embodies a desire for order and meaning in every area of life.[13] In classical

Greek society, which was rigorously controlled and regulated by strict laws, the disciplined body of the athletic urban male provided an important image of social order. The idealized human body acted as a visible affirmation of the power of Greek culture.[14] According to the art historian Alex Potts, the body of the athlete was also seen as the physical expression of a 'free self' and a manifestation of the 'ideal sovereign subject'. Potts has argued that the flawless and serene beauty of the figure of the Greek athlete is 'a sign of its not being in any way disfigured or constrained by the world around it'.[15] In the classical context, therefore, political, cultural and even religious values seem to have been most prominently broadcast through glorified images of athletic bodies. But, whilst the ideal body may have functioned as a paradigm, it was clearly unattainable for any 'normal' person.

The sculpture of the 'Discobolus', or 'Discus Thrower', by Myron (*c.*450 BC) (Figure 3.3) demonstrates how a static image of the body can reinforce and maintain dominant social and cultural values. Although the original bronze sculpture is now lost, the 'Discus Thrower' remains one of the most well-known images from the classical period, with many Roman copies still in existence. This model of the well-proportioned, symmetrical and muscular male body was used to symbolize a regulated, powerful and stable society where wholeness, strength and control are the 'norm'. But, although it has been praised for its realism and dynamic power, this is a highly contrived image. At first sight the sculpture offers a convincing representation of a young athlete in the act of throwing a discus. Its life-like qualities are expressed in the muscular tension of the body and in details such as the depiction of the veins that stand out on the hand and arm supporting the discus. But the artist was not simply concerned with reproducing nature or creating a mimetic replica of the body of an individual athlete. As the art historian Ernst Gombrich has explained, Myron has 'composed his picture of a man's body out of the most characteristic views of its parts'.[16] That is to say, when the torso is viewed from the front, the legs and arms are presented from the side. Yet, although the various parts of the athlete's body are actually shown in an impossible relationship with one another, they work together visually to form an apparently coherent, harmonious and realistic whole. This image of perfected human being, designed to promote the idea of a similarly strong and organized society, is actually an artificial and largely unattainable representation made up of a collection of disparate fragments.

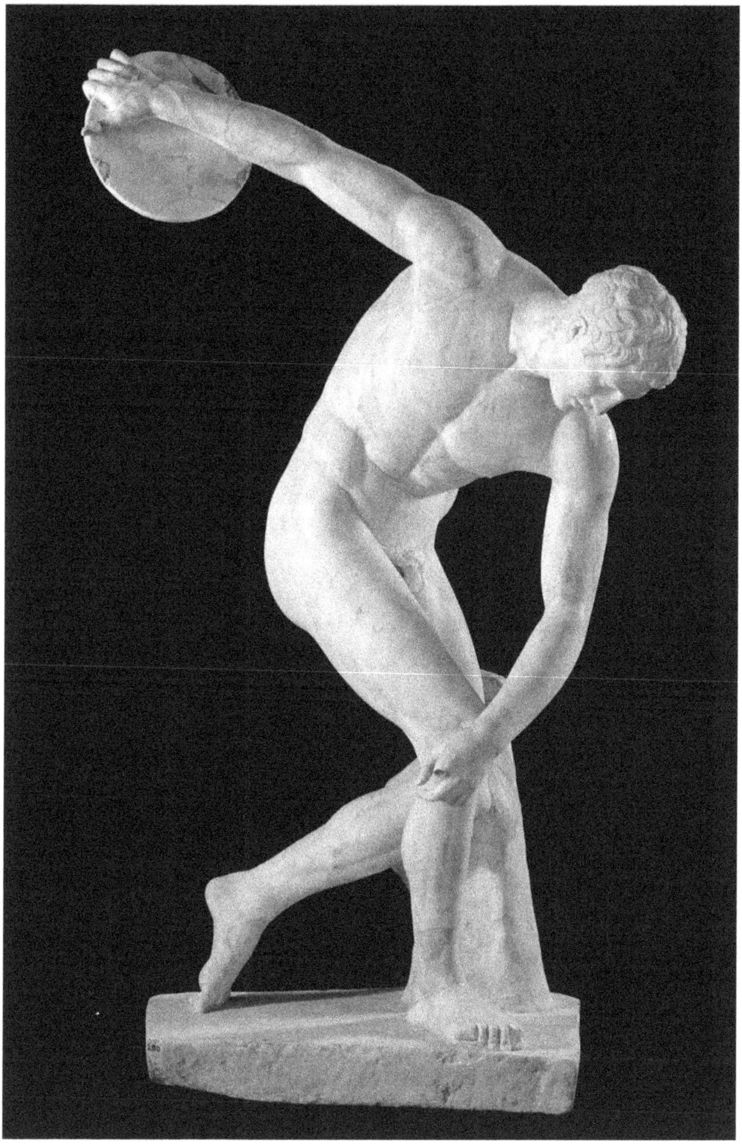

3.3: Roman copy of Myron's 'Discobolus' ('Discus Thrower').[17]

Classical sculptures such as the 'Discus Thrower' show how positive social values can be asserted and maintained through the public display of an idealized body. The strange or deformed body of the human monster has historically performed a similar function, but in a contrary way, by embodying that which perverts the accepted social norm. Like the athletic figure of the 'Discus Thrower', the symbolic bodies of monsters are also composed of an assortment of parts, and yet the combination of these parts has a very different meaning. As a whole, the body of the monster is incomprehensible. It brings unknown or inappropriate elements together with recognizably human components in strange or impossible combinations. Although it is highly significant, the 'unnatural' morphology of the monster makes no sense. Foucault has theorized this combination of incoherence and significance, identifying it as a defining feature of all pre-modern monsters:

> Paradoxically, the monster is a principle of intelligibility in spite of its limit position as both the impossible and the forbidden. And yet this principle of intelligibility is strictly tautological, since the characteristic feature of the monster is to express itself as, precisely, monstrous, to be the explanation of every little deviation that may derive from it, but to be unintelligible in itself.[18]

Here Foucault explains the essentially contradictory character of the monster as it literally takes on the characteristics it is cautioning against. Giving visible form to a state of chaos or uncertainty, the body of the monster is, therefore, simultaneously reassuring and terrifying.

As we saw in Chapter 1, social and ontological confusion was manifested in the abnormal bodies of creatures such as the Monstrous Races from antiquity. But the late fifteenth and early sixteenth centuries saw a massive increase in popular interest in prodigies, or monstrous births.[19] At this time, human identity and the external world were still thought to be so intimately connected that it was not possible to develop a sense of oneself as a separate entity that could be set apart from society or divorced from a religious understanding of the world.[20] This correspondence between 'man' and world is consistent with the classical world-view discussed above, in which the human body is believed to act as a visible and tangible link between society and the cosmos. In this context, babies born with deformities were understood to be an inevitable and irredeemable consequence of the action of astral positions. This conviction was probably based on an ancient idea upheld by the powerful Roman statesman and philosopher Cicero (106–43 BC), who maintained that the future could be read from a deformed body with as much certainty as

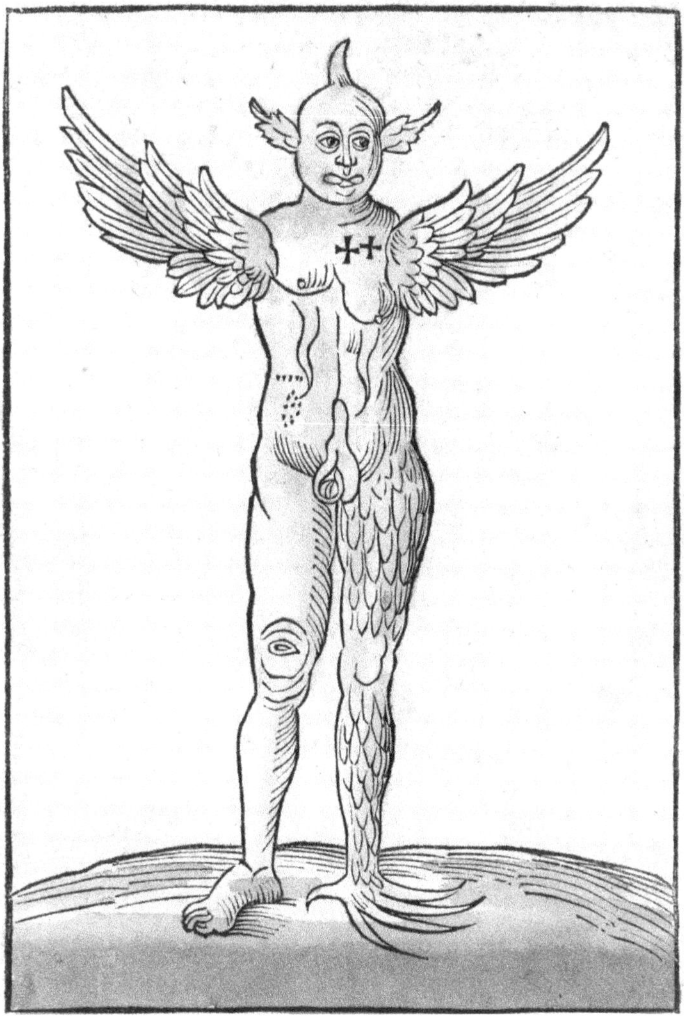

3.4: The Monster of Ravenna (based on an earlier version originally found in Florence) from a German broadside of 1506.[21]

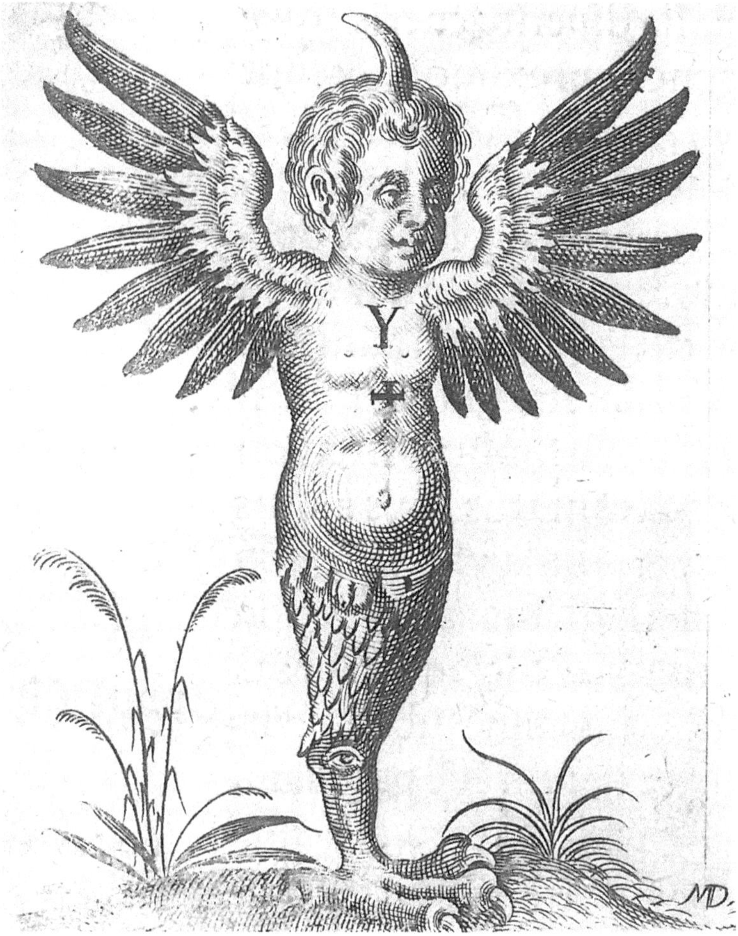

3.5: Licetus, 'The Monster of Ravenna', from *De monstrorum natura, causis et differentis*, 1634, after Ambroise Paré.

from the stars. Cicero proposed that monsters themselves have astrological causes and can therefore be read in the same way as other astrological signs.[22]

The idea that the distorted bodies of monsters could act as direct indicators of religious and social unrest, as well as signifying more general ontological problems, was perhaps most prevalent in the Renaissance. The proliferation of monstrous births in the sixteenth century has been linked to discoveries that challenged the most basic and commonly held beliefs about human identity and the order of the world. For example, it was at this time that the astronomer Nicolaus Copernicus first proved that the earth was not at the centre of the universe. His findings, published in 1543, overturned the previously held belief that the world was organized around 'man' at its centre.[23] Reflecting this reversal in their bodily structure, creatures such as the Monster of Ravenna offered a means of symbolizing the confusion that surrounded this radical shift in understanding.

Monstrous births were also indicative of more localized social and moral instability. For example, the birth of the Ravenna monster in 1512 was believed to have been a sign from God that predicted the sacking of the city of Ravenna during the Italian religious wars.[24] The insecurity of 'man's' position caused by this social and religious upheaval is reflected in every aspect of the monster's oddly configured body. It has a human torso, bird's wings and scaled or feathered legs, with bird-like or reptilian claws in place of feet. It is depicted as a hermaphrodite, sometimes with just one female breast and often with only a single leg. It possesses other significant features, such as an eye in its knee, a horn on its head and religious symbols inscribed on its chest. Even the monster's conception represents a disturbance to the established moral order. It was, according to an early report, born as the result of a forbidden act between a nun and a friar.[25]

At a time when literacy was still a capacity of the privileged few, visual images of monsters must have provided a particularly important means of publicly disseminating and fixing religious and moral ideas. As an object that was structurally equivalent to the society it was found in, the body of the monster enabled the transmission of knowledge or ideas about aspects of life that were normally either invisible, or unrepresentable. But the configuration of this particular monster was constantly in flux. This iconic creature meant quite different things to different people, its mutable body enabling the formation and negotiation of quite contradictory ideas.[26] For example, the Protestant Flemish chronicler Johannes Multivallis (writing in 1512) and the French Catholic writer Pierre Boaistuau (1517–66) each interpreted it according to their own moral and religious beliefs. Both of them treated the monster's body as a text that could be literally translated. Multivallis declared that:

> the horn [indicates] pride; the wings, mental frivolity and inconstancy; the lack of arms, a lack of good works; the raptors foot rapaciousness, usury and every sort of avarice; the eye

on the knee a mental orientation solely toward earthly things; the double sex, sodomy. And on account of these vices, Italy is shattered by the sufferings of war, which the King of France has not accomplished by his own power, but only as the scourge of God.[27]

Boaistuau added a more specifically religious explanation:

But by this figure Y and the cross were two signs of value, because Y signifies virtue and the cross shows that all who return to Jesus and take up his cross will find a true remedy against sin, and a perfect way to health and salvation.[28]

The various forms and interpretations of this one monster demonstrate how its physical properties were directly determined by changing cultural values, and yet each element of its body was always highly significant. Whilst the Ravenna monster's torso and head mutate over time between male and female, human and animal, adult and infantile forms, the symmetry of sexual difference is cancelled out in the double genitals, which appear in every version. The wings attached to a human torso imply a transgression of the boundaries between earth and air, which, according to the Canadian scholar David Williams, represents a challenge to the perceived opposition between physical and spiritual aspects of human being.[29] The animal and birdlike parts present in every version of the monster offer a pictorial reminder of 'man's' bestial nature. The holy cross on its chest draws attention to the idea of the body as a discursive space, where religious and moral problems may be worked out. The single birdlike leg and foot in later versions (Figure 3.5) negates the logic of symmetry and pairing normally associated with the human body. All in all, the complex iconography of this monster illustrates the symbolic power that was attached to its many deformities. Although the potency of this form of physical monstrosity was most evident in the context of the highly religious and magical belief systems of pre-modern Europe, the Monster of Ravenna acts as a reminder of the importance of the symbolic and representational function of all monsters.

In a diary written between 1450 and 1516 the well-known Florentine apothecary Luca Landucci noted the occurrence of many monstrous births, including the Ravenna Monster and the rather less well-known Volterra Monster. This creature was said to have been born with the head of a bull, a female human body and the claws of a lion, and was thought to have prefigured the sacking of the city of Volterra in 1474. Landucci also recorded in his diary the birth of a pair of conjoined twins around Venice in 1489, and a thirteen-year-old boy with a parasitic twin born in Florence in 1513. His accounts of the births of the more obviously fantastic creatures like the monsters of Ravenna and Volterra, and the 'real' births of conjoined twins or the boy with the parasitic twin are equally matter of fact. He even accords the Monster of Ravenna a date, place and time of birth. All of this suggests that this monster was considered to be a real phenomenon. Modern writers have also speculated that depictions of the Ravenna monster were in fact based on the real birth of a severely malformed child on the specified date. And yet images such as those shown in Figures 3.4 and 3.5 are now clearly seen as quaint mythological illustrations rather than depictions of the deformed infant's 'real' form.[30]

Such a lack of discrimination between what we would now consider 'real' and 'mythical' is not uncommon in sixteenth-century reports of monstrous births. For example, in 1493, the German encyclopedist Conrad Lycosthenes wrote, 'In Rome a twin was born conjoined, lived but a few days, not long after that a boy that was half a dog was born – these two prodigies signified the murders and wickedness which were to follow'.[31] In this single sentence the writer makes no distinction at all between the significance of the fantastical dog-headed boy and the more realistic figure of conjoined twins. Whilst these examples clearly demonstrate some interesting historical changes to notions of what can be considered 'real' or 'unreal', in the words of the Renaissance scholar Dudley Wilson, the 'difficulties which normally exist in distinguishing between the real and the imaginary persist strongly in the area of the monstrous'.[32] Any attempt to fully disentangle the 'mythic' from the 'real' in the arena of human monstrosity is fraught with contradiction.

If the forms that human monstrosity can take have altered over time, there have also been historical changes in what it is possible for the monster to signify. In the Middle Ages, for example, the Monstrous Races were still understood as 'moral prodigies', portents, or signs from God.[33] It was not until the early sixteenth century, a time of great religious uncertainty, that the presence of a monster became a signifier of the presence of evil within society. The deformed body was then directly related to the idea of human wickedness, or sin.[34] This concept of evil is inextricably linked to religious thought. It implies something that is harmful or tending to harm, either intentionally or characteristically.[35] It is a complicated idea that, in the Christian tradition, is associated with temptation, with immorality and with what is considered unnatural. The evil signified by Renaissance monsters seems to have been directly linked to various fears surrounding the moral, religious and political unrest that took place throughout Europe. The display of monstrous infants, both 'in the flesh' and, more commonly, in pictures, acted as a way of publicizing and consolidating moral and social problems or catastrophic events. Creatures such as the Monster of Ravenna portended the imminent ruin of the Catholic Church, as well as indicating a more widespread sense of disempowerment for non-Catholics. The disordered body of the monster personified the idea that early sixteenth-century European society was failing to conform to what was believed to be the rational, 'natural' order of things.

Paintings and drawings of transgressive creatures like the Ravenna monster provided a means of broadcasting political or religious propaganda and issuing moral warnings to a largely illiterate population. The importance attributed to pictures of Renaissance monsters is demonstrated in a note Luca Landucci made in his diary on 11 March 1512, where he seems to assume that a painting of the Monster of Ravenna provided living proof of its existence: 'we heard that a monster had been born at Ravenna, of which a drawing was sent here . . . I saw it painted and anyone who wished could see this painting in Florence'.[36] The documentary significance attributed to drawn or painted pictures by writers such as Landucci seems to indicate that they were understood as objective records of the 'truth' in much the same way as photographs would be in the late nineteenth century.

At the beginning of the sixteenth century, the public dissemination of images of monstrous prodigies was significantly enhanced by the new technology of printing. Although books were still quite rare, the publication of small, popular, inexpensive illustrated pamphlets and broadsheets meant that news of monstrous births could be disseminated much more widely. These publications often juxtaposed images with texts that mixed scientific detail with word-of-mouth reports, sometimes mentioning the address at which a monster was supposed to have been born and urging the public to go to see it for themselves. In this case, drawings seem to have been used in the same way as the photographs in modern tabloids – to prove the authenticity of a report and to heighten its emotional effect.[37]

Physiognomy

So far in this chapter we have seen how the 'proper' human body has served as a model of cosmological and social order within the ancient system of astrology, and also in the case of classical Greek sculpture. In the tradition of the astrological or cosmological body, the body of the pre-modern monster functioned as a negative representation of social and moral values. In this context, the sixteenth-century Monster of Ravenna offers an extreme example of the way that a deformed, transgressive or 'wrong' body can indicate moral, social and religious disorder. But, as an image of society, this Renaissance monster was accorded no interiority and no subjectivity. It was entirely emblematic, and could be 'known' only in terms of its physical and visual significance.

The practice of physiognomy, which was highly popular during the eighteenth and nineteenth centuries, is based on the belief that there is a direct correspondence between a person's inner being, or character, and his or her outward appearance. Like astrology, physiognomy is an ancient belief system that spans several cultures. In line with the cosmographic systems referred to earlier in this chapter, it treats the body and particularly the face as a representational image in which symmetry stands for attractiveness, goodness and beauty, whilst physical distortion, disproportion, lack or excess represents unfitness and a deviant or criminal character. The lexicon is similar to that of the Renaissance monster, except that within the discipline of physiognomy the meanings derived from a particular body relate to the character of the individual, rather than to society as a whole.

Historical texts show that physiognomy was popular in ancient China and in the Arab world as well as in ancient Greece, where it was systematically discussed in the *Physiognomonika*, an influential work that has been attributed to Aristotle.[38] Here, the author explains that human character follows physical characteristics, and so when the condition of the mind changes, it changes the appearance of the body: 'an ill-proportioned body indicates a rogue, while a well-proportioned frame is characteristic of upright and brave men'.[39]

The belief that the human body is a significant surface which, when decoded, reveals some deeper truth is common to all astrological and physiognomic systems and is deeply embedded in human culture. So, too, is the idea that symmetry and proportion are desirable and 'proper' qualities, whilst physical deformity, lack or excess is negative and troubling. These same principles have historically informed the work of many artists and scientists. For example, although Leonardo da Vinci was sceptical of what he understood to be the 'unfounded determinism of physiognomics', his physiognomic sketches (*c*.1480–1510) demonstrate an interest in identifying character types using the theory of the four humours: choleric, melancholic, sanguine and phlegmatic, each of which is evidenced by a different kind of physique.[40] In his drawing 'Five Grotesque Heads' (Figure 3.6), da Vinci has systematically linked the morphology of the human face to variations in temperament and character, so that each figure illustrates a different physiognomic type. As the art historian Michael Kwakkelstein has observed, in this work, 'Leonardo drew each different grimace, expressing either laughter, fury, obstinacy or attention in such a way as to conform to the physiognomic type expressive of the prevailing temperament or disposition'.[41]

In 1586 the Italian scientist and polymath Giambattista della Porta published a richly illustrated study of physiognomy, *De humana physiognomonia,* in which he too maintained that human character and physique are based on the four humours. Della Porta was perhaps the first to set out the principles of the physiognomic correspondence between external form and internal character in any systematic way, although his system seems to have been more magical than scientific. Building on earlier ideas that combined astronomy and physiognomy, della Porta maintained that the features of a particular species of animal correspond to its temperament, and that humans who have a similar character will exhibit equivalent physical features. *De humana physiognomonia* contains a large number of illustrations that make a rather exaggerated visual correlation between human and animal physiognomies and character traits.[42]

The idea that physiognomic studies could provide moral information from which a person's character, temperament

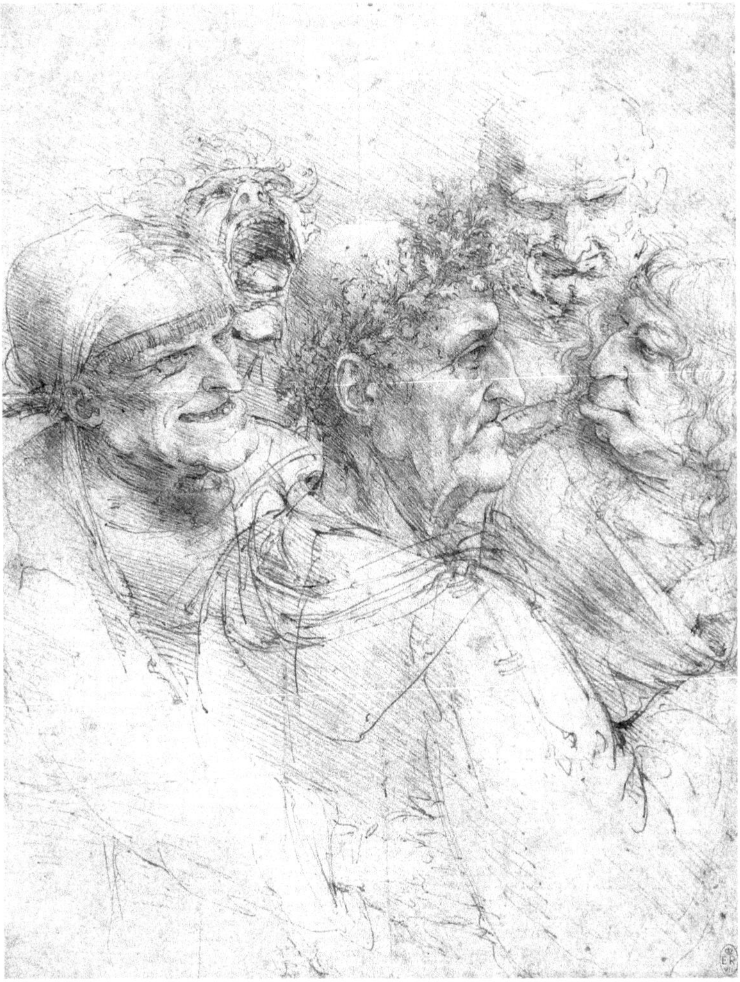

3.6: Leonardo da Vinci, 'Five Grotesque Heads', c.1480–1510.

and capabilities could be scientifically measured was first given credence by the work of the French artist and theorist Charles Le Brun (1619–90).[43] Le Brun believed that there is a direct correspondence between mind and body whereby a person's character is revealed through particular, classifiable facial features.[44] He was especially interested in the physiological expression of emotion through the dynamic features of the face. In the posthumously published *Treatise on Expressions* (1698), Le Brun visualized a theory of facial expression based on the ideas of the philosopher René Descartes, who proposed that the human face directly reflects the workings of the mind. Following della Porta, Le Brun also saw a correspondence between the appearance and disposition of certain animals and particular human characters. In order to illustrate Descartes' physiognomic theories, he developed a geometrical system for measuring and correlating the faces of men and animals

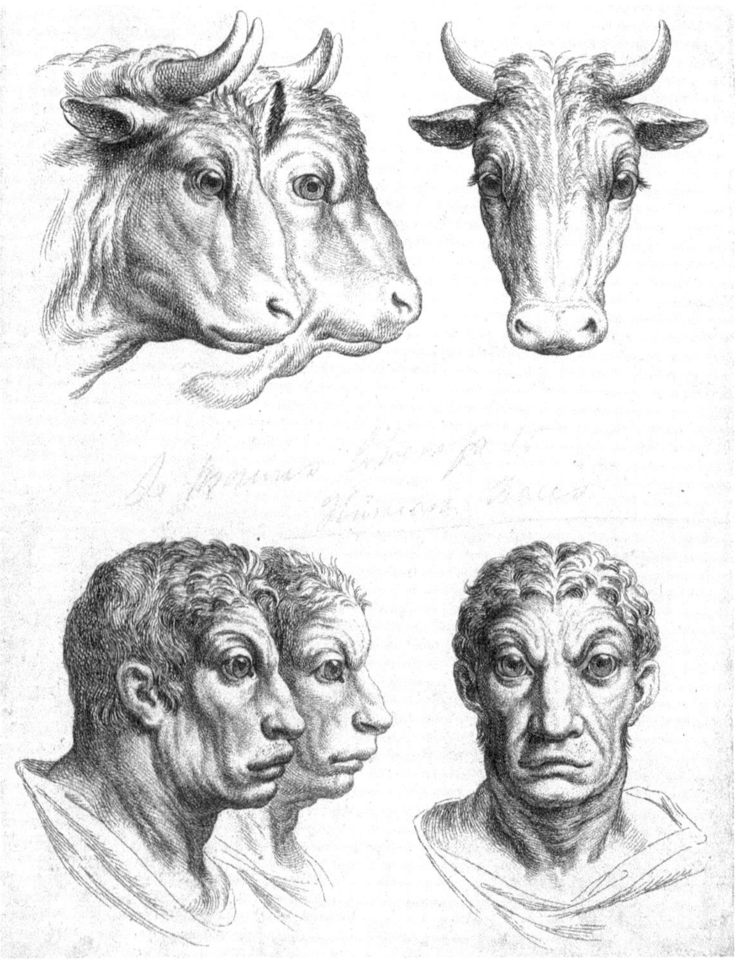

3.7: Charles Le Brun, 'The Head of an Ox and the Head of an Ox-like Man: Three Figures of Each Showing their Physiognomical Relations', c.1820.

(Figure 3.7).[45] Le Brun made a large number of detailed drawings comparing human and animal physiognomy in order to show that a range of human 'passions' could be determined through this analogy.

The eighteenth century saw a resurgence of interest in physiognomic ideas, but the old ideas were somewhat modified. Whereas previously the whole of the body had functioned as an indicator of moral or social values, the work of Le Brun and later physiognomists led to a progressive withdrawal of signification from the body to the face and head. By the late eighteenth century, therefore, attention was focused almost entirely on the face as an indicator of character. It was at this time that one of the most influential modern physiognomists, the Swiss theologian Johann Kaspar Lavater (1741–1801), was attempting to establish physiognomy as a modern science, using geometric methods developed by Le Brun. Lavater focused on the underlying structure of the face and head rather than on its dynamic features. He attempted to assemble an encyclopedia of the human face, the *Physiognomische Fragmente* (1775–8), which remains a key text in the history of physiognomy.[46] In this work, Lavater reaffirms the ancient Greek equation of beauty with goodness: 'the more I reflect the more I am convinced that virtue and vice . . . are beauty and deformity'.[47] For Lavater, to look at a person was to know him or her. He understood a person's anatomical features as immediate indicators of his or her intellectual ability, and moral and psychological attributes. Lavater's writings suggest that he saw the human face as a legible and meaningful surface on which not only a person's character but also a whole range of social and moral conventions could be inscribed.

Lavater's physiognomic analysis of the Greek philosopher Socrates (*c.*399–369 BC), for which he created a series of profiles drawn from a portrait bust (Figure 3.8), demonstrates his belief that physiognomic narrative was best extracted from static images. He thought that the static image would give a more accurate reading because meaning was primarily derived from a person's fixed characteristics. Lavater preferred, therefore, to base his physiognomic readings on drawings, sculptures and even corpses because he believed that the facial expressions and movements of a living person and any interactions with him or her would impede his search for 'true' physiognomic meaning. His work on Socrates demonstrates particularly clearly how images of people and the narratives constructed around them can come together to produce an identity that may or may not

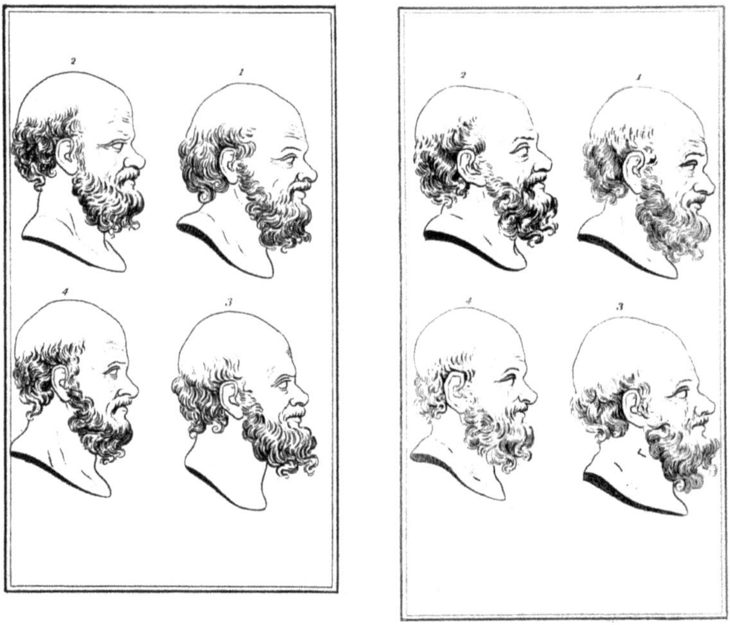

3.8: Johann Kaspar Lavater, 'Eight Ways of Looking at Socrates', from *Essays on Physiognomy, Designed to Promote the Love and Knowledge of Mankind*, vol. 1, London: G.G. & J. Robinson, 1789.[48]

coincide with that of the 'real' person. Socrates was well known for being extremely ugly, and yet he was also known for being a noble, pious and good person. Lavater deals with the problem of this discrepancy by subtly manipulating the visual image of the ancient philosopher, redrawing and softening different features to conform to his highly subjective ideas (Figure 3.8). He justifies this by criticizing all previous representations for their inaccuracy and by suggesting that only an experienced practitioner like him could read the truth of a person's physiognomy. He writes that 'the form of the face of Socrates may have appeared very ugly to inexperienced eyes, while the play of his Physiognomy presented the features of celestial beauty'.[49] Focusing on Lavater's adaptations of the image of Socrates, the American scholar Kevin Berland points to the flexible way in which visual images can be interpreted: 'portraits of Socrates are not simply fixed, objective, factual data; rather, they serve as raw material which can be adapted or refashioned to support a new preconception or theory'.[50]

Although as a physiognomist, Lavater's own intentions may not have been directly racist, his work was used by some of his peers as a systematic means of 'othering' people from non-European races and cultures. For example, Georges Cuvier's notions of racial determinism, according to which inequality was the inevitable result of a person's outward appearance, were informed by Lavater's physiognomic ideas.[51] The work of Francis Galton (1822–1911), another key figure in modern 'scientific' physiognomy, was also used to justify racism. Galton, who was a cousin of Darwin and a leading biological scientist, applied Darwinian theories of evolution and natural selection to human society in order to differentiate between humans and animals, as well as between those who were considered 'civilized' and 'less civilized'. Galton and his contemporaries used what they believed to be new 'scientific' methods of measurement and classification to establish the limits of what was socially acceptable, or acceptably human. In pursuit of this project, Galton founded the discipline of eugenics, which was later used to justify the 'racial purification' programme in Nazi Germany. Inspired by Darwin's ideas of natural selection, the eugenicists believed that the human body is perfectible and that negative attributes such as insanity or criminality are biologically determined. Fuelled by fears of social instability, they therefore thought that it was correct to eliminate from society 'defectives' such as the mentally ill, or those they saw as 'racially inferior'.[52]

By visually identifying a 'norm', Galton and his colleagues established the idea of the deviant individual, and the associated idea of the deviant body.[53] In doing so they made a practical contribution to the association between monstrosity and criminal character that Foucault describes as a feature of nineteenth-century thought: 'starting in the nineteenth century . . . monstrosity is systematically suspected of being behind all criminality. Every criminal could well be a monster, just as previously it was possible that the monster was a criminal'.[54]

Key to Galton's project was the new technology of photography. Although visual images such as Leonardo da Vinci's anatomical drawings had been central to scientific inquiry since at least the early sixteenth century, pictures could only properly be used as scientific evidence after the invention of reproducible photographic imagery in 1839.[55] This new and supposedly 'objective' form of representation had a profound effect on the practice of criminal anthropology by appearing to give it scientific credibility. In fact, in their effort to establish a complete, objective and comprehensive social taxonomy and social order, Galton and his colleagues seem to have used photography as though it offered a direct equivalent to reality.

The invention of photography facilitated the institution of what the artist and writer Allan Sekula has called a 'unified system of representation', or a 'physiognomic code'.[56] The inherently reproducible nature of the photographic image enabled the widespread distribution of pictures of 'ideal', 'abnormal' and 'monstrous' individuals or types to which 'normal' members of society could compare themselves.[57] The photograph enabled people to construct an accurate image of the general and particular marks that distinguished the undesirable 'other' from the 'normal' self. The widespread circulation of these apparently objective images had the effect of fixing the meaning of certain physiognomic traits. Most importantly, they gave reliably recognizable human form to abstract notions such as danger and evil. This dual emphasis on the semiotic meaning of the body and on the photograph as a means of both disseminating and embedding ideas about human character has had a strong impact on modern constructions of human monstrosity.

These nineteenth-century processes have had a lasting effect on the way that photographs are used to locate criminality and deviance.[58] As Sekula has argued, there remains an influential photographic archive of images of the body that contains 'traces of the visible bodies of heroes, leaders, moral exemplars, celebrities and those of the poor, diseased, insane, criminal, non-white, female, and all other embodiments of the unworthy'.[59]

Galton made use of photography to develop his own, innovative methods of visualizing 'abnormalities' such as disease and criminality. He superimposed the photographs of different kinds of individuals to create composite images (Figure 3.9). These composite photographs were intended to give a precise but generalized portrait of the average features of particular groups of people, such as those with identifiable diseases, or specific criminal types.[60] But, in his attempt to construct an entirely visual representation of the criminal type, what Galton actually created was a statistically defined abstraction – an immaterial and non-existent criminal face. This non-existent imaginary figure was arrived at with scientific accuracy and could, therefore, be treated as a scientific subject, providing a kind of 'ideal' criminal body.[61] In the 1880s Galton also took a

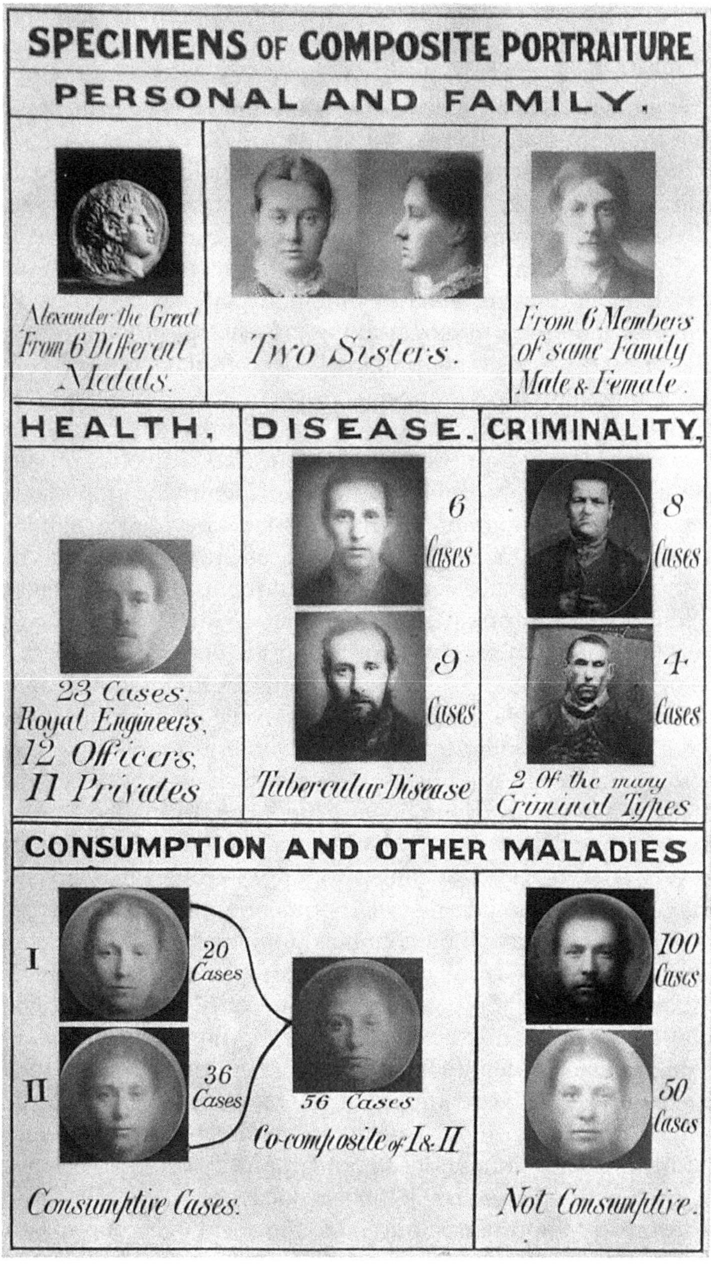

3.9: Composite portraits from Sir Francis Galton, *Inquiries into Human Faculty and its Development*, London, Macmillan and Co., 1883.

large number of photographs of mentally ill patients at Bethlem Hospital with the intention of producing composite images of 'the insane'. This project, which represented an attempt to prove the hereditary nature of mental illness, was unsuccessful and the composites were never made.

Whilst most late nineteenth-century criminologists believed that criminality was genetic and that a person's moral disposition could be determined from his or her appearance, the French policeman and physical anthropologist Alphonse Bertillon (1853–1914) used physiognomic imagery slightly differently. He was the first to systematize the use of photography in criminological identification. His project was a simple pragmatic one of cataloguing, classifying and quantifying the appearance of individual criminals.[62] For Bertillon, whose work has had a lasting impact on criminology, the criminal body expressed nothing. The classification of physiognomic 'types' simply provided a means of identifying individuals.[63] For him, the photograph clearly operated as evidence, although his doubts about the objectivity of the camera eventually led him to create a mathematical system of 'anthropometry' that relied on actual bodily measurements rather than on images of the body.[64] Bertillon's method involved surveying the body of a suspect for recognizable signs of his or her criminal *identity*, rather than his or her character. He made frontal and profile photographs, which were kept on standardized cards in orderly files. These cards systematically recorded measurements, such as head length and breadth, the length of the fingers, the length of the left foot and the length of the forearm. Eye colour was also recorded. Although it was later replaced by fingerprinting, Bertillon had invented the first effective modern system of identification. His controlled method of photographing criminals from the side and full face to create a 'mug shot' is still used by police today. Albeit less ethically problematic than the practices of some of his peers, Bertillon's physiognomic photography also had the more general effect of fixing a person's identity firmly in his or her external image, which eventually led to the widespread use of modern identity cards.[65] Although his project may have had an entirely practical intention, it further demonstrates how a photographic image of a person can be used to fix and reaffirm established values.

Another important figure in nineteenth-century physiognomy was Cesare Lombroso (1835–1909), an Italian professor of criminal anthropology and the founder of the Italian school of positivist criminology. Lombroso, who thought that all human difference is manifested in the face and body, believed that criminal behaviour is biologically and socially determined and that 'criminals are born with evil inclinations'.[66] Lombroso maintained that criminals possess animal instincts which are expressed anatomically and that, along with the related discipline of phrenology, physiognomy could prove that criminality marks a return to a primitive or pre-human state within modern society.[67] He attempted to show that a 'born criminal' could be differentiated from normal, socially well-adjusted people by the degenerative traits visible in his or her physical appearance.

Lombroso revised his treatise several times, perhaps in an attempt to respond to the growing numbers of scholars who contested his theories. In a later summary of his writings, compiled by his daughter Gina Lombroso Ferrero, and first published in 1911, it is noted that 'if we examine a number of criminals we shall find that they exhibit numerous anomalies in the face, skeleton, and various psychic and sensitive functions, so that they strongly resemble primitive races', and 'a high percentage of criminals have small skulls'.[68] In each edition of his work Lombroso remarks that criminals frequently have 'jug-shaped' ears. This is repeated by his daughter, who, perhaps in an effort to be more persuasive, states that, in fact, 'twenty eight percent of criminals have handle-shaped ears standing out from the face as in the chimpanzee'.[69] These strange assertions are in keeping with the earlier ideas of della Porta and Le Brun, who both made correlations between human and animal traits, although Lombroso's conclusions are more moralistic and deterministic than those of his predecessors. In an attempt to give his work statistical and scientific credence, Lombroso made a number of first-hand studies of the demographics of various Italian societies. He also drew on moral readings of the body established by Lavater.

In addition to his work as a criminologist, Lombroso was trained as a medical doctor. He was responsible for psychiatric patients at a number of different hospitals in Italy during the 1860s and 1870s.[70] In 1876 he became professor of legal medicine and public hygiene at the University of Turin, where he wrote his most important and influential work, *L'uomo delinquente* (*Criminal Man*). In this work Lombroso uses modern Darwinian theories of evolution to inform his findings. He associates criminality with a type of madness that he calls 'moral insanity', both of which are visible in the appearance of the criminal: 'the physiognomy of morally insane offenders reveals that they have all the characteristics of the criminal man: large jaws, facial asymmetry,

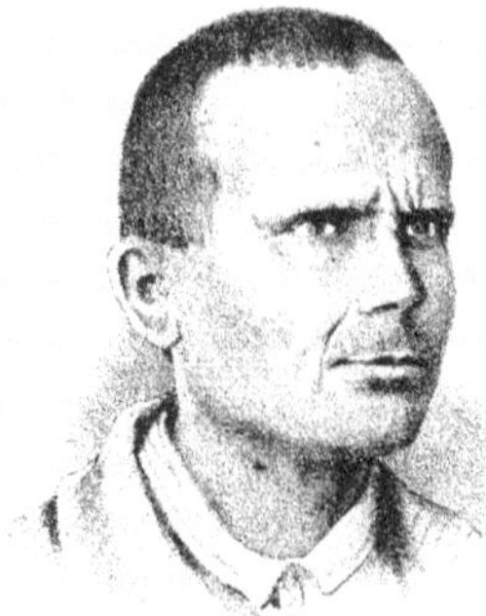

Fig. 1. — SALVATORE A., brigand de la Calabre.

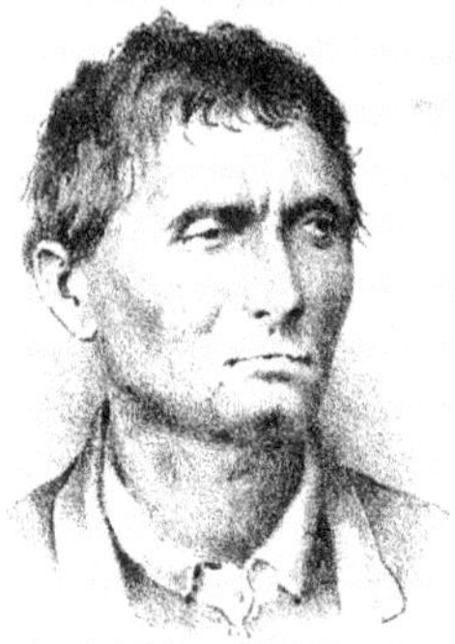

Fig. 2. — G. SANA DE GALLUCCIO, brigand

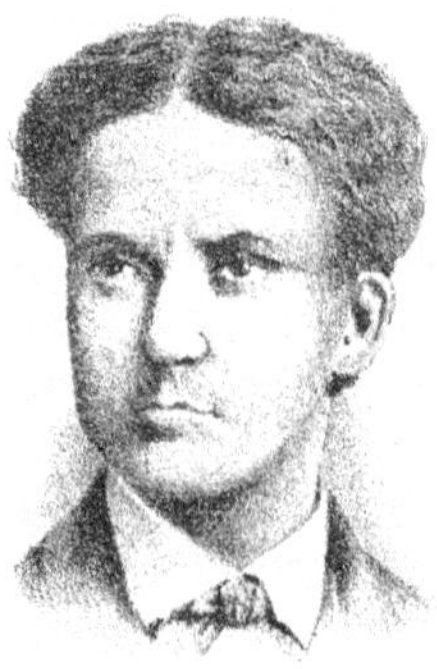

Fig. 3. — CAVAGLIÀ, dit *Fusil*, assassin.

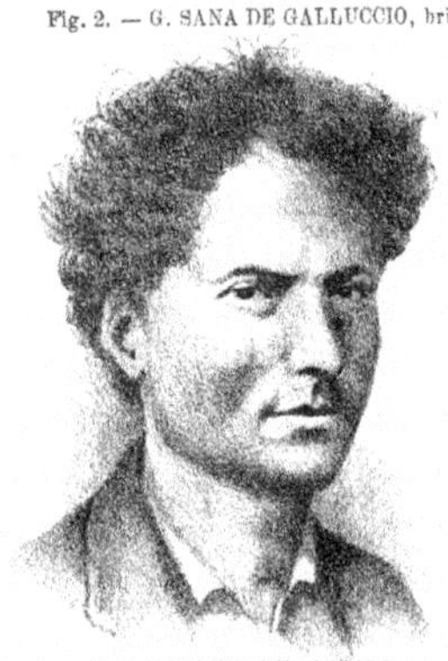

Fig. 4. — G. B. VENAFRO DE CASPOLI, brigand.

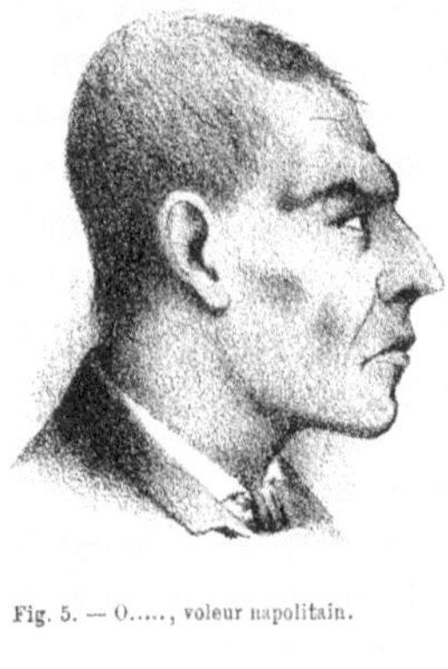

Fig. 5. — O....., voleur napolitain.

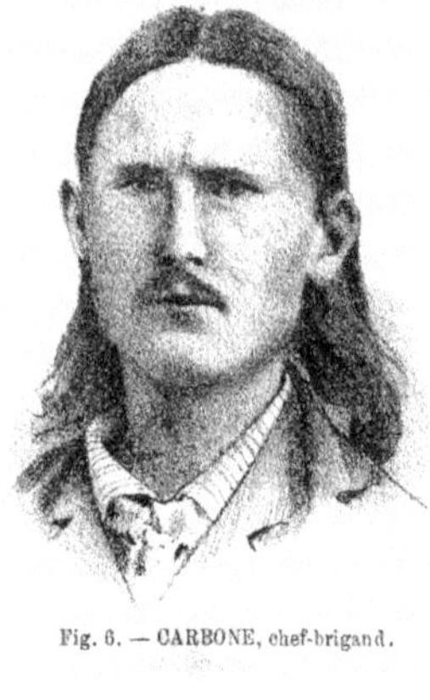

Fig. 6. — CARBONE, chef-brigand.

3.10: Cesare Lombroso, 'Six Criminal Types', from *L'uomo delinquente* (*Criminal Man*), Rome: Bocca, 1888.

unequal ears, scanty beards in men and virile physiognomy in women'.[71] Lombroso goes on to make an even more explicit association between criminality and insanity, writing that, 'while theories of punishment can be debated at great length, experts agree on one point: many criminals are insane'.[72] In his view, the same factors bring about a predisposition towards crime as towards madness, except that criminality is innate, whilst madness is usually an acquired condition.

Lombroso's work in criminal anthropology has, like that of his contemporaries, now been officially discredited because it is deemed unscientific, racist and deterministic. Nevertheless, many of the links he made between criminality and appearance remain implicit in contemporary attitudes, both popular and scientific. For example, his methods still inform modern criminology to the extent that forensic scientists use visual and physical clues to piece together a psychological profile for individual criminals before they are identified.

The belief that the human body and face are visibly marked by a person's state of mind is central to all Lombroso's work. Originally derived from ancient and medieval physiology, this idea was given new significance in the seventeenth century by the philosophical works of René Descartes and the physiognomic studies of Charles Le Brun. Whilst Lavater includes a catalogue of the physical and behavioural signs of what he vaguely terms 'idiocy' in his *Physiognomische Fragmente* of 1775–8, it was not until the early nineteenth century that a more structured physiognomic analysis of the signs of madness appeared. In the nineteenth century the ability to make a connection between a person's state of mind and his or her facial appearance was not only thought to provide a viable means of identifying criminals and 'the insane', but also took on a new status as a tool for the diagnosis of mental illness. Precise visual descriptions of the physical manifestations of insanity were thought to be key to understanding a number of mental conditions.

In 1840, the distinguished psychiatrist Sir Alexander Morison asserted, 'there is no class of diseases in which the study of physiognomy is so necessary as that of mental diseases . . . the appearance of the face is intimately connected with and dependent upon the state of mind'.[73] Whilst his reports do also take a person's overall demeanour and bodily gestures into account, Morison locates the signs of insanity primarily in the face. Morison and his colleagues believed that they could build on the Cartesian idea that the face is the most accurate reflection of the mind because of its proximity to the brain, as well as its capacity for minute changes of expression. They thought that the repeated movements of facial muscles in what they called 'the insane state' would lead to particular, indicative facial expressions:

> the repetition of the same ideas and emotions, and the consequent repetition of the same movements of the muscles of the eyes and of the face, give a peculiar expression, which, in the insane state, is a combination of wildness, abstraction or vacancy.[74]

Morison's book, *The Physiognomy of Mental Diseases* (1840) is a descriptive catalogue of a range of 'varieties of mental disorder' as Morison describes them, richly illustrated with more than a hundred portrait sketches of mentally ill patients. In many cases a second portrait of the same individual 'in a sane state' follows, presumably to help the viewer to recognize the visible features of each particular type of illness.

In 1879 two other leading psychiatrists, John Bucknill and Daniel Tuke, published one of the first and most influential textbooks on psychiatry, the *Manual of Psychological Medicine*. Here, they describe small transient changes in the muscles of the face – particularly the eyes and mouth – that can be read as indications of various mental states.[75] They too assert that 'the mental physician has to be a good physiognomist', because he will then be able to tell whether a patient is insane or not, and even to determine the type of insanity simply from a person's appearance.[76] According to Bucknill and Tuke, 'facial expressions of the insane are often similar to those observable in the sane, but more intense'.[77] They explain that this is because the expressions of 'the insane' are not modified by the presence of intellect, without which 'the facial indications of powerful and unrestrained instincts often profoundly degrade and brutalise the human face'.[78] Despite the fact that attitudes towards mental illness were changing at this time, this curious assertion suggests that the mentally ill patient was still located in the category of the 'uncivilized', the animal and ultimately the monstrous 'other'. Bucknill and Tuke's diagnoses focus on their observations of the dynamic features of the face. They record a 'remarkable peculiarity in the physiognomy of the insane' – that is, 'a want of accord in the expression of different features'. They claim that these contradictory expressions of the mouth and eyes are only observable in 'the insane', and then only in some of them.[79] This is perhaps their way of accounting for the failure of their project to reliably diagnose a person's mental state from his or her facial features or expressions.

In 1858–9 John Connolly, a professor of medicine at the University of London and superintendent at the Hanwell Asylum in Middlesex, published a series of articles entitled 'The Physiognomy of Insanity' in the *Medical Times and Gazette*. In the first of these articles he writes:

> I used to frequently regret the want of the art or of the help of a painter, to enable me to convey to others by pictorial images the strange aspects and facial expressions of mental malady, which were often more forcible than any words that could have been employed . . . Since the time to which I am referring, however . . . the new and important discovery of the art of photography . . . has endowed the Physicians attached to asylums with the power I wished for.[80]

Just as psychiatrists such as Morison and Bucknill and Tuke in the UK and Philippe Pinel and Jean-Étienne Esquirol in France were developing the belief that mental pathologies could be understood by closer and closer scrutiny of a person's appearance, the new technology of photography emerged. This apparently objective, faithful and detailed mechanical process clearly seemed to offer a means of visually identifying, examining and then classifying those 'others' within society – like criminals and 'the insane' – who were not necessarily monstrous, but were certainly social outcasts with incomprehensible behaviours.

Each of Connolly's articles is constructed around a lithograph after a photographic portrait by Dr Hugh Welch Diamond, who, he writes, has made 'curious portraits of the insane', whose 'singular fidelity' enables the recognition of types of diseases from facial appearance.[81] It is ironic that Connolly writes of fidelity, as in many cases the lithographs bear little resemblance to the original photographs. For example, in the lithograph (Figure 3.12) the face of the woman photographed by Diamond (Figure 3.11) has been turned so that her gaze is downward, her bent elbow now rests on two (presumably religious) books, and her right arm lies across her lap, rather than hanging straight down as it does in the original. These changes are perhaps meant to help the viewer to recognize the 'outward marks of a mind which, seemingly, after long wandering in the mazes of religious doubt . . . is now overshadowed by despair'.[82] Connolly provides a list of features:

> the high and wide forehead . . . the slightly bent head leaning disconsolately on the hand; the absence from that collapsed cheek of every trace of gaiety; the mouth inexpressive of any varied emotion; the deep orbits and the long characteristic eyebrows, [her] . . . high wide forehead . . . black hair heedlessly pressed back . . .

Along with the plainness of her dress, these are seen as further indications of the woman's pathologically melancholy state.

Diamond (1809–86), who was also a psychiatrist, pioneered the use of photographic portraits in the study and treatment of

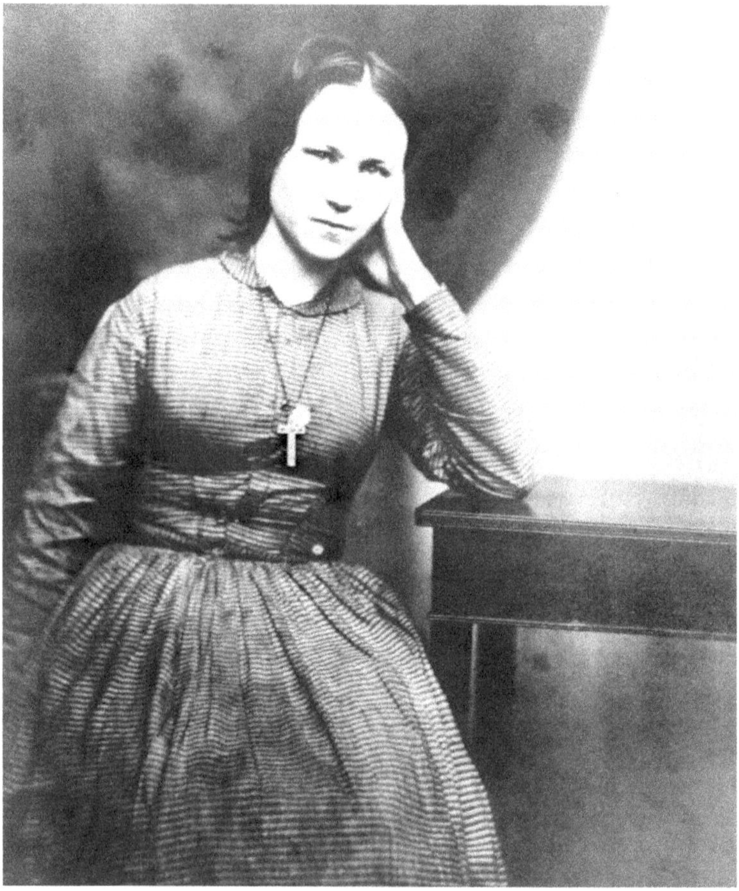

3.11: Hugh Welch Diamond, 'Religious Melancholy', a patient at Surrey County Lunatic Asylum, albumen silver print from glass negative, c.1850–8.

the mentally ill whilst working as a superintendent at the Surrey County Lunatic Asylum in Tooting, South London, from 1848 to 1858. In the asylum, Diamond used photography to build on the catalogue of portraits assembled by his predecessor Sir Alexander Morison, in an attempt to record the particular traits of different psychiatric patients. His techniques contributed to a shift in understanding, from the old idea of the 'lunatic', who was considered a dangerous animal that had to be controlled by constraint, to the more humane image of the 'mental patient', afflicted with a disease of the brain or nerves that could be cured, or at least treated.[83] Enabling psychiatrists to look at patients

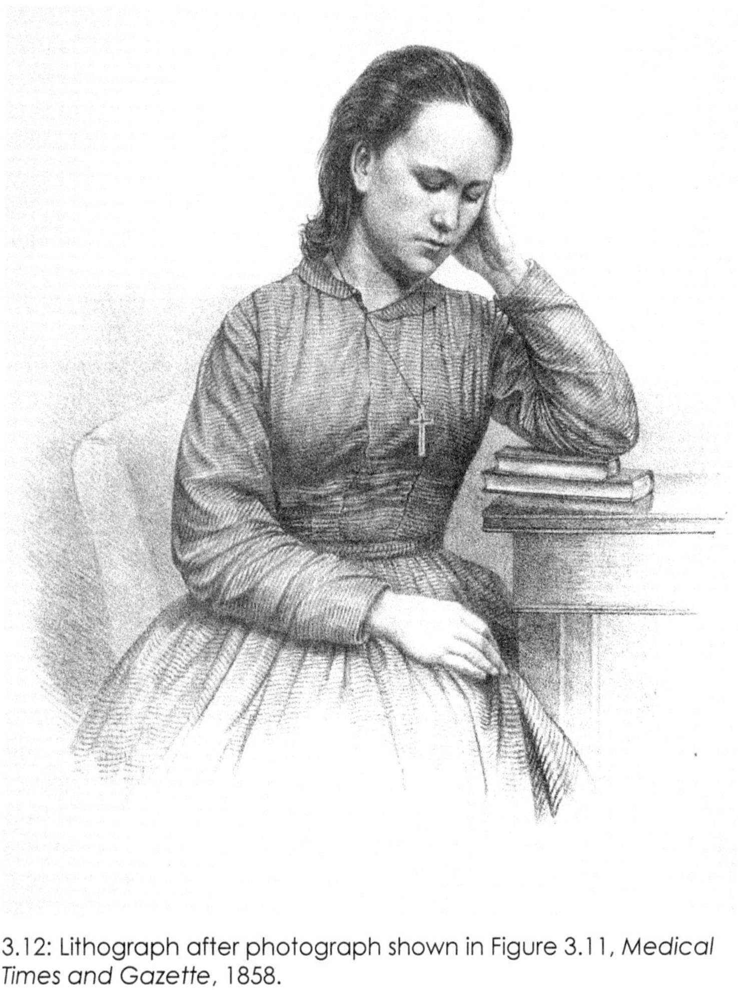

3.12: Lithograph after photograph shown in Figure 3.11, *Medical Times and Gazette*, 1858.

in greater detail, Diamond's photographs were believed to be instrumental in helping to establish a boundary between normal and abnormal mental states.[84] However, as we have seen, this supposedly objective visual evidence was often manipulated to conform to a preconceived idea of the patient's condition.

In the final chapter of his book, *Madness and Civilization*, Michel Foucault writes of the 'absolute observation' at play in the nineteenth-century asylum, where a 'non-reciprocal' relationship existed between 'the mad' and 'men of reason'.[85] Whilst Foucault's image of the culture of the asylum seems inconsistent with the therapeutic intentions of, for example, Tuke or Diamond, the gaze of those considered to be endowed with 'reason' does seem to have played a significant role in the nineteenth-century construction of 'insanity'.[86] The excitement around early psychiatric photography suggests that, at the advent of the modern science of psychiatry, photography appeared to offer a promising means of extending 'the medical gaze' as Foucault puts it, into the psyche. With the transformation of mental illness from a generalized social problem to a newly categorized spectrum of uniquely medical conditions, the appeal of the equally new technology of photography as a means of visualizing, and therefore understanding, psychological abnormalities must have been very great.

In *Madness and Civilization* Foucault recounts some of the earlier attempts, made during the eighteenth century, to describe and classify mental illness according to observable signs. He states that:

> The essential thing is that the enterprise did not proceed from observation to the construction of explanatory images; that on the contrary, the images assured the initial role of synthesis, that their organizing force made possible a structure of perception, in which at last the symptoms could attain their significant value and be organized as the visible presence of the truth.[87]

Here Foucault seems to be arguing that, since the eighteenth century, visual images have played a significant role in the construction of 'madness' as a series of recognizable diseases of the mind. If this is the case, then perhaps rather than offering physiognomists and psychiatrists a new tool for recognizing existing conditions, nineteenth-century photographs of the insane were simply building on an established tradition of constructing 'knowledge' about various psychiatric conditions from outward appearances.

4 | Monsters in Proximity

Freaks and the Spectacle of Abnormality

By the nineteenth century the physiognomic tradition in which unusual, uncertain or exaggerated bodily traits were read as signs of social or moral deviance was well established. Against this background, an unremarkable appearance could be seen as a desirable indicator of normality. This is a quality that Michel Foucault has declared 'the new law of modern society', according to which all forms of bodily difference must be scientifically explained and controlled.[1] Lennard Davis, a specialist in disability studies, has explained this further, remarking that 'the concept of a norm, unlike that of an ideal, implies that the majority of the population must or should somehow be part of the norm'.[2] At times of change, when existing social, cultural or religious norms are overturned, new types of human monster come into view in order to manifest the monstrous disruption that occurs. In modern Western society, the theatrically enhanced deformities of nineteenth-century freaks interrogated new understandings of 'normality'.

The public exhibition of freaks, whose existence depended on the theatrical display of their 'monstrously' deformed bodies, was a popular form of entertainment throughout the nineteenth century. And yet the French philosopher and physician Georges Canguilhem has argued that corporeal monstrosity began to lose its symbolic significance in the late eighteenth century. He attributes this change to the expansion of modern scientific thought, which, he writes, rendered physical deformity 'transparent' by naming, classifying and explaining its causes. Canguilhem believed that once scientists such as Etienne Geoffroy de St Hilaire were able to create monsters in the lab, scientific knowledge could eliminate all correspondence between physical deformity and the threatening force of the monstrous.[3]

Foucault takes up Canguilhem's argument in his lectures on the abnormal, where he maintains that since the end of the eighteenth century the presence of monstrousness is evident in the *behaviour* of an individual rather than in his or her physical appearance.[4] Although a shift of emphasis from appearance to monstrous character undoubtedly did take place in the late eighteenth and early nineteenth centuries, the visible signs of human difference continued to be exploited in the domain of public entertainment as well as in the areas of criminology and mental health. Whilst Foucault and Canguilhem have both argued that the significance of corporeal monstrosity was erased by science after the eighteenth century, this chapter aims to show that on the freak show stage 'monstrous' physical deformity remained an important tool for the negotiation of human difference throughout the nineteenth century.

Concurrent with an increase of interest in reading an individual's character from his or her physical appearance, the freak show, in which strange and unusual bodies were exhibited for profit, emerged as a highly popular form of amusement. Like all monsters, freaks represent the values and concerns of the society that has produced them. In this case, the coincidence of a renewed faith in physiognomy and the theatrical production of the different body as an entertaining public spectacle points to a deep insecurity about who should be included as an acceptable member of society. During the nineteenth century in particular, freak shows and carte de visite photographs of freaks acted as strategies for dealing with the 'monstrous' spectrum of human difference found within modern Western society.

The Emergence of the Freak Show

The display of human monstrosity has a long history that, as we saw in the previous chapter, can be traced back to the Renaissance. By the mid-seventeenth century, 'abnormal' humans were regularly being exhibited on the streets of major cities, along with dancing bears, monkeys and exotic wild animals.[5] In his book *The Shows of London*, the American literary scholar Richard Altick gives a detailed account of many of the human anomalies on display and the social context in which they were received in seventeenth- and eighteenth-century London. Altick notes that 'giants, gigantic children, large men, dwarfs, giants and dwarfs exhibited together, masculine women, persons without arms and legs, monstrous births, strange formations and diseases', some from as far away as China, were amongst the oddities displayed for money, both inside and outside the city's taverns and inns.[6] The practice of exhibiting physically deformed, exotic or unusual people for money seems to have continued throughout the eighteenth century, when the display of 'freaks' became increasingly accepted as a respectable element of travelling fairs. By the mid-nineteenth century, freak shows were an established attraction in circuses, fairgrounds and amusement parks in both Europe and America. The popularity of freaks was greatly enhanced by the opening of showman P.T. Barnum's 'American Museum' in New York City in 1841. The museum housed a spectacular collection of exotic animals, including 'the first hippopotamus in America', 'educated' dogs and seals as well as human 'freaks', amongst which were a bearded lady, 'Siamese twins' and an 'Albino family'. Along with his American Museum, P.T. Barnum's 'Great Travelling Museum, Menagerie, Caravan and Hippodrome' established the sideshow freak as a crucial element of nineteenth-century travelling shows in both North America and Europe.[7]

A freak is, by definition, a monstrosity.[8] The term is probably derived from the early English *freke*, meaning a 'remarkable creature or being, especially an angel, demon or giant'.[9] But the freaks described in this chapter are not 'freaks of nature'; they are theatrically produced freaks of culture whose bodies, like those of earlier monsters, show or demonstrate (*monstrare*) that which is not 'normal'. Like both the classical Monstrous Races and the sixteenth-century Monster of Ravenna, freaks were exotic curiosities that transgressed classifications by exhibiting a mix of races, genders, species or forms in the same uncertain body. Their monstrousness was immediately evident in their strange appearance, which, like that of any other monster, combined 'real' and mythical or fantastic elements. By the nineteenth century, however, scientific explanation was beginning to replace mystical and religious interpretation. This shift in understanding affected the way in which the monstrous body was understood. At this time, as Rosemarie Garland-Thomson has remarked in her introduction to *Freakery, Cultural Spectacles of the Extraordinary Body*, 'monsters shift[ed] into the category of curiosities'.[10] In other words, strange or extraordinary bodies lost their divine or magical significance, instead becoming indicators of secularized social deviance.

A crucial feature that distinguishes freaks from earlier monsters is their proximity to the 'normal' observer. Whilst, like freaks, the strange bodies of the Monstrous Races reflected prevailing social and individual anxieties about the acceptable limits of human being, these earlier monsters were clearly defined as 'other' by virtue of their physical distance from the normal, everyday world of Western society. Like the wild men and women described in Chapter 2, the exotic races remained out of sight, appearing only in drawings and narrative accounts.

Renaissance monsters were located within society, and therefore much closer to 'normal' people, but they too were usually seen in the form of prints and drawings. By contrast, freak shows offered a strategy for the public exhibition of what appeared to be 'real', 'live' corporeal monstrosities.

As public events, accessible to any member of society who could afford to pay a modest entry fee, freak shows remained a legitimate form of entertainment for both middle- and working-class audiences well into the twentieth century.[11] The enormous popularity of freaks during the nineteenth and early twentieth centuries in both Britain and America clearly owed a lot to the marketing skills of P.T. Barnum. They were also culturally significant events. In her book *Extraordinary Bodies, Figuring Physical Disability in American Culture and Literature*, Garland-Thomson links their popularity to an attempt on the part of modern Western societies to come to terms with particular social and cultural changes, such as increased immigration and the gradual emancipation of women.[12] More broadly, freaks emerged out of the processes of industrialization and modernization, which precipitated the formation of a market economy, demanding greater mobility for workers and fragmenting established communities. Garland-Thomson makes an important point when she comments that these rapid social changes 'forced people to rely on bodily appearance rather than kinship or local memberships as indices of identity and social position'.[13] In this climate of uncertainty the freak shows offered a certain sort of reassurance. They responded to the need for an expanded notion of what constitutes a 'normal' or 'acceptable' appearance on the one hand, and a resistance to accommodating different sorts of bodies within the 'norm' on the other.[14]

In the tradition of earlier monsters, any kind of physical or cultural difference that might threaten the established understanding of what was acceptably human could be represented in the freak body. Whilst freaks were recognizably human characters, their exaggerated or distorted bodies typically displayed a lack or excess of 'normal' human attributes, or showed certain strange and 'inhuman' features. For example, very large or small people, or excessively fat, thin or hairy people could be exhibited as freaks, as could people born with too many or too few limbs, or people whose status was ambiguous, such as hermaphrodites, conjoined twins or 'bearded ladies'. The boundary transgressions which were historically thought to have been brought about through a combination of different species, races or sexes in the same individual, the mixture of animal and human, or the merging of two individuals in one body were all represented in the spectacle of the freak show. Like the bodies of the earlier monsters discussed in the previous chapters, freak bodies were presented as objects of contemplation, marked as visibly different to all the other ordinary bodies found within society.

Garland-Thomson has argued that the freak show is 'a cultural performance that gives primacy to visual apprehension in creating symbolic codes . . . [it] institutionalizes the relation between the spectacle and its spectators'.[15] But if we think of spectacle as pure representation, 'a pseudo-world apart, an object of mere contemplation', as the French filmmaker and writer Guy Debord has described it, the freak – whose assumed social role is so obviously fake – is securely located in the realm of the fantastic.[16] He or she is seen to exist outside, or apart from, normal, everyday experience. But, as Peter Stallybrass and Allon White note in their book, *The Politics and Poetics of Transgression*, 'the spectacle is not a collection of images; it is a social relation between people that is mediated by images'.[17] This statement is important because it draws attention not only to the monster or freak as a social construct, but also to the role of the *image* of the different or deformed body as a site of negotiation. In the public space of the sideshow a necessary objectification of 'the other' takes place. The real identity of the person exhibited as a freak is concealed or negated by the spectacle of the deformity he or she is exhibiting. This denial of subjectivity has the effect of removing the freak from the 'real' world of social relations, placing emphasis on what the spectacularly deformed bodies on show can tell the onlookers about themselves.

The 'norm' from which all freaks were seen to deviate was inevitably the 'civilized', self-controlled and rational, middle-class white male. In comparison, the 'wild' racial 'otherness', the indeterminately gendered or inappropriately configured bodies of the freaks were clearly deviant. They manifested all sorts of social and individual anxieties about the size, skin colour, bodily configuration and even behaviour suitable to an acceptable human being living within modern Western society. Freak shows combined narratives of social and cultural difference with those of physical difference to produce forms of otherness that the sociologist Robert Bogdan has divided into two distinct categories: 'normal' but exoticized non-Westerners, whose racial differences are aligned with primitive, animal savagery, and physically 'abnormal' Westerners, who are presented as sophisticated and capable, despite their physical deformities.[18] But, unlike most of the earlier types of monsters, these ambiguous characters were not understood as complete outsiders, rather as manifestations of the strangeness within society itself, and of the individuals that made up that society. The freak show offered a discursive space in which the exaggerated bodies on display could reinforce the 'normalcy' of the spectator and at the same time offer reassurance that anyone with a lesser difference or deformity could fit into society. Although we may now see them as a distasteful form of entertainment, it seems that freak shows did perform an important social role, offering the possibility for the members of increasingly mixed urban societies to see themselves united as 'not-freaks'.

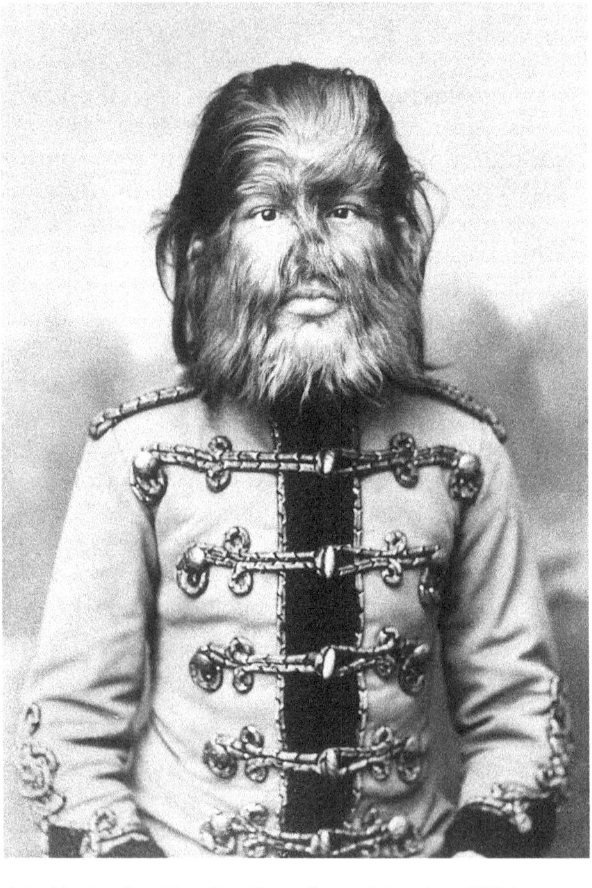

4.1: 'JoJo, the Russian Dog-faced Boy', c.1884.

The exaggerated bodies of famous freaks such as 'Zip', the African 'Pinhead', 'JoJo, the Dog-faced Boy', Madame Devere, the 'Bearded Lady' and Charles Tripp, the 'Armless Wonder' manifest a whole range of spectacular differences. Each of these characters was based on a living human subject whose unusual appearance could be taken to signify a transgression of one or more of the conventional boundaries between male and female, sexed and sexless, animal and human, self and racial other. As freak show exhibits, their individual differences were often visually enhanced by the theatrical use of props, costumes and settings. In addition, exotic and improbable narratives of origin or cause were constructed around each freak in an attempt to further augment his or her strange appearance.

Views of the 'monstrosities' on display inside the freak shows were usually preceded by textual and verbal narratives, all of which were designed to amplify the audience's expectations of what they would see. These narratives often drew inspiration from well-known mythological archetypes such as the wild man, the giant or the dwarf. For example, a notice published in the New York press in 1888 advertising the exhibition of Fydor Jeftichew as 'JoJo, the man with a dog's head', is reminiscent of one of the most ancient and popular types of mythical monster, the dog-headed cynocephalus. Jeftichew, who was born in Europe, was of Russian descent. He had inherited hypertrichosis, a condition that leads to excessive growth of body hair, from his father, who also toured as a sideshow exhibit.[19] Jeftichew, who was exhibited as 'JoJo, the Russian Dog-faced Boy' by P.T. Barnum, had a long and successful career that also took him to Europe and Australia. His dramatic animal-like appearance was exaggerated during performances, where he reportedly wrapped himself in a blanket and yelped like a dog until he was freed.[20] The narrative that accompanied Jeftichew's performances in Barnum's touring exhibitions claimed that 'JoJo' and his father had been living in the wild in the forests of central Russia until they were caught by a party of hunters. According to this classic 'wild man' story, 'JoJo' was then domesticated and taken to America.[21] His fictional heritage as a part-human, part-animal foreigner was supported visually by exotic costumes, such as the Russian cavalryman's uniform he is wearing in the studio portrait shown in Figure 4.1.

Perhaps the most questionable, but also the most interesting of all the freaks exhibited by Barnum is William Henry Johnson, or 'Zip the Pinhead'. Like 'JoJo', 'Zip' conformed to the exotic freak show stereotype of the semi-bestial foreigner. Johnson, who was born in New Jersey, USA, around 1842, was recruited by Barnum in 1860 to play the part of a primitive African freak that had supposedly been found during a gorilla-hunting expedition in West Africa. As a bizarre photograph (Figure 4.2) taken by the famous New York society photographer Charles Eisenmann shows, 'Zip' was portrayed as a creature somewhere between human and animal. Seen in the light of nineteenth-century interpretations of Darwin's new theory of evolution, Johnson's character was depicted as an atavistic throwback, aligned more with the idea of the 'missing link' between human and animal than with the figure of the 'wild man'. He was advertised by Barnum as the 'What Is It?' – an indescribable mixture of man and ape.[22] In accordance with this myth, Johnson never spoke during performances. Dressed in a trademark fur gorilla suit and with his head shaved, except for a small tuft that further elongated its unusual shape, he is said to have simply grunted when addressed or questioned during a show.[23]

Johnson was widely exhibited and extensively photographed, usually against a painted landscape such as that shown in Figure 4.2. In this studio shot, taken around 1885, he is wearing a picture of George Washington around his neck. He is posed as though boxing with Ashbury Benjamin, a young black man with vitiligo, a condition in which patches of the skin lose their normal pigmentation. Apart from the painted backdrop, the only props in the image are the enormous white boxing gloves worn by both men – the accidental inclusion of a posing stand behind 'Zip' only works to emphasize the artificiality of the staged scene. In counterpoint to the strange figure of 'Zip', Benjamin, the 'Leopard Boy' was supposed to represent 'a more evolved type, a negro turning white'.[24]

From the age of about twelve, Benjamin was also exhibited alone, advertised as the likely result of racial mixing.[25] According to the American historian Nadja Durbach, the narrative woven around him represented 'part of the discourse of imperial superiority' that 'helped to establish for a broad British public the normative nature of the "Caucasian" and thus the intrinsic aberrance of all Others'.[26] The socially undesirable or 'abnormal' traits represented by the marginalized 'types' that made up nineteenth-century freak shows were often overlapping and interchangeable. With reference to Johnson, Lennard Davis has observed, 'what is most interesting about this strange phenomenon is that the category of disability defines itself through an appeal to nationalism. The disabled person is not of this nation, is not a citizen in the same sense as the able-bodied.'[27] Davis' comment evokes the ancient Greek idea of the *polis*, where only the 'normal' male citizen living within society and subject to its laws can be fully human. All 'others' are dismissed because to acknowledge them would be to threaten the established definition of what is normal.[28]

Although Johnson's freak show persona was particularly demeaning, it seems that, like many other sideshow entertainers, he personally profited from, and creatively contributed to, his construction as a freak.[29] He originated from an impoverished family of former slaves, yet Johnson became one of the most popular freaks of his era and consequently came to be relatively wealthy. From our contemporary perspective it is impossible to understand how he might have felt about exhibiting himself as an object of curiosity. We can only guess at the degree of exploitation involved in his stage appearances. But it seems clear that in performing as a freak Johnson and others like him supported an industry that 'exploited the public's stereotypes, prejudices and hatred toward people of colour' in a context where black skin represented a highly visible form of cultural difference.[30] In his book *Freak Shows and the Modern American Imagination*, Thomas Fahy even claims that 'showmen had a mandate to mould the presentations of the Africans they exhibited to justify slavery and colonialism'.[31] This suggests that whilst the freak shows were presented as pure entertainment, their messages were in fact highly political.

The picture of Johnson and Benjamin (Figure 4.2) certainly evokes a complex set of prejudices relating to skin colour and to mental capacity, creating an image of 'Zip' as an idiotic primitive, more animal than human. Whilst the shape of his head is consistent with a form of disability that usually involves mental impairment – an association that seems to have been exploited during his performances – Johnson is reported by Robert Bogdan to have been of 'normal' intelligence, and in control of a career that lasted until his death in 1926.[32] But not all writers concur with this. The historian James Cook suggests that, as a young mentally disabled African American, Johnson 'probably had little control over his entrance into show business' and for the first ten years he had 'almost to be forced to mount the platform'.[33] It is difficult to know which version is more accurate, but the overt racism displayed by this image, in which Johnson, as racial 'other' is crudely represented as an uncivilized 'wild man' creature, is

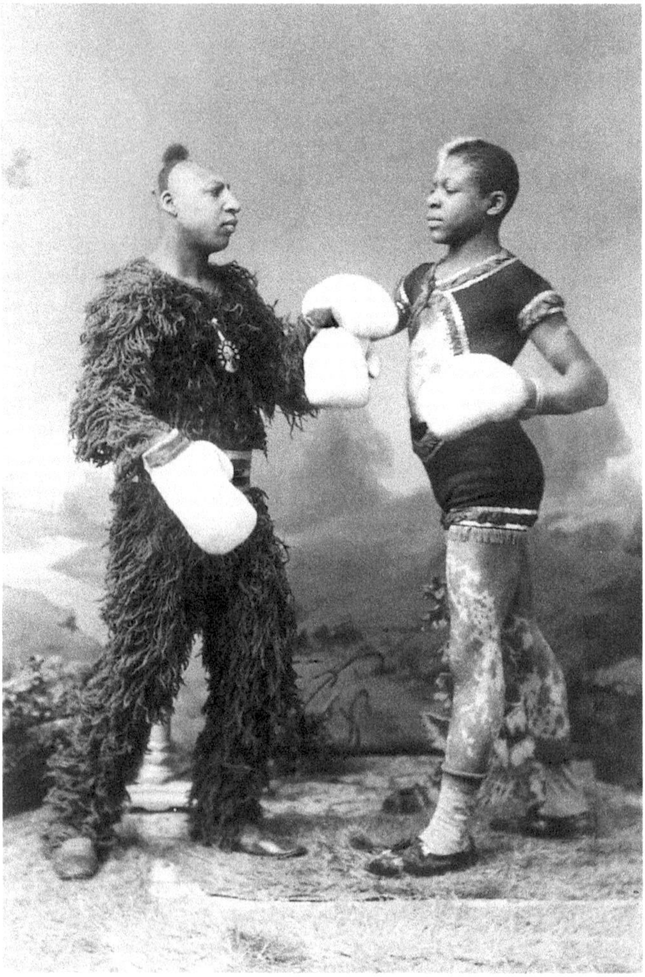

4.2: Henry Johnson as 'Zip' with Ashbury Benjamin, the 'Leopard Boy', c.1885.

offensive. And yet the picture is also humorous. It seems to stage the racial 'other' as a figure of fun, not to be taken seriously. This is emphasized by the fact that 'Zip', who is clearly physically inferior to his more muscular opponent, appears to be trying to hold Benjamin's hand rather than attack him.

This photograph references another form of popular entertainment – the boxing show. During the 1890–1 season Barnum reportedly staged several live boxing matches between 'Zip' and the 'Piebald Boy' (another name for Benjamin), at which this 'calling card' photograph would have been sold as a souvenir.[34] Boxing shows were very popular exhibits in nineteenth-century fairgrounds and would have been visited by the same audiences as the freak shows. As we will see later in this chapter, calling cards or 'cartes de visite' such as this enabled the circulation of the freak show spectacle in the form of a mass-produced, static image. These popular, entertaining images reinforced the stereotypes set up in the freak shows themselves.

The Production of Difference

Rachel Adams' book, *Sideshow U.S.A.: Freaks and the American Cultural Imagination*, offers a thorough analysis of the dynamic between freak show performers and their audiences. Here she argues that 'freak shows are guided by the assumption that *freak* is an essence, the basis for a comforting fiction that there is a permanent, qualitative difference between deviance and normality, projected spatially between the spectator and the body on the stage'.[35] This idea of an absolute difference between monstrous 'other' and 'normal' self is central to the construction of human monsters in any context. But freak exhibits are particularly interesting in this respect because of the way that they deliberately exploited this self/other relationship. The freak show itself seems to have provided a structure that could offer the illusion of a social encounter with another being that both is and is not like the self, whilst at the same time reinforcing the boundaries between the viewing subject and the monstrous object of his or her gaze. In order to enhance the sense of difference, the 'monstrosities' displayed by a particular freak were often exaggerated, or in some cases even manufactured.[36] Within the formalized spaces of shows, museums and fairs, audiences could experience these 'monstrous' differences in close proximity, but set apart from the 'real', everyday world in which they lived. The shows were structured in such a way that freaks were usually exhibited either on elevated stages or lowered into pits. This was significant because it meant that the eye level of the performer was never the same as that of the viewer. People performing as freaks were set apart by the artifice of the stage, the costume, the 'act' and the fact that the audience had to pay to see them. These distancing devices maintained the credibility of some of the more overtly artificial exhibits on the one hand, and offered reassurance that the freaks on display could neither contaminate nor interrogate the spectator's own sense of identity on the other.

Within this structure, the potential proximity between the 'normal' cultured spectator and the freaks that he or she had paid to see was further exploited for dramatic effect. Many freaks sang, danced or played musical instruments. Those with disabilities often demonstrated special capabilities like, for example, Charles Tripp, the 'Armless Wonder' (Figure 4.6), who could eat, write and shave with his feet. In this 'unreal' context the challenge to established identity posed by the human monster could be experienced as cathartic. The freak show provided a physical, visual and narrative structure that safely located the recognizably disordered body of the monster – and all the monstrousness it signified – apart from the spectator. Perhaps in order to further reinforce the idea that they could never share the same social space as the 'normal' onlooker, freaks were not permitted to converse with their audiences. And yet, although first-hand documentation of the atmosphere of freak shows is scarce, it seems that they were, as Adams has suggested, 'hardly spaces of restraint or decorum' and were 'probably far more interactive than critics have acknowledged'.[37] Garland-Thomson has observed that 'freaks were celebrities as well as spectacles, their popularity suggested that audiences simultaneously identified with and were repulsed by the performers', which perhaps helps to explain the emotive and often bawdy atmosphere of the shows.[38]

Part of the allure of freak shows seems to have been the obvious way that they provoked the contradictory responses of recognition and denial, empathy and aversion, inclusion and exclusion that are a feature of any encounter with a human monster. In the illusory world of the show, where monstrous difference was temporarily relocated from the 'real' domain of the everyday to the artificial realm of the spectacle, the impact of racial differences, disproportionate bodies or indeterminate genders could be explored without consequence for the spectator. The different body was staged as an object upon which the viewer could project all sorts of cultural characteristics that he or she personally disowned, or that were deemed socially unacceptable. Freaks themselves were consistently denied the right to respond, or to return the gaze of the spectator.

Freak shows were always highly mediated events. Outside each show a 'talker' persuasively called people in. The exaggerated spoken narratives repeated by these attention-grabbing 'pitchmen' were designed to heighten the public's expectations

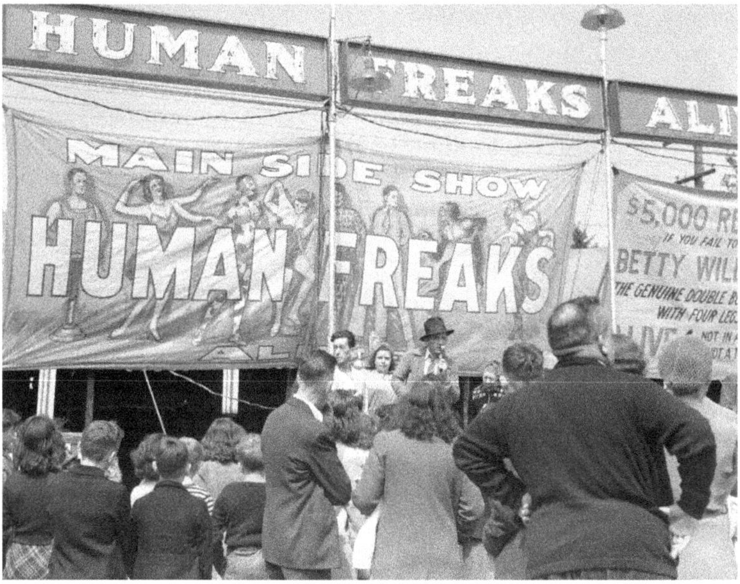

4.3: Freak show at the Rutland Fair, Vermont, 1941.

of the extraordinary nature of the freaks they were about to see. Banners and misleading pictures exhibited outside the show tent were also used to fuel the audience's fantasy about what they would find inside. The main purpose of these sensationalized displays was evidently to encourage audiences to form grossly exaggerated mental images of the monstrosities they would see on the freak show stage (Figure 4.3). The combination of fabulous images and exaggerated narratives available outside the shows gave the freaks exhibited within an almost mythical status, alienating them from the 'real' world of the observer before they were even seen. Here, the visual imagery was limited to evocative and exaggerated drawn or painted pictures. Photographs were not used because it was thought that they would reveal too much.[39] With all these expectations, viewers must have found many of the freaks exhibited inside the show disappointingly close to the 'norm'. And yet it seems that large numbers of people were willing to suspend their disbelief and pay to enter the shows despite – or perhaps because of – the artificially exaggerated nature of the images outside.

Following in the monster tradition, the deformed body of the freak signified the presence of troublesome differences within society. Yet the overt artifice of the sideshows must have acted to reassure audiences that the monsters on display were largely mythical beings, and so their monstrous differences could not be a 'real' problem. If, as the French semiotician Roland Barthes has argued, within the realm of myth signifiers act as reassuring statements of fact, perhaps the mythical construction of monstrosity enables the idea of monstrousness to be presented as an external fact of life.[40]

Cartes de Visite

Whilst photographic imagery was thought to be too 'realistic' to advertise the exhibition of freaks publicly on the posters or banners displayed outside the shows, it nevertheless played a crucial role in their production. The high degree of public visibility achieved by many freaks was supported by the artefacts – such as posters, pamphlets and cartes de visite – that accompanied the sideshows. The most subtle, but perhaps most powerful of these forms of publicity was the photographic carte de visite, which was invented in 1854 by the Parisian portrait photographer André-Adolphe-Eugène Disdéri. Highly popular until the end of the nineteenth century, these small, cheap and easy to mass-produce albumen prints enabled ordinary people to own portraits of themselves and their family and friends. Like most other nineteenth-century portrait photographs, carte de visite pictures were constructed in the artificial setting of the studio. Here illusionary backdrops, drapes and three-dimensional props were arranged to evoke exotic and distant landscapes, or to signify the comfort and culture of a wealthy interior. Cartes de visite were initially used to promote famous people such as heads of state, politicians and actors, but they quickly became a necessity for anyone with social aspirations.[41] To own a picture of oneself was no longer just a private and exclusive privilege of the upper classes. The inexpensive nature of these cards meant that for the first time almost anyone could commission a photographic portrait of him- or herself, copies of which could then be circulated to friends and family.

In line with the ascending social mobility of the mid-nineteenth century, most middle-class homes would have owned an album in which to present their collection. This enabled people to recreate social structures, forming imaginary alliances that defied established social hierarchies. Portraits of celebrities, which had become highly visible and valued commodities, could be placed alongside those of family members.[42] The cards often formed the basis of personal narratives, giving the illusion of a sense of proximity to the subject, whether he or she was a celebrity, a freak or someone the owner knew personally. In seeming to establish a connection between members of the public and 'well-known' individuals, the new, mass-produced photo-cards both contributed to the emergence of the celebrity figure and gave ordinary people a sense of status.[43]

The enormous popularity of cartes de visite points to a nineteenth-century belief that the photographic representation of oneself and one's family was, in the words of the historian of photography Geoffrey Batchen, 'a sign not only of financial and social success, but of moral and intellectual character'.[44] It is interesting, therefore, that pictures of freaks were commonly collected alongside those of celebrities and 'normal' people. The cards of freaks, which often included a description of the subject's 'condition' and a biography printed on the back, could be bought inside freak shows, then taken home and displayed in albums alongside those of family, friends and famous people. They helped to transform individual freaks into celebrities by giving them each a recognizable public image and a name. Although they clearly reinforced many of the narratives set up within the freak shows, these small, inexpensive portrait photographs also offered a different mode of representation for those who performed as freaks.[45] Unlike the sideshow exhibit, the portrait photograph often represents the freak as someone who belongs to a particular time and social context. At the same time it promotes him or her as unique and memorable in various more or less subtle ways, as the examples discussed later in this chapter demonstrate. The highly staged images printed on freaks' cartes de visite seem to have brought something of the dynamic of the sideshow into the home, enabling discourse on human difference to enter the everyday setting of the Victorian parlour. These supposedly realistic mementos of 'real-life' characters allowed the 'normal' spectator to take time to look at and contemplate the physical differences exhibited by a particular freak in the intimate personal context of the parlour.[46]

Although the settings are clearly very contrived, the portraits of freaks generally follow the same conventions as those of 'normal' sitters. In studios such as that of Charles Eisenmann in New York, for example, freaks were photographed against the same kinds of sets as celebrities and 'normal' subjects. The photographs imitated the aesthetics of great portrait painters such as Van Dyck, Rubens and Rembrandt.[47] Techniques of studio lighting, framing and depth of field were combined with pose, costume and accessories to confer a sense of status upon the subject. Within a limited range of established conventions that dictated both pose and setting, many freaks could choose how they wanted to appear and would have commissioned their own photographs in the same way as anyone else. Whilst the convention for racial freaks such as 'Zip' was more rigid – they were almost always depicted as 'outsiders', 'at home' in outdoor settings – Western freaks such as Madame Devere and Charles Tripp were, like 'normal' celebrity subjects, depicted in comfortable Victorian interiors. Some of the narratives of social inclusion and exclusion set up around Western freaks like Tripp and Devere are evident in the individual carte de visite photographs analysed below.

Madame Devere

Jane Devere was born in Kentucky, USA, in 1842. She joined Sells Brothers' circus at the age of forty-two, with a beard measuring fourteen inches in length. In contrast to 'Zip' and 'JoJo', who are depicted in what Bogdan has called 'the exotic mode', 'Madame Devere' was presented in the 'aggrandized mode', which, as Bogdan explains,

> emphasized how, with the exception of the particular physical mental or behavioural condition, the freak was an upstanding, high status person with talents of a conventional and socially prestigious nature . . . the publicity suggested that the exhibit belonged in the same social circle as celebrities.[48]

Unlike either 'Zip' or 'JoJo', Mrs Devere kept her own name, with the addition of the aristocratic title 'Madame'.

Bogdan has pointed out that, except for their beards, ladies like Madame Devere 'represented the quintessence of refined respectable womanhood'.[49] In the individual portrait of Jane Devere (Figure 4.4) this is affirmed by her upright posture, stylish close-fitting dress and lace-edged décolleté, which reveals the figure of an apparently normal female. In this image the subject leans forward slightly towards the camera, but her gaze does not quite meet ours. She is staring introspectively somewhere just beyond the camera, her impassive face giving no indication of character. This sense of detachment seems to make it easier to objectify this woman who, apart from her beard and perhaps the ambiguously male or female arrangement of her hair, appears like any other woman of her time.

Disdéri, who stressed the need for the photographer to capture the 'language of physiognomy' of his subject, stated that the aim of the portrait photographer should be to create a 'pleasing likeness' of his sitter.[50] However, this image suggests that in the case of the 'bearded lady' the aim was not so much to represent

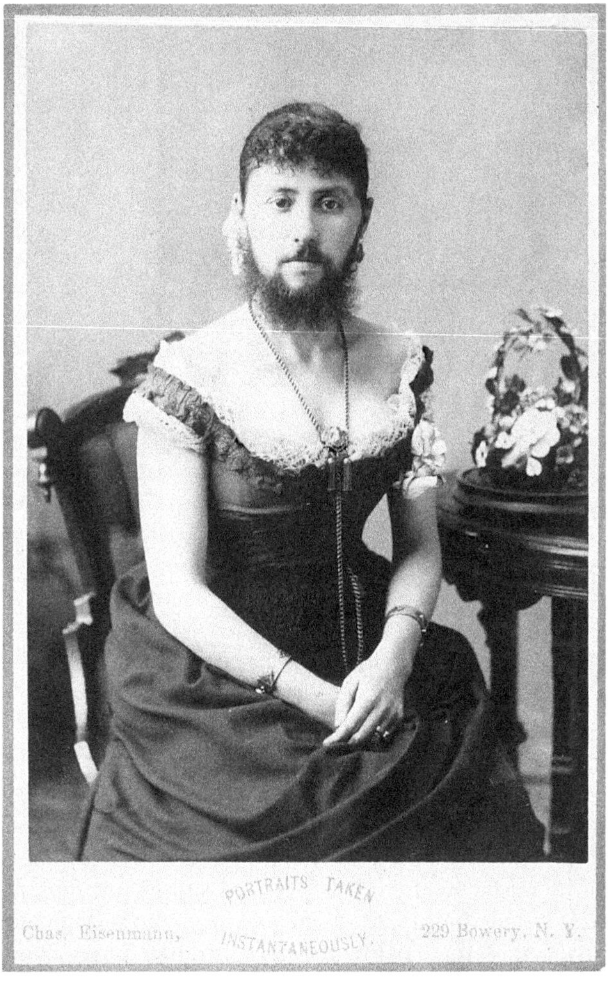

4.4: Bearded lady, Madame Devere, c.1878.

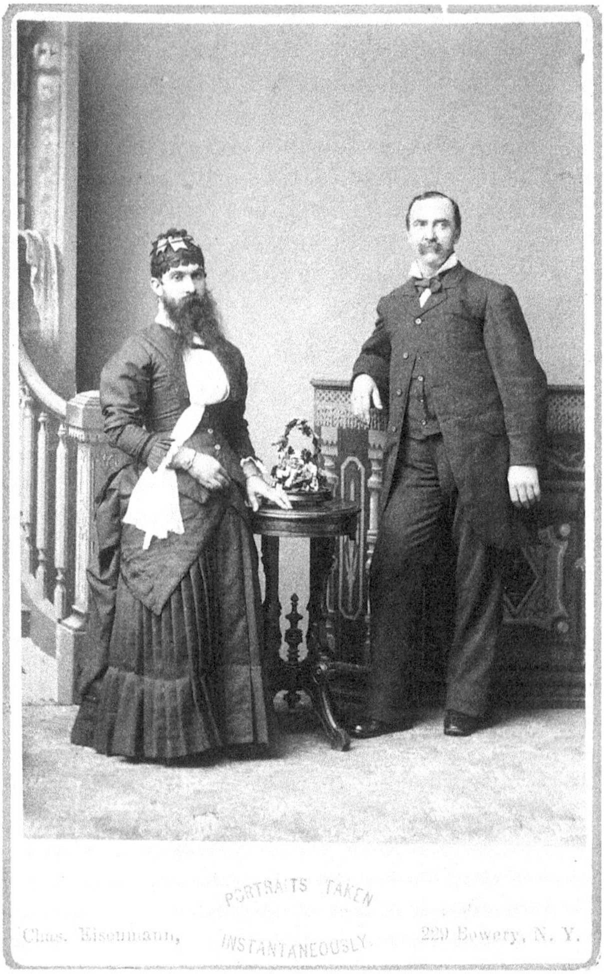

4.5: Bearded lady, Madame Devere, with her husband, c.1878.

the character of the individual depicted as to draw attention to the potential signification of her physical anomaly. Visibly disrupting the rigid categories of male and female, the figure of the 'bearded lady' could be seen as a challenge to the clearly defined social roles of men and women. It is perhaps significant that, at a time of female emancipation, Madame Devere, who is depicted as a perfectly normal female below the neck and like a man from the neck up, was such a popular figure on the freak show circuit. Like all freaks, her deviance from the established 'norm' was manifested as a highly visible phenomenon. However, as Nadja Durbach has commented, bearded women 'could easily be constructed as models of middle-class normative sexuality because they were without exception white Europeans or Americans'.[51]

Non-white hairy women, such as the famous Mexican freak Julia Pastrana (1834–60), were presented as primitive human/animal hybrids, the combination of black skin and unfeminine hairiness placing them in a sub-human category of their own.

Charles Tripp

Charles Tripp was born without arms, in Woodstock, Canada, in 1855. Tripp is a particularly interesting character because he seems to have lived successfully both as a member of mainstream society and as a sideshow performer. This may seem to contradict the notion that a freak could not share the same social space as a 'normal' person. But it is important to remember that Tripp's 'freak' status may well have been cast off once he left the sideshow stage. Although he was exhibited as a freak for over fifty years, Tripp made a living both as a carpenter and as a photographer for the Barnum circus. His lack of arms, which was framed as a monstrosity on the sideshow stage, does not appear to have impeded his 'real-life' role as a productive member of society.[52] In fact, following the death of his father when he was a young teenager, Tripp was able to support his mother and sister from an early age. In this respect he was an exception. Most people who chose to become freaks did so because they were unable to undertake traditional forms of work. In the nineteenth century the ability to work was, for middle- and working-class men alike, a means of establishing their identities as citizens and as men.[53] People exhibited as freaks were almost exclusively from those members of the lower classes who did not, or could not, contribute to modern society through any other form of employment.

The various different portrait photographs of Tripp, such as that shown in Figure 4.6, present him in an elegant but ordinary Victorian setting. Dressed in a dark suit with a white shirt and gold watch chain, he is represented as a respectable, responsible man. Like Jane Devere, he is depicted as entirely normal apart from one anomaly – his lack of arms, which is, apparently, compensated by the remarkable dexterity of his feet. The photographs of Tripp all depict him either drinking tea using his feet or demonstrating 'talents' such as penmanship, painting and paper cutting. The paraphernalia of these crafts are usually arranged on the floor around the chair on which he poses. There is always a silver tea set on a table beside him. The setting in all the available images of Tripp appears to be the same; only his appearance changes as he ages. In the relatively early image shown in Figure 4.6, he gazes directly at us, apparently in complete control of his situation and seemingly enjoying posing for the camera. This image of Tripp embodies several contradictory messages – inviting both identification and rejection. For example, although he is cast as

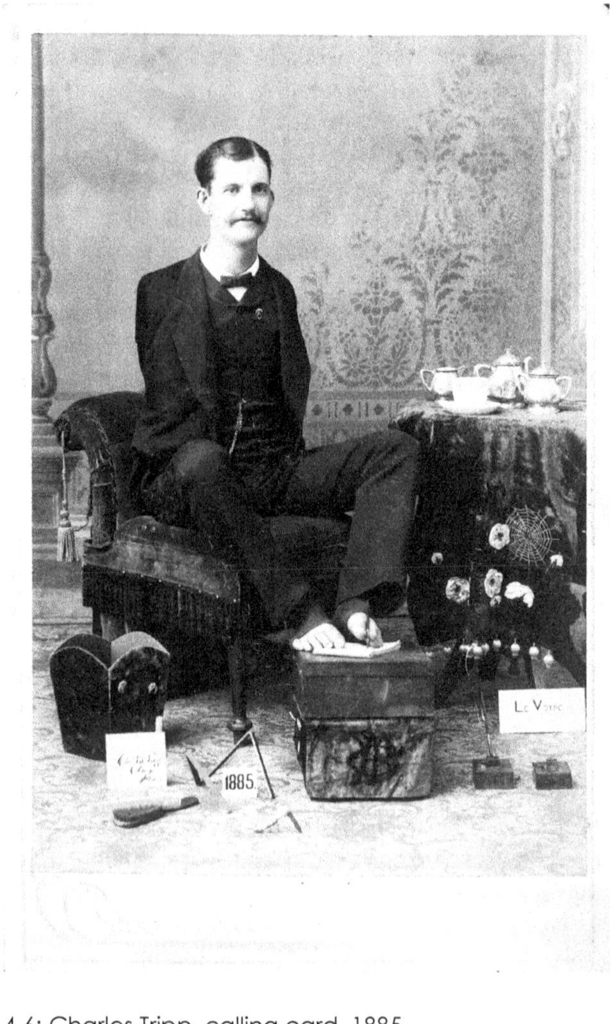

4.6: Charles Tripp, calling card, 1885.

an upper middle-class character, his smart clothes and wealthy setting accentuate his odd body. The everyday setting has the effect of further removing him from the norm and reaffirming the cultural superiority of the onlooker.[54]

The label 'freak' or 'monster' does not necessarily indicate a particular type of physiology, but instead points to a way of thinking about and representing difference. The bodies that appeared in freak shows and in freaks' carte de visite photographs simultaneously challenge and reinforce ideas about gender, race and physical disability. As we have seen, the messages conveyed by disabled freaks such as Charles Tripp, who seems to have led a relatively normal life outside the freak show, are somewhat mixed. The existence of people like Tripp could be taken to indicate that the freak show provided a manageable context within which to introduce the idea that, if a person with a deformity can live an apparently 'normal' life, perhaps he or she is not so different to the observer.

Disability and the 'Norm'

The idea of a 'norm' that underpins the modern construction of the deformed body as monstrous 'other' is relatively new. In the words of Lennard Davis, this idea is 'less a condition of human nature than it is a feature of a certain kind of society'.[55] According to Davis, the modern notion of normality and what he calls 'the social process of disabling' emerged as a result of industrialization in the eighteenth and nineteenth centuries.[56] The category of the 'norm' and the modern concept of the disabled body are, therefore, linked to the same social changes that brought about the popularity of the freak shows. Davis argues that the idea of 'normality', or 'normalcy', emerged in the nineteenth century as a result of the processes of modernity, giving rise to new understandings of notions of nationality, race, gender and sexual orientation – all of which can be related to an increased emphasis on bodily appearance.[57]

Davis explains that the idea of the 'norm' was originally a mathematical concept that the French statistician Adolphe Quetelet (1796–1847) then applied to human beings to establish the concept of 'the average man'. Quetelet developed a set of medical statistics that could determine what and who should be considered physically and morally average.[58] A whole range of nineteenth-century practices and discourses, including physiognomy, anthropology, criminology, photography and medicine – all of which rely on observation and measurement of the body – acted to define and maintain the 'norm' by describing and visualizing what was 'abnormal'.

In her essay 'Constructions of Physical Disability in the Ancient Greek World', Martha Edwards maintains that the notion of a 'norm', to which all deformed or different bodies are compared, did not exist in the classical world. Although disability and deformity were common in classical Greece, it seems that people with disabilities were integrated into society to the extent that there was no clear division between able-bodied and disabled people.[59] If, as Edwards suggests, the general concept of disability did not exist in ancient Greece, perhaps the visibly disabled body had no moral or social significance. This idea is supported by Davis, who has shown that in ancient Greece disability was not just a physical feature of the body, but was based on a person's functional capacity, particularly his or her ability to contribute to society through work.[60] Yet, accounts of the status of physical deformity in the ancient world are contradictory. For example, Robert Garland has noted that in classical Greece it was a legal requirement to abandon an infant born with a deformity.[61] He goes on to point out that in the fourth century BC Aristotle even recommended that there should be a law 'that no deformed child should live'.[62] But the motives for this infanticide were based on utilitarian and economic considerations. Deformity had no moral associations.[63] Ancient Roman law was even more categorical, decreeing that 'a father shall immediately put to death a son recently born, who is a monster, or who has a form different from that of members of the human race'.[64] There is a suggestion in this statement that monstrosity is a matter of degree rather than of absolute difference. But if the deformed bodies of monsters are not always visibly or structurally different from disabled bodies, how is it possible to distinguish between a monstrosity and a disability? Foucault maintains that Roman law, which provides a background to the question of the monster, 'carefully, although not entirely clearly, distinguished two categories: that of deformity, disability and deficiency . . . and then the monster in the strict sense'.[65] While he does not explain how this was done, he does go on to make a clear conceptual distinction between the effects of disability and monstrosity:

> Disability may well be something that upsets the natural order, but disability is not monstrosity because it has a place in civil or

canon law. The disabled person may not conform to nature, but the law in some way provides for him. Monstrosity, however, is the kind of irregularity that calls the law into question and disables it.[66]

And yet in practice monstrosity and disability are culturally encoded terms that often appear to overlap and are frequently confused. All different or deformed bodies challenge the accepted relations between mind and body, character and form. The irregularity of a deformed body is disconcerting because it does not conform to the symmetry of the 'proper' body and is therefore not as immediately 'legible' as a 'normal' body. But, as Georges Canguilhem explains, if this distortion can be explained and understood it is no longer threatening and need not be considered monstrous. As we saw earlier in this chapter, Canguilhem believed that, in the nineteenth century in particular, corporeal monstrosity was reduced, or 'normalized' through scientific explanation.[67] But even when bodily difference can be understood within existing knowledge systems, the disabled body is often seen to lack symbolic power and status.[68] In situations where physical deformity is not well understood, disabled bodies are assigned negative value and are set apart from the 'norm'. Even now, images of people with physical deformities are sometimes considered 'upsetting' or 'disturbing'. This suggests that the distinction between monstrosity and physical disability is still not always entirely clear.

Whilst the disabled body is often treated as insignificant, the monstrous body is by definition meaningful, although it is also, paradoxically, unintelligible. As we have already seen, the bodies of human monsters have historically manifested social and moral disorder as physical deformity. But, as Robert Garland has pointed out, any symbolic interpretation of deformity is 'partial and subjective'.[69] A body that is categorized as disabled in one context can be considered monstrous in another. For example, the conjoined twins included in Luca Landucci's early sixteenth-century list of monstrous births mentioned in Chapter 3 would now officially be framed as spectacularly disabled, not monstrous.[70] Neither disability nor monstrosity is a concrete condition. Monstrosity is a social construct that arises out of the need to represent social and political problems. It also signifies a lack of comprehension. As Davis has shown, disability is a culturally and historically specific concept, which was first brought into general use in Britain in the early twentieth century to refer to those wounded in war. Durbach explains this distinction: 'the category of "the disabled" did not replace either "the cripple" or "the freak" because it was coterminous with the war-wounded . . . [who] could demand preferential treatment in employment, housing, medical care and other social services.'[71]

The shifting understanding of what constitutes a monstrosity seems to suggest that the source of the confusion between monstrosity, deformity and disability lies in the observer, not in the body that is being observed. It depends on the context in which the body is seen and on the social and moral values of the 'normal' onlooker.

The Legacy of Freaks

Although freak shows were a predominantly nineteenth-century phenomenon, the photograph of a mid-twentieth-century American exhibit (Figure 4.3) clearly demonstrates an ongoing fascination for the spectacle of the different body. By the 1950s, however, the live exhibition of freaks for money was formally discredited and freak shows disappeared from view in both Europe and America. And yet, even though people with physical disabilities are now generally accepted as valid members of mainstream society, there is still a widespread and enduring fascination with looking at extreme physical difference. This is demonstrated by the popularity of television documentaries such as the *Extraordinary People* series shown on Channel Five in the UK, and *Extraordinary Humans* on the American channel National Geographic, both of which were first aired in 2003. Programmes such as these have simultaneously humanized their subjects and presented them as freakish curiosities in a way that is reminiscent of nineteenth-century freak shows.

One episode in the *Extraordinary People* series first shown in 2008 features a thirty-three-year-old British woman, Mandy Sellars, who was described in advance publicity as 'a woman with a bizarre condition that has left her with legs four times larger than those of the average person'. Whilst this may be a factual statistic, it is also sensationalist – inviting audiences to 'see for themselves' in a similar way to the freak show publicity described above. The title of this episode, 'The Woman with Giant Legs', is in itself reminiscent of freak show rhetoric. Nevertheless, the documentary reveals Mandy to be a well-adjusted, intelligent person who can speak eloquently about her disability and who manages her life well despite the evident difficulties presented by her legs, which continue to grow. Her own enthusiasm and her ease in front of the camera make Mandy appear completely human and very likable. But this is to some extent undermined for the viewer by the dehumanizing effect of statistics such as 'Mandy weighs twenty stone, fifteen of which are her legs', which are repeatedly given throughout the film. The message of the programme is, therefore, ambiguous. Whilst apparently aiming to be inclusive and to indicate that the strange deformities of the subjects do not diminish their 'humanness', earlier episodes in the series also stage the people involved as freakish curiosities. In the case of Mandy, the viewer is caught between empathy with her as a person and a voyeuristic fascination that surely echoes that of freak show audiences as they watched Charles Tripp drinking tea with his feet.

On the one hand such documentaries frame their subjects as ordinary and capable people with loving families and normal human aspirations, yet on the other hand they tantalize audiences with bizarre visual imagery and sensationalist descriptions. *Extraordinary People,* which – now in its ninth season – has been enormously popular, traverses between reiterating freak show stereotypes and cleverly forcing the viewer to face his or her own prejudices and preconceptions. The series was initially entitled *Extraordinary Bodies* – a denial of subjectivity that clearly echoed the dynamic of the freak shows. The change of name to *Extraordinary People* and a slight shift of emphasis to a more person-centred approach that focuses on the search for a scientific 'cure' points to a move away from the dehumanizing aspects of the freak shows. Yet the success of such programmes continues to rely on the same sort of voyeuristic fascination. If, as Foucault has argued, bodily deformity has lost its symbolic significance, why is it that audiences are still so compelled to watch people with unusual or extreme bodily traits living 'normal' lives?

5 | A Monstrous Subject

Representations of Joseph Merrick, the 'Elephant Man'

In the second half of the nineteenth century Joseph Merrick, the 'Elephant Man', exhibited himself as a freak before becoming both a medical curiosity and a social subject. Merrick's grossly deformed body clearly represented a significant challenge to the prevailing notion of what was acceptably human. But crucial to the narratives surrounding this intriguing individual is the discovery of his refined character, which to some extent came to efface the monstrous effects of his physical deformities. The acceptance, within a particular context, of Merrick as a socially developed human being could be seen to indicate a shift of emphasis from the morphology of the body to the character of the individual. And yet this is contradicted by the fact that Merrick was never able to show himself in public without provoking extreme and unwanted reactions.

Michel Foucault's argument that, by the end of the eighteenth century, monstrosity was transposed from the domain of somatic and natural disorder to that of criminality is key to this study of the visual significance of human monsters. In Foucault's view, it was during the nineteenth century that 'monstrous criminality' or 'a monstrosity that does not produce its effects in nature and the confusion of species, but in behaviour itself' began to supersede morphological monstrosity.[1] It is clear that at this time advances in medical and forensic sciences and the development of new imaging technologies such as photography did contribute to the discourses that began to uncouple physical deformity from what is monstrous. And yet the transition from corporeal to behavioural monstrosity has not necessarily been straightforward or even complete, even within the formal domains of science and law. Some of the contradictions that point to a shift away from the notion of monstrosity as somatic disorder on the one hand, and towards the enduring power of the body as a visual signifier of monstrousness on the other, will be investigated in this chapter.

The case of Joseph Merrick is particularly interesting because he clearly existed as both a real person and a mythical character (the 'Elephant Man'). The original documentation of his life has subsequently fuelled numerous more or less romanticized and fictionalized accounts that make it difficult to distinguish between 'the myth of the Elephant Man' and the 'facts' of his story. For example, contemporary perceptions of Merrick are undoubtedly influenced by subjective accounts, such as *The Elephant Man and Other Reminiscences*, published in 1923 by Frederick Treves, the surgeon who claimed to have 'rescued' him from his life as a freak exhibit. Treves' narrative, which presents Merrick as a refined but dependent and emotional, childlike character, clearly inspired more recent fictionalized accounts such as the well-known film *The Elephant Man*, made by David Lynch in 1980. This in turn informs the public image of Merrick today.

Several original documents relating to Merrick are preserved in the archive at the Royal London Hospital. These include the letter written in 1886 by F.C. Carr Gomm, the chairman of London Hospital Management Committee, to the editor of *The Times* newspaper, appealing for public donations towards Merrick's upkeep at the hospital; a copy of Merrick's visiting card; his birth and death certificates and a number of medical photographs and drawings. Other items such as the letter written by Merrick to one of the society ladies who befriended him (Figure 5.1) are held at the Record Office in Leicester, Merrick's birthplace. Along with the records of eyewitness accounts and factual details such as his date and place of birth and death, these artefacts act as reminders that Merrick was a real person. Living from 1862 to 1890, he is the most recent of the 'monsters' described so far. He is also spatially and emotionally proximate – the act of handling his original, personal documents gives a sense of intimacy with Merrick as a person. His own handwriting is especially evocative. The fact that we know Merrick lived in London for much of his life at a specific, identifiable location further enhances the feeling of familiarity. But, whilst we know when, where and, to some extent, how he lived, the 'Elephant Man' is still a predominantly mythical figure. The various ways in which this one unique individual was characterized offer an interesting insight into the contradictions inherent in the transition from physical to behavioural monstrosity that Foucault describes. The identity that has been constructed for him seems to have emerged out of a particularly nineteenth-century preoccupation with establishing a distinction between physical difference and what is monstrous. Perhaps more than any other individual, Merrick has acted as a locus for a renegotiation of the perceived relationship between morality and physical deformity.

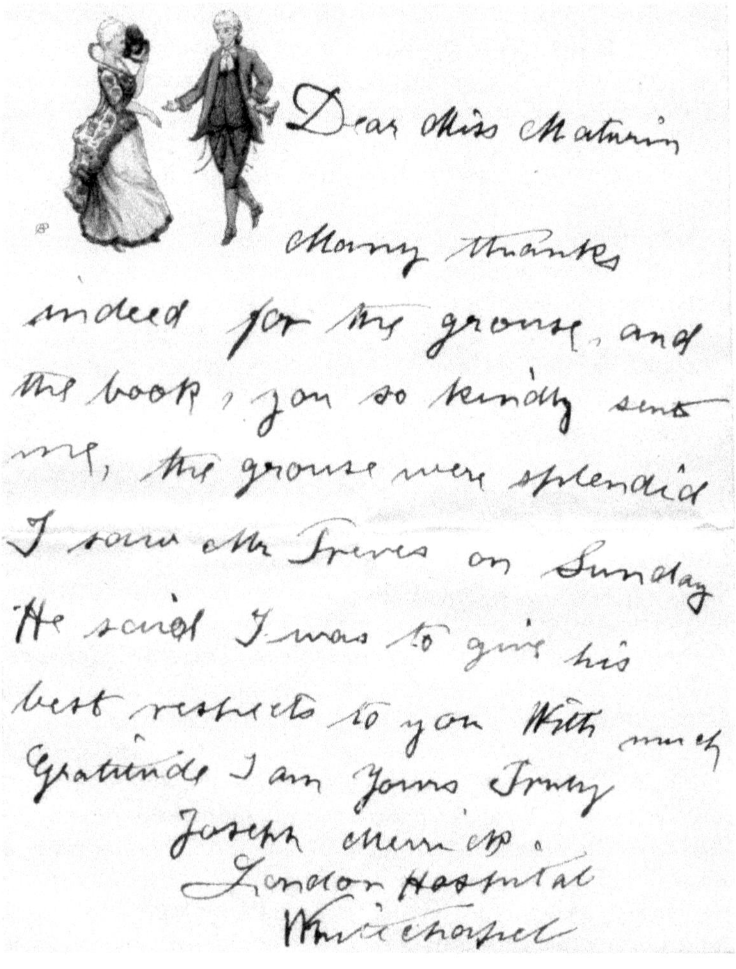

Dear Miss Maturin

Many thanks indeed for the grouse, and the book, you so kindly sent me, the grouse were splendid I saw Mr Treves on Sunday He said I was to give his best respects to you With much Gratitude I am Yours Truly

Joseph Merrick.

London Hospital

Whitechapel

5.1: Letter written by Joseph Merrick to Leila Maturin, 7 October 1889.

The Story of the 'Elephant Man'

Although it is known from his birth certificate that Joseph Merrick was born to a working-class family in Leicester in 1862, the documentation of his earliest years reads rather like a fairy tale.[2] According to narratives based on his own account, his mother, who was also disabled and – according to Merrick – beautiful, died when he was around eleven years old.[3] Merrick was then placed in the care of a cruel stepmother, who he ran away from to join a freak show operated by promoters Torr and Ellis at the 'Gaiety Palace of Varieties' in Leicester. Merrick's early life was reportedly one of poverty and deprivation.[4] His unfortunate circumstances were the kind to which contemporary forensic psychologists might attribute the 'bad character' of a criminal monster, and yet his character was always found to be good.

Between the sixteenth and eighteenth centuries in particular most people believed that maternal imagination could affect a foetus, to the extent that the object of a woman's thoughts was imprinted onto her child.[5] In this tradition, Merrick's deformities were initially given a mythical explanation. In an account attributed to Merrick himself, his appearance is explained like this:

> The deformity which I am now exhibiting was caused by my mother being frightened by an elephant; my mother was going along the street when a procession of animals was passing by, there was a terrible crush of people to see them, and unfortunately she was pushed under the elephant's feet, which frightened her very much; this occurring during a time of her pregnancy was the cause of my deformity.[6]

In the early 1880s the British showman Tom Norman, alias the 'Silver King', exhibited the 'Elephant Man' as a travelling spectacle that eventually occupied an empty shop at 123 Whitechapel Road in the East End of London in 1884. The shop was opposite London Hospital. Merrick's presence was noticed by some junior doctors, who brought their mentor, the surgeon Frederick Treves, to see him.[7] On describing this encounter, Treves' language is filled with disgust. His declaration that 'at no time had I met with such a degraded or perverted version of a human being as this lone figure displayed' suggests that his judgement of Merrick was, at this time, a moral one based on appearances.[8] Initially he:

> supposed that Merrick was imbecile and had been imbecile from birth. The fact that his face was incapable of expression, that his speech was a mere spluttering and his attitude that of one whose mind was void of all emotions and concerns gave grounds for this belief.[9]

If Merrick was not a monster in Treves' opinion, this statement suggests that at this time Treves considered him barely human, perhaps because the thought that such a creature might have a subjectivity that mirrored that of a 'normal' human being was initially too threatening. On one hand Treves describes this early encounter with Merrick emotively, portraying him as a disgusting and degraded quasi-human subject living an animal-like existence. But he also writes that, as a medical doctor, he was 'anxious to examine him in detail and to prepare an account of his deformities'.[10] Merrick was, therefore, taken to London Hospital, where Treves scrutinized him in the anatomy lab before displaying him as a medical curiosity at a meeting of the prestigious Pathological Society of London. As a scientist, Treves was clearly interested in attempting to 'make sense of' Merrick's abnormalities through meticulous observation in the anatomy lab.

Shortly after his presentation to members of the Pathological Society, Merrick resumed his life as a freak. In an unpublished manuscript Tom Norman, who acted as Merrick's manager, wrote that he had refused to return to London Hospital because he preferred to be exhibited in a freak show where he was paid, rather than 'over there [in the hospital where] I was stripped naked, and felt like an animal in a cattle market'.[11] It is impossible to know whether this is a true account of Merrick's feelings, but it poses an interesting challenge to Treves' story that his relationship to Merrick was entirely philanthropic. His original motive for taking Merrick in certainly seems to have been one of scientific renown. Whatever Merrick's own feelings, documentation suggests that it was considered acceptable and 'proper' for him to be scrutinized within a scientific context, whilst his deformities were thought to be too sensational for public display. Norman's exhibition of Merrick was closed down by police because it was regarded as an offence to public decency.[12] In her recent book, *Spectacle of Deformity: Freak Shows and Modern British Culture*, Nadja Durbach supports Norman. She argues that as a freak Merrick had largely been in control of his own bodily display and was therefore able to see himself as an independent working-class man, but that under Treves' care in the hospital he was completely reliant on the good will of his patrons. In Durbach's words, 'In return for this care and support [Merrick] was required to surrender his right as an independent man to govern his body and to determine its uses.'[13] In fact, she argues, the freak show continued in the hospital as Merrick's high-society visitors had, in effect, paid to see him through their charitable donations.

Whilst both Treves' and Norman's accounts are open to interpretation, it is known that Merrick returned to Treves for help in

1886, following a difficult time attempting to survive as a freak in Belgium.[14] Treves' version of the story of Merrick's 'rescue' is somewhat romanticized and was fiercely contested by Norman, but it is certainly the case that rooms were found for Merrick at London Hospital, where, according to Treves, his socialization began.[15] Although he was born into a working-class family and the extent of his education is unclear, it seems that in the hospital Merrick acquired middle-class social skills and was also able to maintain some sort of intellectual life. In his *Reminiscences* Treves expresses excitement over Merrick's ability to converse and to read, and marvels at his good nature.[16] He states,

> to secure Merrick's recovery and to bring him, as it were, to life once more, it was necessary that he should make the acquaintance of men and women who would treat him as a normal and intelligent young man and not as a monster of deformity.[17]

The story follows that, as people were encouraged to treat Merrick as a human being, 'he began to change . . . from a hunted thing into a man', developing a range of refined social and craft skills.[18] The theme of salvation from a state of bestiality whereby the deformed monster is shown to have an empathetic and very human character is the central to well-known nineteenth-century literary works such as Mary Shelley's *Frankenstein* (1818) and *The Hunchback of Notre Dame* by Victor Hugo (1834).[19] Part of the reason for his popularity amongst cultured society ladies must have been Merrick's status as a living manifestation of this popular nineteenth-century narrative. In keeping with the emergent museum culture that was gradually taking over from that of travelling shows, Merrick had clearly become a curiosity for the upper- and middle-class people who visited him, as well as for the scientists who studied him.

In April 1890 Merrick was found dead in bed, asphyxiated by the weight of his head.[20] Treves attributed his death to an experiment in which Merrick was trying to fulfil his wish to sleep lying down like other people, whilst Norman identified it as an act of suicide.[21] Again, we can only guess what really happened, although Durbach argues that Merrick's death was a wilful bid for freedom:

> According to Norman, Merrick's suicide was not the result of his failure to measure up to 'the norm'. It was instead his

last expression of bodily control, an act of manly defiance that was ultimately an explicit refusal to be further objectified and pathologized by modern science.[22]

After his funeral Merrick became a medical specimen once again – his body was transferred to the London Hospital medical college, where casts were made. It was then dissected. His skeleton remains in the Royal London Hospital archive, where it is now accessible only to medical specialists.

Scientific Context

To contextualize the re-evaluation of Merrick's physical difference during his transition from freak show spectacle to medical specimen and society figure it is perhaps useful to consider some developments in the scientific understanding of monstrosity that took place in the nineteenth century. The work of the French zoologists Etienne Geoffroy de St Hilaire (1772–1844) and his son Isidore (1805–61) seems to have had a particularly profound effect on perceptions of what is monstrous. Their findings would certainly have been studied by medical practitioners such as Frederick Treves, and would consequently have influenced the way that Merrick was perceived and treated.

Ideas developed by Etienne and Isidore Geoffroy de St Hilaire also informed the theoretical work of both Georges Canguilhem and Michel Foucault. Canguilhem makes frequent reference to St Hilaire in both *The Normal and the Pathological* and his 1962 lecture, 'Monstrosity and the Monstrous'.[23] For example, when in 'Monstrosity and the Monstrous' Canguilhem asserts that 'it was really in the nineteenth century that the scientific explanation of monstrosity was elaborated, and with it the correlative reduction of the monstrous', he is primarily referring to the work of St Hilaire and his son.[24]

In the early nineteenth century Etienne Geoffroy de St Hilaire, who was concerned with the function of monstrosity rather than its cause, began to categorize monsters in terms of characteristics such as excess, lack or displacement of organs.[25] He advanced the idea that monstrosity is not unnatural, but results from the arrested development of a normal organism. Foucault is following this idea when he maintains that 'the monstrous forms of some individuals are only the product of a disturbance in the action of natural laws'.[26] According to scientists like St Hilaire, therefore, there was nothing inherently different about monsters – they were simply errors of nature.

Writing in the mid-nineteenth century, Isidore Geoffroy de St Hilaire, who also saw monstrosity as part of a natural process rather than as a significant phenomenon, proposed that it was 'no longer a random disorder, but another order, equally regular and equally subject to laws'.[27] He reinforced the idea that, once physical deformities are rationalized within scientific discourse, their moral significance is removed. By refusing to see the human monster as a failure of normality or as a social reject, Geoffroy de St Hilaire reduced the negative associations of physical deformity. And yet it seems that he had not quite abandoned the idea of monstrosity as a morphological condition.[28] In his treatise on teratology, he describes monstrosity in terms of a number of complex and serious anomalies that result in severe physical malfunctions or malformations, rendering those suffering from them visibly different to the rest of their species.[29] By contrast, Canguilhem maintained that: 'the transparence of monstrosity to scientific thought henceforth deprives it of all relationship to the monstrous. Realism systematically condemns the monstrous to be nothing more in kind than the imprint of monstrosity'.[30] In this view, once a scientific language is established to explain physical deformity and account for its causes, the relationship between monstrosity (which is an effect of the monstrous) and the monstrous (which is an infraction of the law that results from monstrosity) breaks down completely, and the monster disappears.

The theories developed by Etienne and Isidore Geoffroy de St Hilaire undoubtedly contributed to Canguilhem's argument that nineteenth-century scientific discourse had banished all previous forms of monstrousness to the realms of myth and imagination.[31] Isidore in particular demonstrated that if a physical deformity can be named, classified and understood it need no longer be considered monstrous. It is, as Canguilhem has suggested, 'domesticated'.[32] But, in practice, complex cases such as Merrick's resist this process. From the time he was first exhibited, doctors have been fascinated by his obscure and unclassifiable condition and by the challenge of trying to identify it.[33] The various diagnoses of his disorder have included elephantiasis, a tropical disease; leontiasis, a disorder which causes overgrowth of the facial and cranial bones; neurofibromatosis, a genetic disorder that produces deformities of the bones and skin and, more recently, another genetic disorder, 'Proteus syndrome'.[34] However, according to the Royal London Hospital archivist, Jonathan

Evans, Merrick's grossly deformed body continues to confound definitive scientific classification.[35] His deformities were displayed, depicted and described, but they could not be classified or made to signify anything. And yet the fact that, despite his profound and inexplicable deformities, Merrick himself was 'domesticated', and humanized, by the acquisition of social skills and a more socialized appearance seems to support the idea that 'monstrosity of character' has replaced 'monstrosity of nature'.[36]

The ancient belief that an irregularity in the natural formation of the human body signifies moral or social disorder was exploited by the freak shows, and yet it lies in direct contradiction to the discourses of modern science. Etienne and Isidore Geoffroy de St Hilaire and Georges Canguilhem all interpreted monstrosity as a physical phenomenon that could be rationalized by subjecting it to a medical gaze and defining it using medical terms. This new transparency, Canguilhem concludes, is the end of naturally occurring monstrosity – what is monstrous is now what can be man-made in the science lab by 'experimental teratologist[s]', who transgress the laws of nature by producing unacceptable hybrids that threaten established classifications.[37] Foucault relates to the scientists' findings rather differently. Whilst he acknowledges that Etienne de St Hilaire had 'demonstrated that the monstrous forms of some individuals are only the product of a disturbance in the action of natural laws', for him human monstrosity was not eliminated once the techniques of visualization and classification had severed the link between physical deformity and monstrousness.[38] Instead, he claims, monstrosity shifted from the physical to the psychological. This type of monstrosity is not readily accessible to the gaze. It resists visual representation, is difficult to regulate and, most disturbingly, difficult to categorize as 'other' in terms of social or medical pathology.

Representing the 'Elephant Man'

The story of Merrick's 'domestication' in spite of his appearance marks a crucial shift in attitude that initially seems to support Foucault's proposition that by the nineteenth century human monstrosity was no longer manifested in a person's physical form, but in his or her character. In many of the narratives that surround Merrick, he is depicted as a 'good person' – an unfortunate individual trapped in a grotesque body. Written accounts emphasizing his good character and refined social skills appear on the surface to present him as a kind of anti-monster, someone to be accepted into society in spite of his appearance. Although the limited social status that he enjoyed could only be possible in a context where monstrosity is no longer directly aligned with appearance, on closer inspection the texts and visual images that represent Merrick and his complex transition from freak to medical curiosity and social subject are ambiguous and contradictory.

In a text that has been attributed to Merrick and which first appeared on the 'Elephant Man's' freak show pamphlet, he describes his own appearance as follows:

> The measurement around my head is thirty six inches, there is a large substance of flesh at the back as large as a breakfast cup, the other part in a manner of speaking is like hills and valleys, all lumped together, while the face is such a sight that no one could describe it. The right hand is almost the size and shape of an Elephant's foreleg, measuring twelve inches round the wrist and five inches round one of the fingers; the other hand and arm is no larger than that of a girl ten years of age, although it is well proportioned. My feet and legs are covered with thick lumpy skin, also my body, like that of an Elephant, and almost the same colour, in fact, no one would believe until they saw it, that such a thing could exist.[39]

Whether it was actually written by Merrick himself or by a copywriter, this description is significant.[40] It mixes factual information such as the circumference of his head and hand with more evocative similes and sensationalist statements to create a vivid image of a strangely fragmented or formless body. Images such as the flesh which is 'as large as a breakfast cup'; the right hand which is 'the size and shape of an Elephant's foreleg' and the claim that 'no one would believe it until they saw it' all echo the rhetoric of the freak show talker.

The troubling nature of a creature that appears to be simultaneously animal and human is evidenced in Treves' emotive account of his first encounter with the 'Elephant Man' at 123 Whitechapel Road.[41] The actual meeting was prefigured by a view of a life-size painted banner, hung outside the shop, which Treves describes like this:

> This very crude production depicted a frightful creature that could only have been possible in a nightmare. It was the

> figure of a man with the characteristics of an elephant. The transfiguration was not far advanced. There was still more of the man than of the beast. This fact – that it was still human – was the most repellent attribute of the creature. There was nothing about it of the pitiableness of the misshapened or the deformed, nothing of the grotesqueness of the freak, but merely the loathsome insinuation of a man being changed into an animal.[42]

Although Treves is actually describing the painted image of the 'Elephant Man', it appears that he is also referring to the ambiguities displayed by Merrick himself. As Merrick's self-appointed stage name suggests, his appearance indicated a transgression of the most sacred of all boundaries – that between humans and animals. At this initial meeting Treves seems to have been most disturbed by the suggestion that Merrick was apparently taking on animal characteristics. The transmutation from human to animal, which clearly troubled the Victorian imagination, forms the subject of many Gothic horror stories, such as H.G. Wells' tale of fabricated human/animal hybrids, *The Island of Doctor Moreau* (1896). Merrick's developing condition, which was not evident at birth but was growing increasingly severe, presents a powerful image of monstrosity as a process – an affliction that could affect any normal body. Perhaps in the light of the new theories of evolution taken up by the Social Darwinists, the fact that Merrick was apparently a man turning into an animal was particularly frightening because it could offer living proof that an atavistic return to an animal state was possible.[43]

The first of Mr Carr Gomm's letters to *The Times*, published in December 1886, probably did more than anything else to raise public awareness of Merrick's existence at the hospital. This letter describes his circumstances and gives a brief account of his life so far. In general it is sympathetic and sensitive, according Merrick the status of a disadvantaged person rather than a monster. Carr Gomm introduces Merrick to the public by emphasizing the separation between his appearance and his character:

> terrible though his appearance is, so terrible indeed that women and nervous persons fly in terror from the sight of him, and that he is debarred from seeking to earn his livelihood in an ordinary way, yet he is superior in intelligence, can read and write, is quiet, gentle, not to say even refined in his mind.[44]

As a result of this letter, sufficient funds were donated to support Merrick at the hospital for the rest of his life. But the incentives behind the donations were not entirely altruistic. For the benefactors, this act of charity would have offered a public demonstration of their own good fortune, reinforcing their status as 'normal' and useful members of society. However, the public display of acceptance of Merrick is also significant in that it suggests some level of disavowal of the connection between physical deformity and 'bad' character.

In a later letter Carr Gomm casts Merrick in a passive role, as recipient of goodness and care, stating that he:

> was a great reader and was well supplied with books through the kindness of a lady . . . he was taught basket making, and on more than one occasion he was taken to the play, which he witnessed from the seclusion of a private box.[45]

Carr Gomm and Treves, who tells us that Merrick received many distinguished visitors such as the actress Mrs Kendall and Alexandra, Princess of Wales, both frequently emphasize his refined character. In this sense he is shown to be proximate to 'normal' people. But Treves also infantilizes Merrick, writing: 'Merrick still remained in many ways a mere child. He had all the invention of an imaginative boy or girl, the same love of "make-believe", the same instinct of "dressing up" and of impersonating heroic and impressive characters.'[46] Merrick's letters were described as 'the letters of a delighted and enthusiastic child'.[47] Overall, the written narratives that describe and document Merrick's life are contradictory. Carr Gomm and Treves publicly claim to accept him as a human subject, and yet they simultaneously undermine his status as an adult human.

Pictures of Merrick

Whilst the banner advertising the exhibition of the 'Elephant Man' at 123 Whitechapel Road no longer exists, it is quite possible to imagine from Treves' description and from images of similar freak show banners and freak photographs like those discussed in Chapter 3 the extraordinary visual impression it would have given of a man literally being changed into an animal. In this context Merrick was portrayed as a true freak – an unreal, exaggerated creature whose function was to embody monstrous difference so it could be set apart from the 'normal' body of the spectator. Like other freaks, the fictionalized and fantastic persona of the 'Elephant Man' perpetuated the pre-modern idea of the monster as an unnatural physical phenomenon whose strange and different body represents moral and social disorder. Merrick's early representation as a freak would have reinforced historically entrenched popular assumptions, such as the idea that monstrosity is an essential quality and that there is an inherent and permanent distinction between deviance and normality.

The way that Merrick might have been portrayed in the imaginative picture described by Treves is certainly very different to the way he is represented in a set of four medical photographs taken at the time of his admission to London Hospital in 1886 (Figure 5.2). These four images, which show Merrick from the back, the front and both sides, are uniformly shot from a low angle in relatively flat light. The photographs were probably taken in Treves' room at the hospital by a professional medical photographer.[48] This is significant because, as Martin Kemp has pointed out, many medical photographers were trained in the standard genres of professional photography and would, therefore, have brought the conventions of studio photography to the hospital.[49]

Medical photographs such as these reflect the balance of power between patient and physician. As the object of the camera's gaze, the patient had to be passive and remain motionless for as long as the shutter was open, whilst the physician would direct both the subject and the photographer. Consistent with its function in nineteenth-century physiognomy and criminology, the medical photograph was understood to provide an objective document that would enable doctors to discover 'the truth' of a condition such as Merrick's. As Sander Gilman has pointed out, the introduction of images, and photographs in particular, into medical textbooks gradually replaced the display of 'real', live patients for medical scrutiny.[50] For those doctors who were not able to view Merrick 'in the flesh', these photographs, with their documentary appearance of realism, authenticity and authority, would have provided the most comprehensive visual access to his 'condition' available.

As we saw in Chapter 2, photography offered a newly objective form of medical representation in the late nineteenth century.[51] And yet, as Kemp argues, it followed a long tradition of medical illustration that brought with it certain conventions and expectations. These existing standards could not automatically

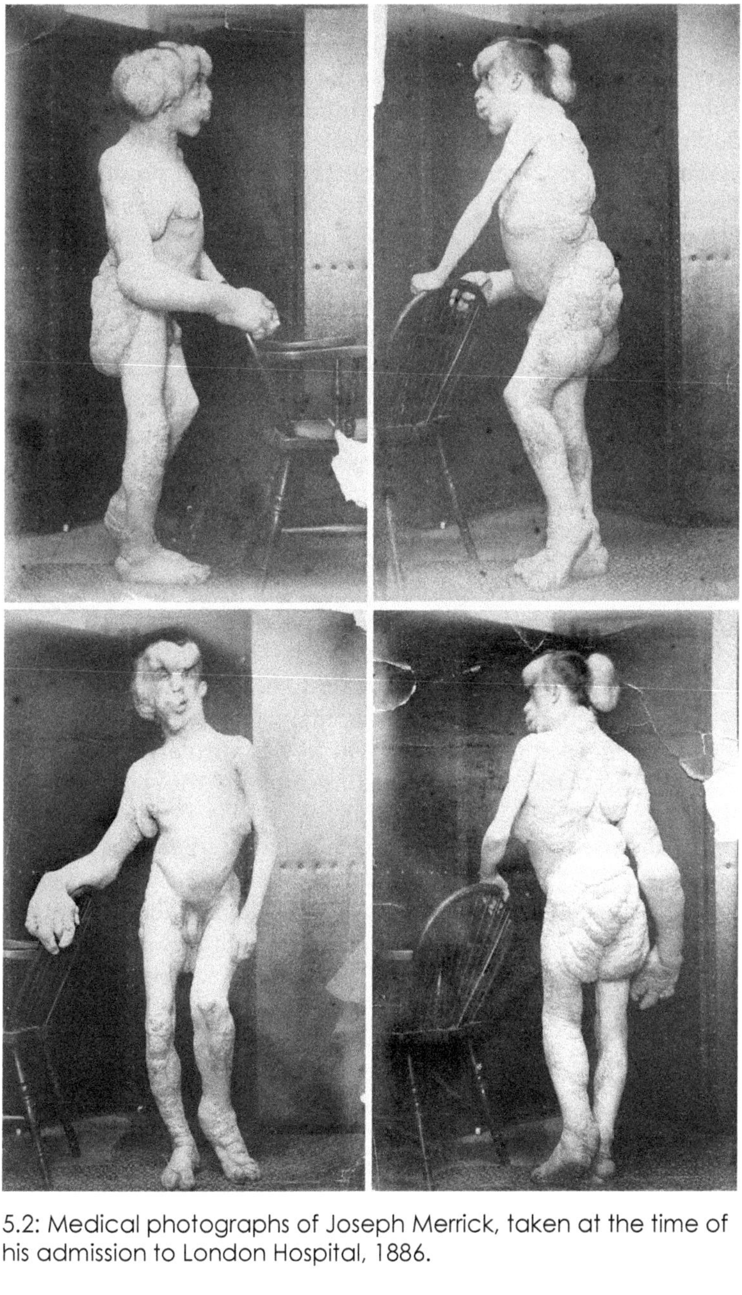

5.2: Medical photographs of Joseph Merrick, taken at the time of his admission to London Hospital, 1886.

be met by the camera, which is not selective, but reproduces everything in its field of view. Therefore, careful choices had to be made about what was and was not included in the image.

In the context of the long description of Merrick's appearance published in the *Transactions of the Pathological Society* a year earlier, the photographs were probably intended to contribute to Treves' attempt to form an understanding of Merrick's condition through detailed visual analysis of his body. In this regard the pictures reflect the idea that photography has a direct relationship to its subject that renders it useful as an analytical tool capable of revealing objective, scientific 'truths'.

In these photographs the attention of the camera is clearly focused on Merrick's naked body as a subject for scientific analysis. In each case the intention seems to have been to depict his deformities as objectively as possible, without sensationalizing them, but with little regard for the man inside the misshapen body. Whilst by contemporary standards the surroundings may appear far from clinical – the inclusion of the wooden chair and patterned rug give the photographs a domestic feel – this was a standard hospital setting in the late nineteenth century. In contrast to Merrick's brightly lit flesh, the shadowy rug and chair would have been sufficiently familiar to be disregarded by those seeking answers to this medical anomaly.[52]

Unlike the painted banner, which was displayed in public and clearly made for public consumption, the photographs shown in Figure 5.2, which depict Merrick's body as a 'case study' for analysis, were meant for a limited audience of medical professionals. They have frequently been published in books written by doctors 'for medical purposes', but broader publication has been restricted 'for ethical reasons'. This is allegedly in order to prevent exploitation of the images as a spectacle and to 'protect' the public from the possible effects of seeing such deformities. But in reality the original small, creased and torn sepia-toned prints are neither spectacular nor shocking.[53] Despite their clinical purpose, these medical photographs actually seem to represent Merrick in a more intimate and personal way than his carte de visite portrait (Figure 5.3). This is partly because in the medical photographs Merrick is naked, whilst in the portrait photograph he is dressed in his 'Sunday-best' suit. But his relationship to the camera is also significant. In the four medical pictures Merrick's pose is relatively relaxed. The 'normal' and deformed parts of his fragmented body are afforded equal status. In one of these pictures Merrick gazes directly into the lens in

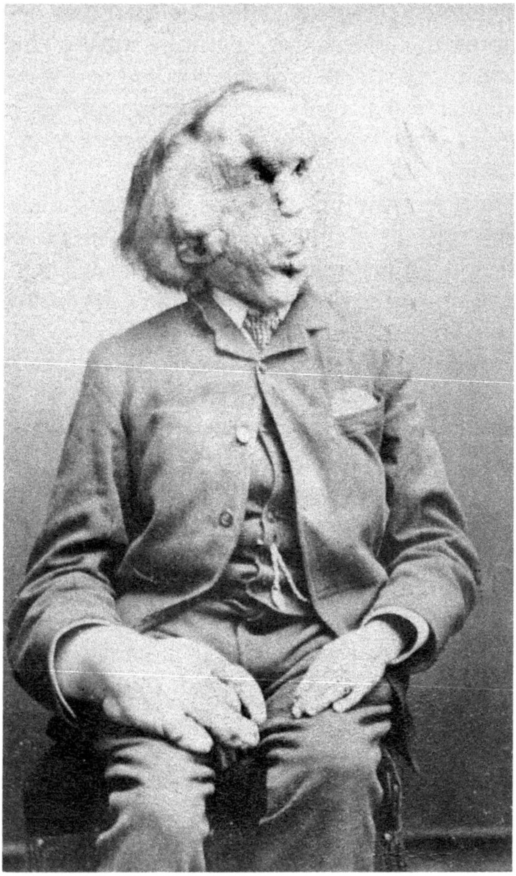

5.3: Carte de visite portrait of Joseph Merrick in his 'Sunday-best' suit, c.1887.

a way that seems both comfortable and confident, whilst in the carte de visite photograph his pose looks both self-conscious and artificial. Although the aim of the medical photographs may be to objectify Merrick's deformities, they are devoid of artifice, and as a result seem to represent his humanity more directly than the carte de visite picture, in which he appears much less relaxed.

For many nineteenth-century sitters the attraction of a carte de visite photograph was not its realism, but its ability to create an illusion of wealth or status.[54] For Merrick, however, it was surely the possibility it offered to create an illusion of apparent ordinariness. It is interesting that he is not photographed against a painted backdrop. He is without any of the theatrical props normally used in a photography studio. This photograph, which was probably taken at the hospital in a style that to some extent emulates that of a studio photograph, is quite different to the more elaborate carte de visite portraits of freaks discussed in Chapter 4.

As we saw in Chapter 3, the new medium of photography emerged at a time when interest in physiognomy was at its height. Both disciplines have been used to categorize, archive and control any type of body that deviates from the social 'norm'. In his book *Photography, Vision and the Production of Modern Bodies*, Suren Lalvani explains how the nineteenth-century portrait photograph was constructed to create an image of 'normality' and to secure the social status of its subject:

> the nineteenth-century construct of personality, solely predicated on outward appearances, was taken as an index of inner feeling and character . . . the body outfitted in a careful repertory of gestures and clothed with a circumspect sense for detail, became an elaborate signification system – a text to be both coded and decoded with infinite care if one was to avoid being ostracized.[55]

Like medical and forensic photography, nineteenth-century portrait photography also functioned to establish and define the 'other'.[56] Merrick's carte de visite photograph is no exception.

Although at first glance this picture may appear to 'humanize' Merrick by representing him as a civilized individual, on closer inspection it becomes clear that the image actually sets its subject apart from 'normal' citizens in several subtle ways. If a portrait usually functions to affirm an individual's status and to reinforce dominant social values, the visual language of Merrick's carte de visite photograph directly contradicts the narratives it is supposedly setting up. For example, whilst the customized suit Merrick is wearing should function to 'normalize' his strange body, it actually draws attention to his abnormalities. These are further emphasized by his relation to the camera. Merrick is not looking into the lens. His head is turned to the side so that the part of his face unaffected by deformity is almost entirely concealed, whilst his misshapen head and displaced ear are clearly visible. Likewise, his enlarged, deformed hand is positioned in front of his 'normal' hand. To have a portrait of himself wearing a suit and tie might have seemed to Merrick to permit him entry into 'normal' middle-class society, affording him a respectable place within the social and moral hierarchy, but this foregrounding of his deformity recasts him in the role of the freak.

Although Treves credits himself with being the 'saviour' of Merrick by facilitating his socialization and rendering him acceptable as a human being, the ambiguity of this photograph suggests that Merrick's social transformation was not as complete as Treves claims. The written narratives relating to Merrick tend to emphasize his refined character, but this highly coded picture, made for public consumption, visually reinforces his status as an 'abnormal' outsider. This seems to suggest that, whilst Merrick's

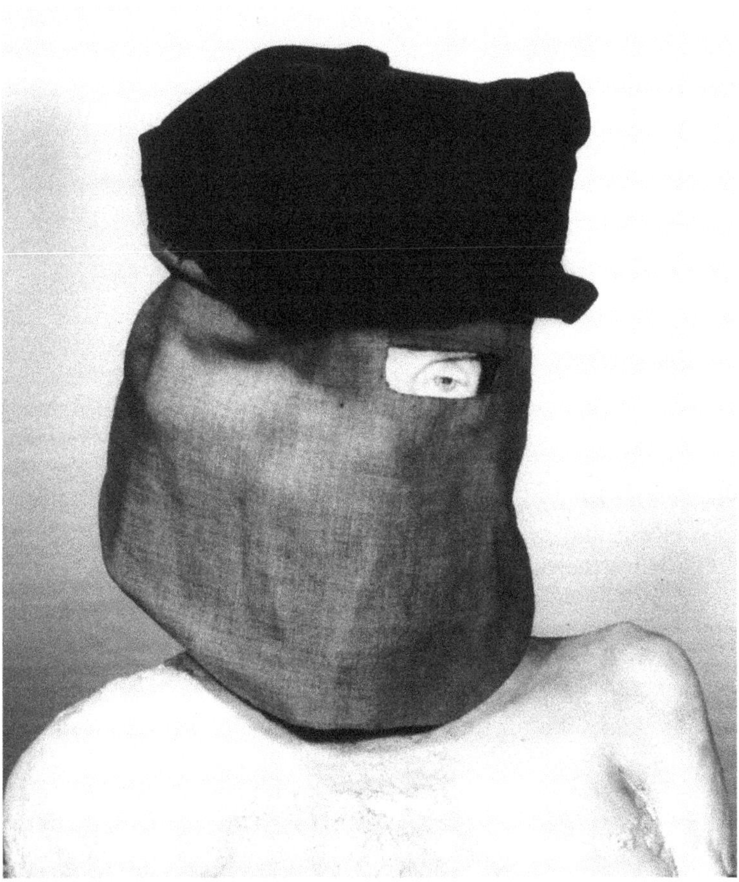

5.4: Merrick's cap and veil, date unknown.

good character clearly proved him not monstrous for those who knew him, his visible features, which could not easily be categorized or understood, were still found to be profoundly challenging when seen out of context. No matter how he was photographed, therefore, Merrick's image would not be fully normalized.

This is further evidenced by his invisibility in the public domain. Although he received many curious visitors to his rooms at London Hospital, the carte de visite portrait was all that most people would have seen of Merrick beyond the walls of the hospital. On the rare occasions that he did go out in public, he adopted a 'disguise' consisting of a full-length black cloak and a black hat with a veil or hood that covered his entire head. Only his left eye, which was unaffected by deformity, remained visible (Figure 5.4). This disguise apparently had the twofold function of protecting Merrick from unwanted attention and protecting the public from the horror they might experience on catching sight of him.[57] The veil provided another strategy for keeping Merrick and his monstrous deformities away from 'normal' individuals. The fact that he could not be seen in public seems to suggest that, at the end of the nineteenth century, the sight of severe physical deformity was still 'monstrously' challenging to most people, even if the idea of it was less so.[58]

Merrick Face to Face

Even within the domain of the hospital, where he was framed as a 'socialized' human subject, Merrick's role was still to some extent that of a freak whose excessive deformities presented a fascinating and horrifying spectacle of 'otherness'. And yet in many ways the relationship between Merrick and his visitors at the hospital would have been very different to that of freaks and their sideshow audiences. Firstly, whilst freaks were subjected to the gaze and the comments of anyone who paid to enter the show tent, Merrick must have had a degree of control over who was permitted to enter his private rooms. Unlike freaks, who were not usually permitted to communicate with their audiences, Merrick is known not only to have conversed with his visitors, but also to have shaken hands with them. Whilst this clearly provided a 'feel-good factor' for his benefactors, for whom he was an ideal object of charity, Merrick could literally meet his visitors at something approximating eye level. It seems, therefore, that in this context he was not entirely devoid of power. As a not-monstrous but still somewhat freakish individual, Merrick could interrogate any façade of politeness put on by his visitors simply by returning their gaze: a social exchange that would never have been possible if he was still unambiguously categorized as a monster.

Although he is often described by his contemporaries in a way that seems patronizing, in the latter part of his life Merrick is represented as a person with 'real' human emotions, desires and aspirations. Treves notes that Merrick wanted to travel in order to 'improve his mind' and enlarge his knowledge of the world.[59] In the hospital and with the help of Treves, it seems that, to some extent at least, Merrick was able to 'revise himself' from the status of freakish monster to human being by demonstrating normal human desires and ambitions despite his disturbing appearance.[60] By acquiring social skills and a comprehensible language he became a person with whom others could, on some level, identify. Treves depicts him as a sociable and romantic young man who reads love stories, falls in love with every woman he meets and dreams of being a lover.[61] He explains in his *Reminiscences* that Merrick's 'bodily deformity had left unmarred the instincts and feelings of his years. He was amorous'. He then asks us to 'imagine the feelings of such a youth when he saw nothing but a look of horror creep over the face of every girl whose eyes met his.'[62] It was fashionable for charitable society ladies to appear to get close to Merrick, but not too close.

One factor that must have figured strongly in Merrick's socialization, but which seems to have been largely overlooked, is the smell of his 'fungous' skin. In his initial description of the 'Elephant Man', Treves notes:

> one other feature must be mentioned to emphasize his isolation from his kind. Although he was already repellent enough, there arose from the fungous skin-growth with which he was almost covered a very sickening stench which was hard to tolerate.[63]

Dr Halsted, the junior doctor who first discovered Merrick, wrote that at this time 'it was hard to see how even the most morbidly curious spectator could feel anything but disgust at the sight and smell of him'.[64] Once Merrick was resident at the hospital, however, a bathroom was added to his rooms because for him a bath was 'not merely a luxury but, from the nature of his affliction, a daily necessity'.[65] This must have contributed greatly to his social acceptability for those who met him face to face.

In their various writings, Carr Gomm and Treves established that Merrick's physical deformity was not accompanied by 'a deformed personality'.[66] He is someone whose ability to communicate with 'normal' people, to behave appropriately and to show that he had 'human feelings' led to the revision of his status in their eyes. In this sense Merrick has come to represent the inverse of what we now understand as a monster. His empathetic character was not monstrous, despite his deformed body. But the visual and narrative accounts that surround the figure of the 'Elephant Man' are often contradictory. The way Merrick is represented in his carte de visite photograph, for example, seems to undermine the narratives which suggest that his physical deformity was no longer understood as a signifier of monstrousness. The different depictions of Merrick provide some evidence of the transition from physical to moral or behavioural monstrosity that Foucault has documented. But they also suggest that this transition was by no means complete at the end of the nineteenth century.

6 | Monstrous Images of Evil

Picturing Jack the Ripper and Myra Hindley

Throughout the history of Western culture the human image has consistently provided a vehicle for the expression and communication of social, political and religious beliefs. Although neither the cosmological associations of astrology nor the physiognomic interpretation of the human body and face are given much credence today, there is, as the historian Ludmilla Jordanova has argued, 'still an urgent search for the meaning in people; this is often assumed to lie below the surface, but with the surface holding the key to it . . . the desire to know people by scrutinizing their appearance is still there.[1]

This process is particularly evident in the field of criminality. Since the nineteenth century, images and textual or verbal narratives have been used within the regulatory disciplines of science and the law as well as in the popular media to construct anatomies for monstrous criminals. One particularly well-known example is the unidentified Victorian serial killer 'Jack the Ripper', who remains an enigmatic figure despite numerous attempts to discover his 'true' identity. The ongoing search for a face for this nineteenth-century killer reveals the extent to which monstrousness that is manifested in a person's behaviour rather than in his or her appearance provokes anxiety when it cannot be assigned an identity that visibly contains it in the place of the other.

This chapter will argue that pictures of monstrous criminals disseminated in the mass media can be made to perform a similar role to the bodies of pre-modern monsters by providing a locus for 'evil' that has occurred within society. A notable example is the police 'mug shot' photograph of Myra Hindley, the British woman convicted of child murder, taken at the time of her arrest in 1965. For a significant proportion of the British public, even those too young to remember the original case, this image has come to be a signifier of iniquity. The iconic status it has acquired suggests that even if, as Foucault has argued, monstrosity is no longer a visual phenomenon in itself, visualization still plays a key role in the effort to contain and limit what is monstrous. But visual images of modern criminal monsters cannot, in themselves, adequately signify the presence of monstrousness. Textual or verbal narratives or captions are necessary to assign particular meanings to pictures, especially since monstrousness is no longer tangibly manifested in a person's physical appearance.

Narrating Monstrous Criminality

In legal and scientific contexts as well as in the popular media, images of criminal suspects are usually constructed and disseminated using a combination of drawings or photographs and narrative accounts. In order to 'reveal' the identity of an individual criminal 'monster' and to uncover the 'true story' of the events that have occurred, pictures are assembled, together with textual or verbal accounts of his or her actions. Before an offender is caught, for example, police often seek to visualize him or her by creating a photo-fit based on verbal or written eyewitness accounts. In many cases, techniques such as criminal profiling and statistical analysis of a crime scene are also used to piece together the identity of an unknown criminal.[2] As the American writers Ronald and Stephen Holmes have explained: 'inherent within the premise of the validity and reliability of a profile is that the person who commits these crimes has a personality that reflects pathology', or in other words, that the criminal can be identified as a monster based on his or her character.[3] Once an offender has been named, methods employed in disciplines such as psychology and anthropology are drawn on to try to account for the actions that have taken place. 'Warning signs' are sought in the form of childhood behaviours such as arson or cruelty to animals.

According to the conventions of modern profiling, the social stereotype of the criminal monster is of someone who comes from a dysfunctional background involving sexual or physical abuse, drugs or alcoholism.[4] Without actually labelling him or her insane, a criminal profiler might depict the 'sickness' of a convicted person as an individual phenomenon with a particular social cause that could not affect ordinary members of society.[5] The American scholar Richard Tithecott explains this mechanism: 'it is not conviction which brings the illusion of closure, only that which we really seek: origins of the story of *his* violence, origins which we figure as belonging solely to the individual, to *a* life'.[6] The narrative process, which ascribes each crime to a particular and unique set of circumstances, is important because it provides a means of identifying the criminal monster as categorically and demonstrably different from us, 'normal' people, even if he or she is ordinary looking.

Without a narrative context for the criminal's actions there is an absence or refusal of meaning. To return to Tithecott:

> the search for the serial killer is the search for visual identification rather than explication. However, when he is caught, we cannot look at him for long. We feel the need to turn away. He is taboo. His image says everything and nothing, for it is 'normality' which stares back at us . . . It is ourselves that we see.[7]

Visible signs alone cannot account for the events that have occurred, but the narratives that replace them are not always reliable. Meanings constructed around monstrous criminal behaviour are sometimes mistaken for 'reality', which is not constructed, but represents an intrinsic 'truth', waiting to be discovered.[8] For example, the identification of Peter Sutcliffe, the 'Yorkshire Ripper', who killed at least thirteen women in the north of England between 1975 and 1981, was obstructed by the fact that police imagined him as a reincarnation of his Victorian predecessor, Jack the Ripper. It was initially thought that, like those of his predecessor, Sutcliffe's victims were all prostitutes. This meant that, even though there were clear connections with the murders of several women who were not prostitutes, police failed to connect Sutcliffe to many of these until after his arrest.[9] In this case, narratives based on what was 'known' about Sutcliffe obscured the facts.

The French philosopher and semiotician Roland Barthes has argued that 'the function of narrative is not to represent, it is to constitute a spectacle'.[10] Here Barthes aligns narrative with a theatrical or performative visual display, which, as exemplified by the freaks described in Chapter 4, has historically provided a strategy for setting monstrous difference apart from the 'norm'.[11] The idea of the spectacle is linked not only to visual phenomena, but also to affect, evoking emotions such as curiosity, contempt, marvel and admiration, all of which come into play in the production of human monsters of all sorts. Following the disappearance of 'the great spectacle of physical punishment' in the early nineteenth century and the more or less coincident transition from physical to moral monstrosity that Foucault has described, images of the body must be re-inscribed with meaning. The sensationalized narratives attaching to modern criminals in the media are certainly, in Barthes' terms, spectacular. In combination with a picture of the ordinary-looking but instantly recognizable face of a criminal monster, these spectacular narratives can help fix monstrous criminality in place, apart from the 'norm'.

Evil Monsters

Several different types of criminal monster emerged during the twentieth century. These include a number of 'dangerous outsiders' such as serial killers, drug dealers, terrorists, pornographers and child-molesters, whose actions are understood to be both a cause and an indication of instability and 'evil' in modern Western culture.[12] Any of these characters could be seen to provide an appropriate expression of the anxieties of a post-modern society where, divorced from a sense of historical continuity, social and cultural identities are commonly experienced as uncertain and abstracted.

If what is monstrous is that which defies the laws of nature and of society, 'evil' may be understood as a harmful negative effect of monstrosity. The concept of evil as an irrational and destructive force has become particularly common since 9/11. In the language of politicians it is synonymous with the threat of terrorism.[13] Commonly seen as an outsider who invades Western society from elsewhere with an extreme religious or political agenda, the stereotypical image of the terrorist is well established. The figure of Anders Breivik, a white, Western terrorist, will be examined in Chapter 7, but an extended discussion of terrorism is outside the scope of this study. Instead, this chapter focuses on an analysis of the 'ordinary-looking' figure of the serial killer, who has no fixed typology and is therefore able to live anonymously amongst 'normal' people in society.

The notion of evil as a moral concept is, even in a modern secular context, associated with religious thought and with ideas of what is 'natural' and 'good'. For example, when 'human nature' is considered originally good, evil is thought to be a result of corruption. Alternatively, when humans are believed to be barbaric by nature, their potential for evil is moderated by culture. In this case, evil is understood to result from a lack of control. According to another, dualistic, view, human nature contains aspects of both good and evil, and evil behaviour results when 'the good part of our nature does not sufficiently dominate the bad part'.[14] The notion that someone is evil generally implies that the person is thought to be aware that what he or she is doing is wrong – the 'evil' killer, for example, is considered both corrupt and out of control. But a question often posed by journalists in relation to killers such as Myra Hindley or Peter Sutcliffe, the 'Yorkshire Ripper', is whether they are 'mad or bad'. If the verdict is that the killer is 'mad', one implication is that he or she is possessed by an 'unnatural' force that is beyond his or her control. In this case the individual is characterized as sick rather than evil. He or she can be dismissed as intrinsically different, and therefore less threatening than the 'evil monster', who is seen to be in possession of a rational mind and so is, in this sense, just like anyone else.

What is a Serial Killer?

The term 'serial killer' is relatively new and quite specific.[15] It is normally used to refer to a definite set of ideas about a particular type of murder. The American sociologist Philip Jenkins claims that the concept of the serial killer is understood to relate not only to repetition of the act of killing, but also to 'a whole demographic profile of both offenders and victims'.[16] In an essay entitled 'Catch Me Before I Kill More', Jenkins provides a review of what he calls 'the new officially-inspired mythology of serial murder', which presents a very specific image of serial killers as 'men, virtually all white, who kill repeatedly for obviously sexual motives', and who prey upon defenseless victims, mostly women and children.[17] But the prevalence of this particular type of murder is open to exaggeration and sensationalism. For example, the American psychologist Joel Norris has made the provocative claim that in the late 1980s there were five hundred serial killers active in the United States at any one time, and that they took five thousand victims a year.[18] These statistics seem unlikely, especially as Norris does not support them with any evidence. His claim demonstrates that, like any other type of monster, the criminal monster is a spectacular construct that is directly related to the moral values and social needs of a particular society.

Serial killing has been described by the feminist scholars Deborah Cameron and Elizabeth Frazer as a 'specifically American phenomenon', and by Richard Tithecott as a product of

'American influenced societies'.[19] Norris portrays it as though it were a kind of disease that is spreading from America to the rest of the world.[20] But there are numerous well-known examples of British killers, including Peter Sutcliffe; Dennis Nilsen; Ian Brady and Myra Hindley; Fred and Rose West; Harold Shipman; and, more recently, Steve Wright. Nevertheless, the perceived 'Americanness' of serial murder draws attention to the link between the construction of the 'monstrous serial killer' as a criminal type, methods of policing and the principles of the mass media in any particular context. One reason we might think of North America as the country with the highest number of serial killers is because it has such a powerful media industry in which crimes such as murder are grossly sensationalized.

Mediated Monstrousness

Human monsters are, by nature, highly mediated creatures. In fact, a defining feature of the modern criminal monster is his or her status as a well-known media figure. It is significant that the mythical character of Jack the Ripper, who is commonly thought of as Britain's first serial killer, was also the first multiple killer to generate, and perhaps also to be generated by, extensive media interest. The 'Ripper' is believed to be responsible for the murder of at least five prostitutes in Whitechapel, East London, in 1888, although no one was ever caught and the identity of the perpetrator of these crimes remains a mystery. The pseudonym 'Jack the Ripper' was formulated in a letter received by a London news agency on 27 September 1888 that was supposedly from the killer himself, but which police later dismissed as a hoax. The imagined 'monstrous' character of the Ripper was – and still is – a construct based on the actions that are attributed to him.

Although a range of new regulatory practices, including modern policing and forensic photography, emerged during the nineteenth century, the most significant technical advances with respect to the Whitechapel murders were surely in the areas of printing and communication. Newly available cheap, illustrated newspapers and magazines enabled the mass circulation of textual and visual accounts of the killings. The story of the Ripper was sensationalized and commercialized, particularly in tabloids such as the *Pall Mall Gazette*, the *Star* and the *Illustrated Police News*. In these publications, the myth of the monstrous killer was disseminated through serial narrative accounts and 'artist's impressions', all created as part of an urgent attempt to assign an identity to the anonymous 'criminal monster'.

The competition between newspapers to produce the most compelling descriptions of the murders, propose the latest theories or publish details of possible suspects meant that the Ripper case was consistently and dramatically brought to the attention of the public. Even the more serious broadsheet newspapers sensationalized the story. The tone of this excerpt from an article published in the *Daily Telegraph* on 1 October 1888 is typically melodramatic:

> London this morning will talk and think of nothing else except these new proofs of the continued presence in our streets of some monster or monsters in human form, whose desperate wickedness goes free and undetected by force of its own terrible audacity, and by an as yet unrebuked contempt of our police and detective agencies. There is, in truth, reason enough for the public anger and even for the public panic, which cannot fail to arise when the details of these latest links in the frightful catena of slaughter have become known to the community. The more hapless and abandoned the victims of such ever-repeated atrocities the more pitiable is their fate, and none the less abominable the cruelty and brutality of this nocturnal slayer, whose infamies scandalize our civilization and bring law and order into contumely and paralysis. There must be, and there will be, a prodigious emotion caused throughout London by the terrible information which we furnish this morning.[21]

Impressionistic images of the supposed appearance of the Ripper were published in newspapers such as the *Illustrated Police News*, a widely circulated weekly penny tabloid that featured sensational and melodramatic reports of murders and hangings. Pictures such as the 'sketches of the supposed murderer' shown in Figure 6.1 were displayed on the cover of the paper as a means of enticing viewers to read the narratives inside. Whilst the Ripper was allocated a variety of potential identities, these visual images instated and then reinforced the idea that all the Whitechapel murders were performed by one person.[22]

In the nineteenth century a literature of criminality first came into view. In addition to the sensationalized stories that appeared in the popular press, the genre of 'true crime' emerged, along with fictional stories such as the Dupin tales written by Edgar Allan Poe in the 1840s, or the Sherlock Holmes novels written by Sir

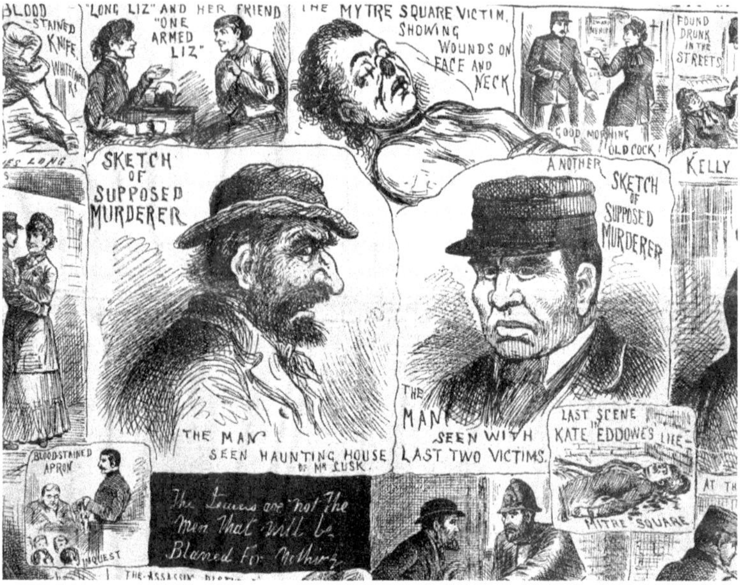
BLOOD-STAINED KNIFE
"LONG LIZ" AND HER FRIEND "ONE ARMED LIZ"
THE MYTRE SQUARE VICTIM, SHOWING WOUNDS ON FACE AND NECK
FOUND DRUNK IN THE STREETS
GOOD MORNING OLD COCK!
SKETCH OF SUPPOSED MURDERER
ANOTHER SKETCH OF SUPPOSED MURDERER
KELLY
THE MAN SEEN HAUNTING HOUSE OF MR LUSK
THE MAN SEEN WITH LAST TWO VICTIMS
LAST SCENE IN KATE EDDOWES LIFE
MITRE SQUARE
BLOODSTAINED APRON
INQUEST
The Juwes are not The Men That Will be Blamed For Nothing

6.1: Sketches of Jack the Ripper from the cover of the *Illustrated Police News*, 20 October 1888.

Arthur Conan Doyle between 1887 and 1915.[23] From the time they first appeared, these different genres have informed one another to the extent that factual information is often indistinguishable from fictional account. For example, the idea promoted by the Victorian media of Whitechapel as a place of disorder, darkness and savagery in which the 'monstrous' Ripper represents an unknown threat lurking in the streets is clearly informed by the imagery of Gothic fiction.[24] The boundaries between the known and the unknown, reality and fantasy seem to have become completely blurred in the various news reports, documentaries, books, plays and films about the Ripper published since the Whitechapel murders occurred. These interpretations have collectively compounded the problem of separating the myth of the Ripper from any known 'facts'.

A television documentary, *Jack the Ripper's Face Revealed*, first shown on Channel Five in November 2006, offers a particularly striking illustration both of the enduring sense of fear provoked by 'evil' that has no recognizable form, and of the inability on the part of the police to distinguish between myth and 'fact'. The documentary shows how police used modern techniques to analyse Victorian witness statements in order to construct a face and a profile for Jack the Ripper almost one hundred and twenty years after the murders took place.[25] In 2006 Laura Richards, head of analysis for Scotland Yard's Violent Crime Command, claimed that she had definitively visualized the nineteenth-century murderer. Richards, who has also studied the serial killer Fred West and child murderer Ian Huntley, stated, 'for the first time we are able to understand the kind of person Jack the Ripper was . . . We can name the street where he probably lived, we can see what he looked like, and we can explain, finally, why this killer eluded justice'.[26]

The fact that police dedicated extensive resources to attempting to visualize a single perpetrator for these crimes so long after the events occurred seems significant. It reveals the high level of anxiety provoked by a monstrous character who remains both invisible and unknowable. Richards employed a team of experts, including pathologists, historians and a geographical profiler to put together what has been described as 'the most accurate physical, geographical and psychological portrait of the Ripper'.[27] She claims that the photo-fit assembled by her team provides an accurate picture of the murderer who, she believes, was between the ages of twenty-five and thirty-five, between five feet, five inches and five feet, seven inches tall and of stocky build. This constructed image (Figure 6.2) depicts a man whose appearance is, like that of all other well-known serial killers, unremarkable, except perhaps for his dark skin. The swarthy and yet unrealistically symmetrical face assembled from Richards' research into Victorian eyewitness accounts reinforces assumptions made at the time of the murders. Embodying the fear and confusion provoked by increased immigration of 'foreigners' into the East End at the time of the killings, the photo-fit is not so different to the sketches of the killer shown in Figure 6.1.[28] And yet it has recently been promoted by police and in the media as a credible likeness of the Ripper.

The purpose of visually identifying a criminal monster at the time he or she is active is clear. But why, when it is still possible that the crimes attributed to the Ripper may have been committed by a number of different people, have police attempted to visualize a character that is, in the words of the writer and activist Joan Smith, 'permanently unknowable'?[29] Perhaps it is because the mythical figure of Jack the Ripper has come to personify the generalized fear of an anonymous threat, which is amplified in the imagination because it has no identifiable object. In the television documentary, Metropolitan Police Commander

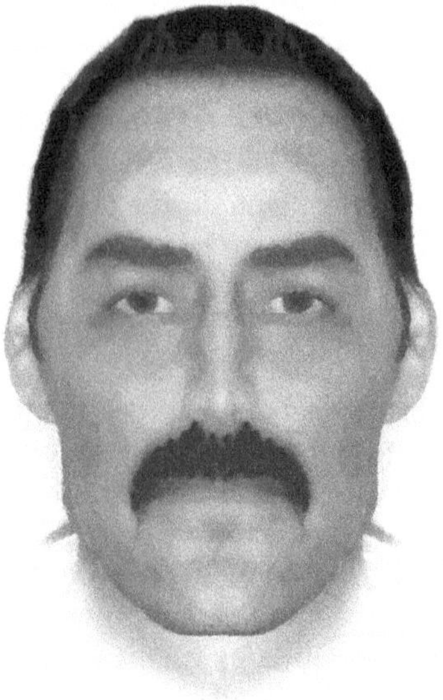

6.2: Photo-fit of Jack the Ripper, compiled for police at Scotland Yard in 2006.

John Grieve, who worked with the team that created the photo-fit, expresses certainty that the Ripper would have been caught if modern profiling techniques had been available at the time he was active. This suggests that the project represents an effort to offer reassurance that although the murders occurred here in London, they are a historical phenomenon which could not happen now.

Serial Killing and Gender

Whilst Jack the Ripper is depicted as a dark-skinned 'foreigner', the twentieth-century stereotype of the serial murderer is that of a white male. This construction has been seen by feminist writers to represent 'a crisis of white masculinity' in contemporary culture, where masculinity is expressed through violence.[30] One feminist critic, Jane Caputi, sees serial murder as sex crime that is rooted in a system of male supremacy. For her, 'the murders of women and children by serial killers are . . . the ultimate expression of a sexuality that defines sex as a form of domination/power: it, like rape, is a form of terror that constructs and maintains male supremacy'.[31] The associated assumption that those who murder repeatedly are motivated by a specifically male form of lust has been used to justify the idea that no woman could ever be a true serial killer.[32] But Philip Jenkins, who identifies a gap between the myths that surround serial killing and the 'scientific' reality of statistics, disputes this idea. He claims that 'at least a quarter of serial killers are women'.[33]

The American scholar David Schmid highlights the power of the gender stereotype in his book *Natural Born Celebrities: Serial Killers in American Culture*. Here he argues that women and violence are traditionally assumed to be mutually exclusive, so that 'when women do act violently they are often rhetorically excluded from womanhood'.[34] Schmid cites the example of Aileen Wuornos, who, convicted in the USA in 1990, was labelled the first female serial killer. Although many women had previously been convicted of multiple killings, Wuornos was believed to be the first woman to kill 'like a man' because she killed strangers rather than people known to her and because she killed outside the home without a clear motive. As a gay woman who is supposed to have acted like a man, Wuornos does not disrupt the stereotype of the male killer because she is not perceived as a 'real' or 'normal' woman.

Myra Hindley and the Role of the Visual Image

In 1966, at the age of twenty-three, Myra Hindley was found guilty of the murders of two children and of being an accessory to a third. Contrary to the stereotype, she has become known as one of the most notorious modern British serial killers. And yet the murders Hindley was convicted of could not easily be attributed to her – there was no obvious causal narrative and, more importantly, she was a woman. At the time of her arrest she was described in the media as a 'normal' young woman who acted under the influence of her boyfriend, the 'evil' Ian Brady. The tabloids reported that Hindley had become 'a changed girl' when she met Brady.[35] The perceived corruption of her feminine status is emphasized in a 1965 press report, in which her sister claimed that before she met Brady, Hindley went to church and liked children, but after she knew him 'she didn't believe in marriage, she said that she hated babies and children'.[36] A remark made by the sentencing judge, Fenton Atkinson, on 8 May 1966, two days after the culmination of the trial in which Hindley and Brady were both sentenced to life in prison, further reinforces the stereotype of the male killer. He said: 'though I believe Brady is wicked beyond belief without hope of redemption, I cannot feel that the same is necessarily true of Hindley once she is removed from his influence'.[37] But the idea that Hindley was a vulnerable and susceptible young woman who had been duped by Brady was not to last. In 1985 Brady was diagnosed as criminally insane and sectioned under the Mental Health Act. He has since remained at Ashworth High Security Hospital, where he has been on hunger strike since 1999, campaigning for the right to die.[38] As the journalist David Jones has recently commented, for Brady 'the ultimate penalty is not death, it is life'.[39] Whilst his case is still emotively reported in the media from time to time, the diagnosis of insanity diverted public interest away from Brady. With the knowledge that he had been identified as a psychopath and would be incarcerated until death, the public's need to find an explanation for what he did was perhaps no longer so urgent. By contrast, Hindley became a national hate figure. As a 'sane' woman who participated in the sexual assault and murder of young people instead of fulfilling her maternal role, she was portrayed as a doubly transgressive character.[40]

Even though Hindley herself was concealed from public view within the prison system, she remained in the public consciousness. An iconic photograph (Figures 6.3 and 6.4), taken just a few days after the murder of Hindley and Brady's last victim, seventeen-year-old Edward Evans, came to represent 'the face of evil'.[41] Taken by a police photographer at the time of her arrest in 1965, this photograph was clearly intended for the practical purpose of identification, and yet it quickly took on a much greater significance. In the words of the writer Helen Birch, this is an image that 'strikes at the heart of our fears about unruly women, about criminality and about the way gender is constructed'.[42] With her blank, sullen expression and bleached blonde hair, the powerful but ultimately normal-looking face of Hindley seems to have offered a particularly timely means of symbolizing the dissolution of traditional gender roles that cast women as domestic, nurturing, morally responsible and above all, natural figures. As Birch, writing in 1994, put it: 'in recent years, in tandem with the growth of second-wave feminism and its principles of self-determination for women, the argument [that Hindley was simply the victim of her lover, Brady's sick, male mind] has all but died'.[43]

In Chapters 4 and 5 we saw how, in the nineteenth century, photography was believed to offer an objective tool for medical and anatomical illustration and for the identification of criminals. Yet it was also used to reinfoce physiognomic ideas. These processes are surely still at play in more recent interpretations of criminal mug shots, like that of Hindley. Whilst her face is, in fact, unremarkable, showing none of the deformities of pre-modern monsters, the narratives that accrued around this image have invested Hindley's features with the signs of evil. For example, whilst Hindley herself reportedly claimed that the brooding expression caught in this image (Figures 6.3 and 6.4) was due to fear and lack of sleep, it has been construed by the media as a mark of defiance and wickedness.[44] The processes by which particular meanings have attached to this image are complex. Firstly, it is a police identification photograph, a type of image that has been seen as indexically linked to 'the truth' since Alphonse Bertillon systematized the process in the late nineteenth century.[45] Another important, and contradictory, factor is the style of the image itself. This striking, well-composed black-and-white photograph could almost be a studio portrait. There is something glamorous about Hindley's seemingly provocative gaze, bleached and backcombed hair and fashionable clothing which, combined with the narratives of deviance that surround her, renders that particular picture simultaneously intriguing and monstrous.

The police photograph is reproduced in the media in a number of different forms. Some close-cropped versions show only Hindley's face, whilst others show the full frame of the original negative, which includes part of her clothing. In this more commonly used high-contrast version (Figure 6.3) the subtlety of Hindley's expression is lost. The hard shadows seem to render her face invulnerable and determined. Another version of the same photograph (Figure 6.4), reproduced on the *Daily Telegraph* website, tells a slightly different story.[46] Here the image is softer. Closer in tone to the original negative, it seems to depict a gentler, more vulnerable character, with a look of fearful apprehension on her face. In this particular case the photograph is asymmetrically cropped, which adds to the sense of vulnerability. This presentation could be deliberate as the image accompanies an article entitled 'The Letter that Made Myra Hindley Cry', which is about Hindley's emotional response to a letter from the mother of one of her victims.

Despite these variations in presentation, the image of Hindley has become fixed in the public imagination through the act of repetition and reproduction, both visually and metaphorically.

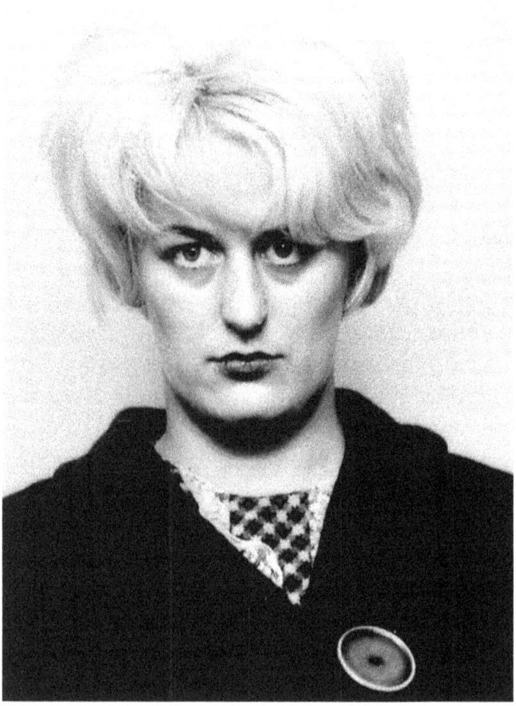

6.3: Widely distributed version of the police mug shot of Myra Hindley, taken at the time of her arrest in 1965.

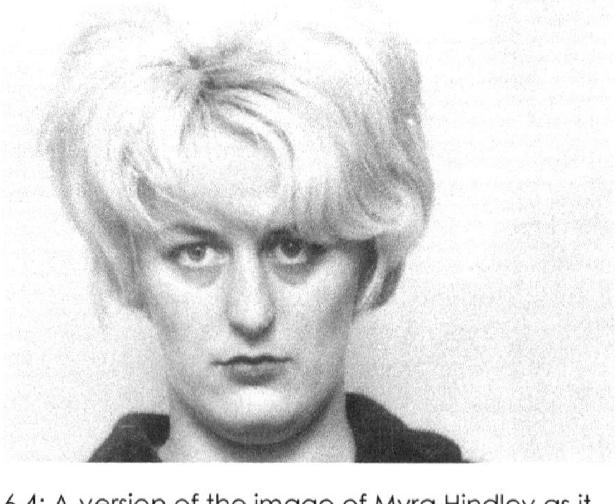

6.4: A version of the image of Myra Hindley as it appears on the *Daily Telegraph* website.

Replication has rendered the picture increasingly solid, diminishing any signs of more 'human' or 'female' qualities that might have been conveyed by the original. The popular reading of this image of Hindley as a visible articulation of evil has also become fixed through persistent repetition. There are obvious discrepancies between this iconic police photograph and less memorable, private images of Hindley as an ordinary middle-aged woman taken at Cookham Wood Prison in the 1990s (Figure 6.5). The later, more human, pictures appear to belong to another unrelated person and are largely ignored. Even though there is nothing particularly abnormal in Hindley's appearance, in repeatedly seeking to publish a picture that everyone recognizes, news editors have, in fact, created a monster. Whether she was responsible for the murders or not, the image of Myra 'the monster' that is fixed in the public imagination is a mythical one generated by repeated publication of the police photograph and the narratives that surround it.

The idea of Hindley as monstrous child-murderer that this image helped to establish was sporadically reinforced by the outrage that surrounded reports that she might be released from prison in the mid-1980s, in the 1990s and again just before

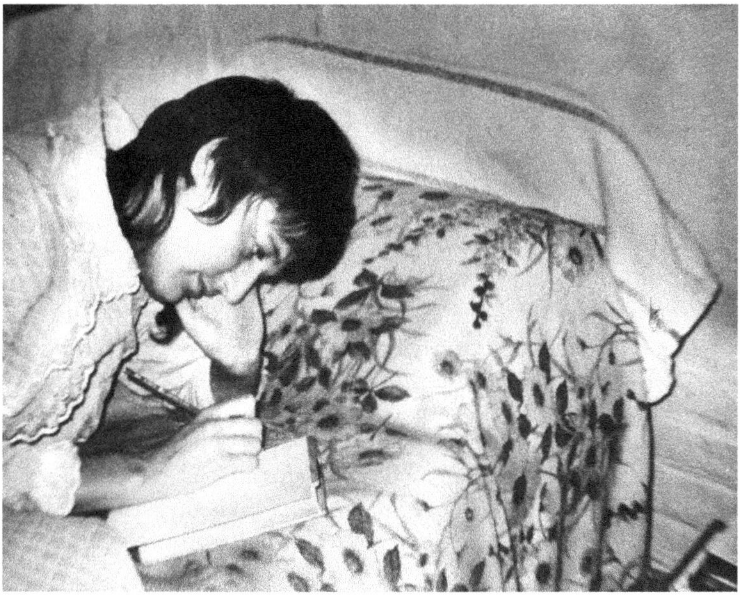

6.5: Hindley in prison, c.1993.

her death in 2002.[47] The emotive reactions of the public, which were strongly encouraged by the tabloid press, were unaffected by reports that Hindley had become a reformed character who was no longer a threat to public safety. It seems that, for those who could not countenance her release into society, it was the static image of Hindley as a young woman that was publicly condemned to a life in prison, rather than the living subject herself.[48]

The unforgettable power of the police mug shot of Hindley is further evidenced by media-generated condemnation of an enormous painting by the artist Marcus Harvey, which was shown as part of the *Sensation* exhibition at the Royal Academy of Art in 1997 (Figure 6.6). The 11ft x 9ft painting, composed of thousands of children's handprints, which collectively reproduce the image of Hindley, provoked intensely emotional reactions. Whilst it was on show at the Academy, the painting was vandalized with ink and then with eggs, before being protected behind perspex and with two armed guards. Four academicians resigned in protest at a decision not to withdraw it from the exhibition.[49] For some, the painting itself clearly became an incarnation of evil, which was all the more provocative because it was deliberately done. The attacks on the picture, therefore, represented a perpetuation of the fantasy of attacking the 'real' Myra.[50] The painted portrait stands in for the photograph, which in turn stands in for the body of Myra, 'the monster'.

The heightened emotional reactions to the *Myra* painting demonstrate the enduring role of this image as an 'icon of evil'.[51] More recently the painting caused another furor when it briefly appeared in video footage of an official party celebrating London's status as host city for the 2012 Olympics. According to a BBC news report broadcast on 25 August 2008, the mayor of London was 'deeply disturbed' by the use of the image, whilst the Conservative MP Ann Widdecombe is reported to have said, 'I do find it utterly extraordinary that if we're trying to promote Britain, we should do so with an image of a mass child murderer.'[52] Widdecombe's comment perpetuates the exaggerated myth of Hindley the monster and in doing so seems to make the actual crime seem less 'real'. Harvey has claimed that he 'always regarded the painting as a sombre critique of the media's exploitation of the Hindley story in general and that image in particular'.[53] But, by bringing it back into the public consciousness, the painter seems to have reignited the moral

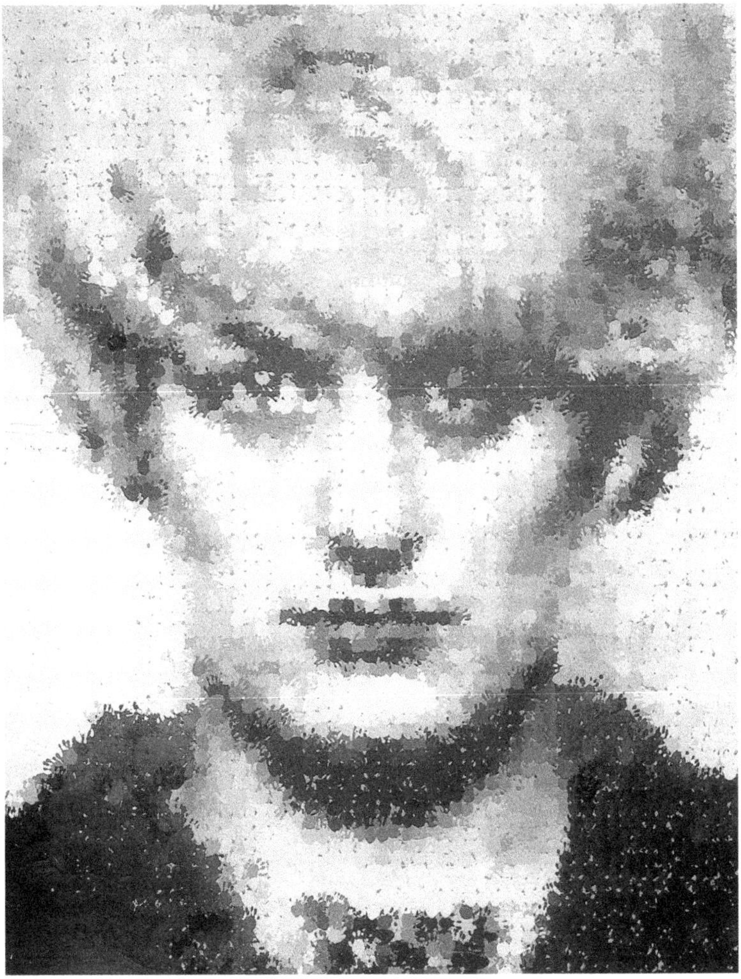

6.6: Marcus Harvey, *Myra*, 1995.

indignation that surrounded the original photograph. In doing so he has reinforced the function of the Hindley image as an incarnation of modern monstrosity.

Tithecott has suggested that 'in an age when the value of images perhaps exceeds the value of words, the search for the serial killer is the search for visual identification rather than explication'.[54] But images and language must work together. In itself, a picture of a normal-looking criminal monster is meaningless unless it has already been associated with an emotive narrative.

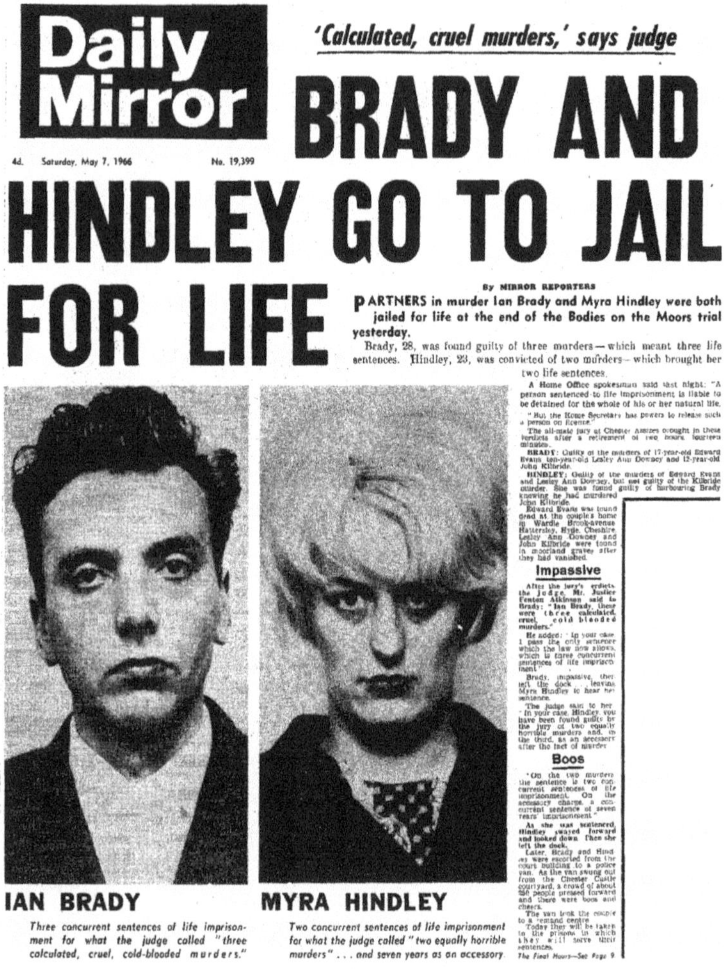

Daily Mirror

4d. Saturday, May 7, 1966 No. 19,399

'Calculated, cruel murders,' says judge

BRADY AND HINDLEY GO TO JAIL FOR LIFE

By MIRROR REPORTERS

PARTNERS in murder Ian Brady and Myra Hindley were both jailed for life at the end of the Bodies on the Moors trial yesterday.

Brady, 28, was found guilty of three murders—which meant three life sentences. Hindley, 23, was convicted of two murders—which brought her two life sentences.

A Home Office spokesman said last night: "A person sentenced to life imprisonment is liable to be detained for the whole of his or her natural life.

"But the Home Secretary has powers to release such a person on licence."

The all-male jury at Chester Assizes brought in these verdicts after a retirement of two hours fourteen minutes.

BRADY: Guilty of the murders of 17-year-old Edward Evans, ten-year-old Lesley Ann Downey and 12-year-old John Kilbride.

HINDLEY: Guilty of the murders of Edward Evans and Lesley Ann Downey, but not guilty of the Kilbride murder. She was found guilty of harbouring Brady knowing he had murdered John Kilbride.

Edward Evans was found dead at the couple's home in Wardle Brook-avenue, Hattersley, Hyde, Cheshire. Lesley Ann Downey and John Kilbride were found in moorland graves after they had vanished.

Impassive

After the jury's verdicts the judge, Mr. Justice Fenton Atkinson, said to Brady: "Ian Brady, these were three calculated, cruel, cold blooded murders."

He added: "In your case I pass the only sentence which the law now allows, which is three concurrent sentences of life imprisonment."

Brady, impassive, then left the dock . . . leaving Myra Hindley to hear her sentence.

The judge said to her: "In your case, Hindley, you have been found guilty by the jury of two equally horrible murders and, in the third, as an accessory after the fact of murder.

Boos

"On the two murders the sentence is two concurrent sentences of life imprisonment. On the accessory charge, a concurrent sentence of seven years' imprisonment."

As she was sentenced, Hindley swayed forward and looked down. Then she left the dock.

Later, Brady and Hindley were escorted from the court building to a police van. As the van swung out from the Chester Castle courtyard, a crowd of about [illegible] people pressed forward and there were boos and cheers.

The van took the couple to a remand centre.

Today they will be taken to the prisons in which they will serve their sentences.

The Final Hours—See Page 9

IAN BRADY

Three concurrent sentences of life imprisonment for what the judge called "three calculated, cruel, cold-blooded murders."

MYRA HINDLEY

Two concurrent sentences of life imprisonment for what the judge called "two equally horrible murders" . . . and seven years as an accessory.

6.7: Police mug shots of Hindley and Brady on the front page of the *Daily Mirror*, 7 May 1966.

In his analysis of the function of press photographs, Roland Barthes describes the communication between image and text, which work together to form a 'totality of information'.[55] He assigns text the role of sublimating, patheticizing or rationalizing the image.[56] By this he means that an image no longer illustrates a text; instead, the text 'loads the image, burdening it with a culture, a moral, an imagination'.[57] Barthes explains how, in relation to a press photograph, the caption seems to become part of what is

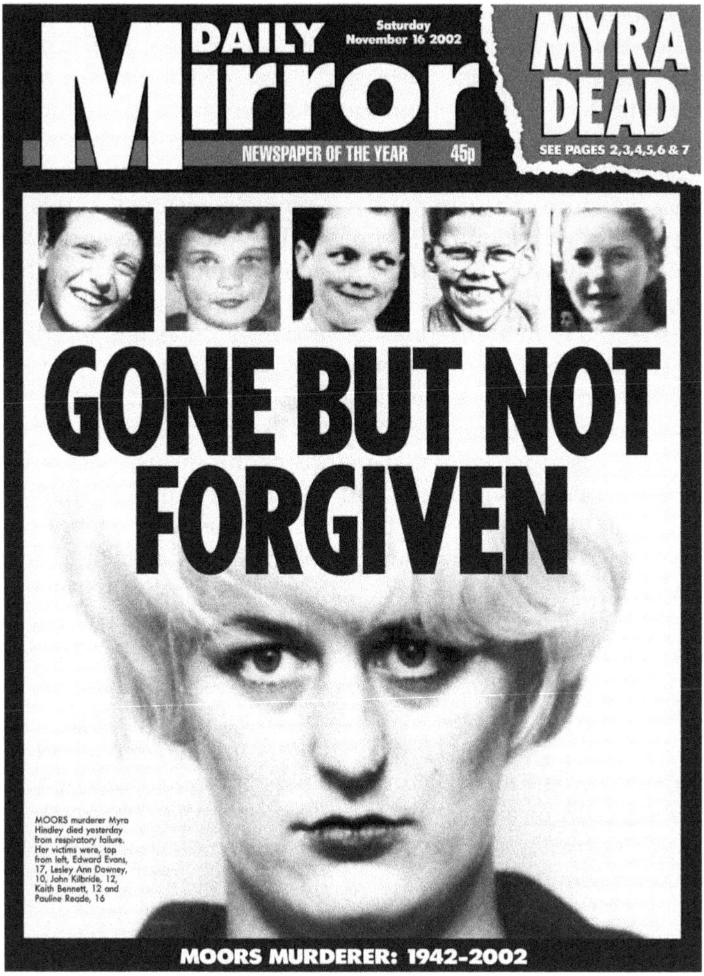
DAILY Mirror
Saturday November 16 2002
NEWSPAPER OF THE YEAR 45p

MYRA DEAD
SEE PAGES 2,3,4,5,6 & 7

GONE BUT NOT FORGIVEN

MOORS murderer Myra Hindley died yesterday from respiratory failure. Her victims were, top from left, Edward Evans, 17, Lesley Ann Downey, 10, John Kilbride, 12, Keith Bennett, 12 and Pauline Reade, 16

MOORS MURDERER: 1942-2002

6.8: The photograph of Hindley on the front page of the *Daily Mirror*, 16 November 2002.

denoted by the image, to the extent that it appears transparent. The iconic police photograph of Hindley offers an example of this process. In tabloid news reports, for example, the lack of signifying features in Hindley's seemingly normal appearance is countered by association with emotive labels such as 'terrorized', 'horrific crimes', 'grotesque', 'brutal' and 'cruel' (Figure 6.7). These captions, which have repeatedly been associated with that single picture of Hindley for almost fifty years, have become inscribed into it to the extent that their meaning remains, even when the words themselves are no longer present (Figure 6.8). The meanings of that particular image of Hindley's face now seem to derive directly and automatically from the photograph in such a way that the published image of the face replaces the face itself as visible evidence of monstrousness. It seems that, once a picture of a criminal has become 'monstered' in this way, repeated publication of the image gives the impression that the monstrousness it represents is identifiable, even though the appearance of the person depicted is unremarkable.[58]

The role of modern 'monster' images such as the photograph of Hindley is in many ways consistent with the role played by medieval drawings of the Monstrous Races or sixteenth-century prints of the Monster of Ravenna in their historical contexts. In each case, the mediated nature of the picture seems to be largely unacknowledged. And yet the process of mediation is crucial to the meanings conveyed by the body or face of the 'monster'. Photographic images of criminals published in the media contribute to the perpetuation of the myths that surround modern criminal monsters. They provide a publicly recognizable identity for some of the challenging monstrous or 'evil' forces that are present within society, assigning to them a 'face of evil' which 'normal' people can feel good about condemning.

The ubiquity of the Hindley photograph demonstrates how a publicly recognizable picture of a person can still function as an embodiment of what is monstrous, even if the person depicted looks 'normal'. But can the 'monstrosity of character' of the modern criminal always be held in place by a static visual image?

7 | Modern Monsters and the Image of Normality

Ted Bundy and Anders Breivik

At the beginning of *Discipline and Punish* Michel Foucault describes the public spectacle of the brutal execution of a French criminal, Robert Damiens, who was convicted of regicide at the beginning of the eighteenth century.[1] The body of this criminal character, who was publicly tortured before being drawn, quartered and burnt to ashes, was staged as both a highly visible warning, and an assurance that social order would be maintained by the state. Like the body of this criminal, the monsters discussed so far in this book have all existed as prominent visual spectacles. The various contraventions of social 'norms' represented by the Monstrous Races, the Monster of Ravenna, nineteenth-century freaks and even the photographic image of Myra Hindley are all manifested in the appearance of the 'monster' in question. In its own context, each of them has acted as a public warning of the presence of social, moral or ontological disorder or confusion, either within society or in the wider world.

In Foucault's account, the offender's body was seen to bear responsibility for social and moral evil on one hand, and to provide a site for the visible endorsement of legal standards on the other. In order to reassert the power of the monarchy and thus to re-establish social order, the body of this eighteenth-century criminal was materially and symbolically torn apart and reduced to nothing in full public view. Even though torture and public execution have long been abolished as an accepted form of punishment, the symbolic figures of more modern criminal 'monsters' such as Myra Hindley occupy a similar place to the publicly disgraced body of the eighteenth-century criminal. In Chapter 6 we saw how members of the public symbolically enacted a form of physical punishment as they attempted to destroy or deface the picture of Hindley. Even after her death, the iconic police photograph of her remains synonymous with the idea of evil. But what happens when the monstrousness behind the modern monstrosity of character that Foucault describes resists representation of any kind?[2] Taking the American serial killer Ted Bundy as its main example, this chapter explores some of the contradictions that arise when the perpetrator of monstrous criminal acts cannot be recognized as a monster. The chapter ends with a discussion of the Norwegian mass murderer Anders Behring Breivik, whose monstrous behaviour has given tangible form to a particular set of social and cultural dilemmas. The debate surrounding Breivik's actions suggests that he might emerge as one of the most significant human monsters of the early twenty-first century.

Monstrous Psychology

In 'The Dangerous Individual', a lecture given in 1978, Foucault refers back to a historical change in the notion of what constitutes criminality that he documented in *Discipline and Punish*. He outlines a shift of attention that took place in the nineteenth century from the crime to the criminal – from the criminal act to the character of the individual.[3] As a result of this change, writes Foucault, direct, corporeal punishment was replaced with a technical knowledge system that was 'capable of characterizing a criminal individual in himself and in a sense beneath his acts'.[4] Only within this knowledge system could the 'criminality' of an individual, his dangerousness, his potential or future behaviour and the threat he posed to society be rationalized and therefore diffused. The nineteenth-century system of knowledge that Foucault is referring to here incorporates the disciplines of criminology, psychology, criminal anthropology and, most importantly, psychiatry. All these areas of expertise were used to account for the behaviour of a particular individual by attempting to explain the causes of his or her monstrously incomprehensible actions within a psychological and social context. The symbolic performances of hanging and torture that publicly enacted retribution on the criminal body were replaced by institutionalization of the offender. Foucault describes this process as the 'psychiatrization of criminal danger'.[5] He explains that early nineteenth-century criminal psychiatry 'first proclaimed itself a pathology of the monstrous', and that it aimed to show that 'monstrous' crime or crime without apparent reason was a disease of the mind.[6]

Nineteenth-century psychiatry was initially promoted as a medical science that could respond to 'dangers inherent in the social body' by recognizing the signs of criminal insanity.[7] It was used to justify a modern criminal justice system that aimed in particular to control the threat of aberrant or deviant human behaviour. Physicians such as Philippe Pinel and Henry Maudsley sought to prove that more serious 'crimes without reason' such as motiveless murder occurred as a result of 'insanity'. They believed this to be an innate condition, the signs of which could only be 'read' by experts like physicians or physiognomists. If, as Canguilhem proposed, nineteenth-century science offered sufficient explanation for physical anomaly to break down the correspondence between monstrosity and the monstrous, perhaps the new discipline of psychiatry represents an effort to extend this process to the internal monstrosity of the criminal character.[8] More recently, emphasis has been placed on explaining a person's monstrous actions according to certain psychological 'abnormalities' that predispose him or her to criminal behaviour. Although – or perhaps because – the mind remains a largely uncharted territory, the causes of monstrous criminal behaviour are largely sought within an individual's psyche, rather than in society as a whole.

At the beginning of 'The Dangerous Individual' Foucault tells the story of a man who, when accused of multiple rapes, refused to answer any of the questions put to him in court. Notably, he failed to respond to the question, 'Who are you?'[9] Foucault uses this example to illustrate the change of emphasis that occurred in the eighteenth and nineteenth centuries from the nature of the crime to the character of the criminal. He goes on to quote a French lawyer who, in defending a child murderer, asked: 'Can one condemn to death a person one does not know?'[10] With this story Foucault is attempting to show how, in the modern context, it is the silence of the criminal monster, or the refusal of the individual to reveal his or her identity that is most threatening. For Foucault, this refusal of identity is of consequence primarily because it renders the law impotent. But it is also interesting because it prevents a categorical distinction being made between the monstrous 'other' and those 'normal' individuals living within society.

The serial sex murderer Dennis Nilsen is a typical example of a quiet, nondescript criminal monster. Whilst maintaining a career as a civil servant at a job centre in North London, Nilsen murdered and dismembered sixteen men at two different suburban flats between 1978 and 1983. Apart from a certain remoteness, he appeared unremarkable and the murders he committed remained undetected until blocked drains at the house where he lived were investigated, revealing a number of human body parts. Concealed behind a veneer of ordinariness, Nilsen's monstrousness is very much of its time. In his book *Killing for Company*, Brian Masters has suggested that Nilsen murdered out of loneliness, combined with feelings of impotence following the break-up of a long-term relationship and a frustration with his own 'ordinariness'.[11] Such experiences of alienation could be considered 'normal' symptoms of twentieth-century urban or suburban life, and yet in Nilsen's case they led to extraordinary, monstrous acts, which seem more chilling because the perpetrator looks so average. If, as Richard Tithecott has written, 'the construction of society's monsters reflects upon the fears and anxieties of a particular historical period', the late twentieth-century figure of the serial killer represents a monstrous eruption within the 'abstract, faceless, colourless, genderless, sexless "middle"', as Tithecott puts it.[12] Although Nilsen is a homosexual and the murders he committed had a sexual element, his anonymous, bland public persona revealed nothing of his inner life.

Ted Bundy

The twentieth-century American serial murderer Ted Bundy is perhaps the most fascinating and extreme example of this seemingly ordinary, indecipherable type of criminal character. Labelled a 'minus man' and 'a type of non person', he typifies Foucault's 'criminal character' who refuses to answer the question, 'Who are you?'[13] Bundy, who eventually confessed to having murdered at least thirty young women across America between 1974 and 1979, is said to have attributed his own success in killing to what he called 'the anonymity factor'.[14] He was first arrested in 1977, but twice escaped from prison, committing more murders whilst on the run. He was finally convicted in 1979 and, after ten years on death row, was executed by electrocution in Florida on 24 January 1989.

Bundy was a young, successful, ambitious, handsome, white, straight, Republican, middle-class American. He described himself as: 'an average-looking person with a family, a job and a home just like yourself'.[15] But, at the same time, we know that he brutally murdered many young women.[16] The figure of Bundy is both horrifying and compelling precisely because his appearance and his day-to-day performance of normality are so completely at odds with the accounts of his monstrous behaviour. Whilst on one hand he has been described as 'terrifyingly normal', Bundy was also diagnosed as a psychopath. This is a clinical construct for a person who exhibits behaviour that remains morally incomprehensible to 'normal' people and which cannot be explained by any of the modern sciences. It is described as a personality or character disorder that leads to a lack of conscience. As an 'inhuman' psychological state that cannot be accounted for, the modern idea of psychopathy seems to have emerged out of the nineteenth-century category of the 'morally insane'.[17] But psychopathy is not synonymous with serial killing. People described as psychopaths are not all physically violent, and those who can keep up a consistent outward appearance of being 'normal' are able to pursue successful careers within mainstream society.[18] Whilst they are not necessarily murderers, people described as psychopaths are commonly referred to as 'social predators' who violate the rules of society for self-gratification. In the context of this study, psychopathy constitutes a form of monstrosity because, in the words of the feminist scholar Judith Halberstam, it 'makes evil into a local effect, not generalizable across a society or culture'.[19] Like 'monster', 'psychopath' is a label that sets certain unacceptable human traits, primarily the lack of empathy and conscience, apart from the 'norm'. In doing so it absolves society of any responsibility for the monstrous events that have occurred.

Even though they knew about his crimes, it seems that many who met Bundy were convinced by, and even attracted to, his façade of humanness. During his incarceration, for example, he received hundreds of fan letters from female admirers. When Ralph Munro, the former secretary of state for Washington, was questioned about his reaction to Bundy's arrest, he stated, 'we were shocked, we couldn't believe it, we tried to raise money for a defence fund for him and tried to protect him . . . they had to have the wrong guy'.[20] It seems that Bundy was able to appeal to almost everyone he met by displaying a credible appearance of normality that profoundly contradicted what was known about his activities. Most bizarrely, the judge who sentenced him said:

> It's a tragedy for this court to see such a total waste of humanity as I've experienced in this courtroom. You're a bright young man. You'd have made a good lawyer, and I'd have loved to have you practice in front of me, but you went the wrong way, partner. Take care of yourself. I don't have any animosity to you. I want you to know that.[21]

Was Judge Cowan's curious endorsement of Bundy perhaps motivated by a problem with condemning someone who appeared to embody many of the qualities that he personally upheld as 'good'? Even in the media Bundy was often described in positive terms. In the British press, for example, references are made to his 'film-star looks', his 'army of female admirers' and his 'charisma'. He is described as 'debonair', 'smooth talking' and 'a handsome, intelligent, sociopathic murderer'.[22] In only a few cases is his image associated with words such as 'evil', 'monster' or 'devil'.[23] However, when negative associations are made, these are usually very forceful. During his trial, for example, Bundy was characterized by investigators as 'the devil himself'.

Bundy's persuasive charisma is most powerfully demonstrated in video documentation of an interview that took place in Florida State Prison the day before he was executed.[24] Dr James Dobson, the right-wing Christian evangelist psychologist who interviewed him, has subsequently said he believed that Bundy was remorseful. When asked whether he felt the interview

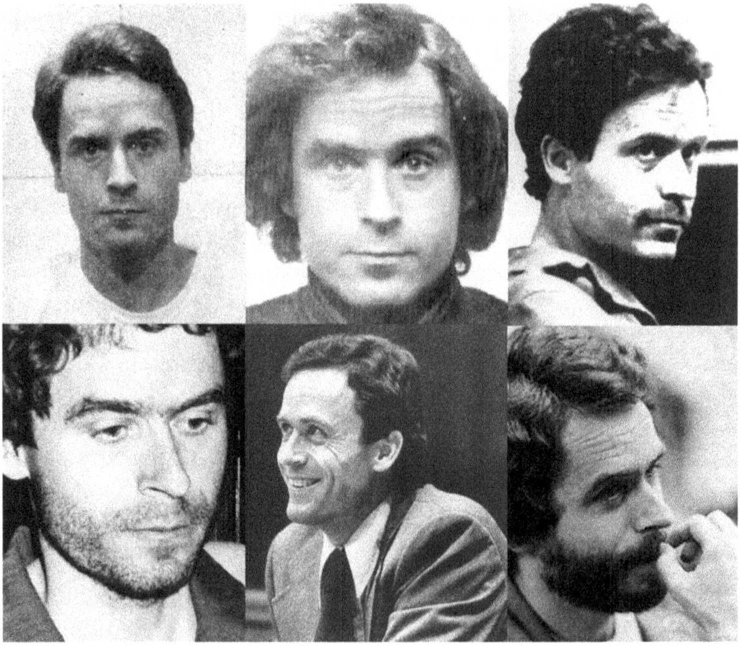

7.1: Some of Ted Bundy's various guises.

represented 'the last honest statements of a condemned man', Dobson replied, 'the answer to that will come from watching the video [of the interview] – listen to the man's voice, look into his eyes, and draw your own conclusions'. This statement is interesting for two reasons. Firstly, because in placing the viewer in the active role of juror, Dobson invites us to reflect on the processes that come into play as we evaluate Bundy's performance. It also seems to imply that Dobson believed the video footage acted as evidence of Bundy's humanity. If this is the case, it functions in the opposite way to the photograph of Hindley, which is commonly promoted as evidence of her inhumanity. How is it that a picture of a frightened-looking young woman can become an icon of evil, whilst the image of a clean-cut all-American boy remains intact, despite the narratives of deviance that attach to it?

Even 'Jack the Ripper', who was never identified, was assigned an appearance that clearly indicates the evil nature of the actions that were attributed to him. Whilst the narratives that surround Hindley are contradictory, her image continues to act as an embodiment of transgression, even after her death. But Bundy, who 'never looked the same from photograph to photograph' (Figure 7.1) remains an enigma.[25] Although there are a large number of still and moving pictures of him in the public domain, his image refuses to take on negative values. This is perhaps partly because there is no one definitive image of him, but also because the various available pictures only seem to endorse his apparent normality – it is impossible to see beyond the mask of the all-American boy. In this sense Bundy is different to the other examples described in this book. His appearance, in all its guises, seems to signify what is 'good' and even 'desirable' in a modern man to such an extent that, when narratives of evil are associated with him, they are not always taken seriously.

The final interview with Dobson was set up at Bundy's request, because he wanted to make a public statement – one in which he claims that pornography and alcohol were 'central to the violent behaviour that I engaged in'. Bundy ingeniously lays the blame for his deviance on the media – the very mechanism by which public opinion is forged:

> those of us who are . . . so much influenced by violence in the media, in particular pornographic violence, are not some kind of inherent monsters. We are your sons, and we are your husbands and we grew up in regular families.[26]

Here he insists that he is not a psychopath, but is as he is because of the kind of society he grew up in. Elsewhere in the interview Bundy talks about being possessed, about having to follow through his violent urges before 'I became myself again'. He claims that 'basically I was a normal person', and he frequently repeats, 'I want you to understand this'. He refers to his own unremarkable appearance: 'I wasn't a pervert in the sense that people look at someone and say I know there is something wrong with him'. Bundy's façade of excessive normality is paradoxical. On the one hand it seems like an empty mask, concealing an inhuman and unreachable character absorbed with his own internal psychotic fantasies. On the other hand it signifies 'nothing but the social determination of the individual within, something like the mass in person', as Mark Selzer has put it.[27] In other words, Bundy is a product of a particular society, and is, therefore, acting as a representative of that society. In the interview he seems to be speaking on behalf of society when he calmly condemns his own behaviour. In the televised court case he plays two parts – he is the accused, but strangely, as an ex-law student, he is also able to act as his own defence attorney, and thus as a representative of the law. In video documentation of one court appearance, Bundy, wearing a suit and tie, is walking freely around the courtroom, carrying a box of papers and conversing with officials as thought he is just another colleague.[28] This does not appear to be the figure of a monstrous criminal.

The dislocation between Bundy's image and what is known about him is intensified by the nature of his confessions, all of which were made in the third person, as though he were an intimate witness to crimes perpetrated by someone else. Bundy describes one murder in this way:

> As he came up behind her, she heard him, she turned around, he brandished a knife and grabbed her by the arm and told her to do what he wanted her to do. And she began to argue with him so he placed his hands around her throat just to throttle her into unconsciousness so that she wouldn't scream any more . . . and then he removed her clothes and raped her. He put his own clothes back on and at about that time he began to notice that the girl wasn't moving.[29]

When asked by Dobson what the emotional effect of his first murder was, Bundy's face and voice appear entirely expressionless. He seems to be a bad actor mechanically repeating a learnt script as he replies:

> I can only liken it to coming out of some kind of horrible trance or dream. I don't want to over dramatize it, but to have been possessed by something so awful and so alien and then the next morning wake up from it, remember what happened, and realize that basically in the eyes of the law, in the eyes of God you are responsible.

Throughout the interview Bundy repeatedly implies that he does not hold himself responsible, and perhaps does not even consider himself to have been present when the murders took place. What is interesting is not so much what he says as he repeatedly asserts his lack of responsibility, but the complex web of contradictions that arise between his words, what his body language refuses to reveal and what we as individual observers bring to our interpretation of him. Watching him on video, it is possible to see how confusing a 'real-life' encounter with Bundy might have been.

Although for most of the interview he appears emotionless, Bundy does manifest a very human sense of fear when he talks about his own impending death. Witnessing his apparently genuine reaction, it is difficult not to empathize with him. This spontaneous, visceral identification with the monstrous killer is disturbing. It suggests that he is closer to us than we might like to think, even though the video, which should give some insight into the character of Bundy and offer some motive for his actions, reveals nothing. The emptiness behind his performance of normality is perhaps what renders him simultaneously so compelling and so monstrous. There is a feeling that we cannot quite reach Bundy, but there is nothing in his appearance, his gestures or his body language that hints at the violence he was capable of. No one was able to detect the signs of monstrousness within his psyche.

Television footage of Bundy's trial was repeatedly aired over the ten-year period between his conviction and his execution. During this time he became a media celebrity in the USA. In fact, according to the American sociologist Philip Jenkins, 'Bundy was already a figure of national notoriety when he carried out his final series of murders in Florida in early 1978.'[30] How could someone who had violently murdered a large number of young women achieve this status? Whilst there is no simple answer to this question, there do seem to be many contributing factors.

As Rosemary Jackson has commented in her book, *Fantasy: The Literature of Subversion*, 'in a culture which equates the "real" with the "visible" and gives the eye dominance over other sense organs, the un-real is that which is in-visible'.[31] Bundy's many crimes left no visible mark on him. For those with no direct experience of the consequences, the reports of his actions, therefore, can easily seem unbelievable. More significantly, as Richard Tithecott has remarked, 'The serial killer character is a very powerful figure, almost like a mythical figure – half real, half fictional, omnipotent, omniscient and omnipresent . . . For parts of our culture, the power that the character represents can be exciting and compelling.'[32]

For most people, the experience of criminal monsters such as Bundy is a mediated one. Bundy was clearly a showman who liked being in the spotlight. He enjoyed performing, and he courted media attention. In the video documentation of his court appearances he often looks towards the camera with a clear and confident gaze. The final interview, recorded on video, seems to represent a calculated ploy to maintain his presence in the public eye long after his death. All in all, Bundy appears to have been very conscious of his public image, which he carefully controlled. But there is also a sense of unreality to his story. Today's pervasive 'literature of criminality' has fostered a reciprocal relationship between invented accounts based around 'real-life' stories, and the activities of actual killers who, according to Mark Seltzer, may even model themselves on fictional villains.[33] Over time, serial killers can also be influenced by media reports of their own crimes, which may seem to turn them into celebrities.[34]

Seen in the context of a ubiquitous popular culture in which murder mysteries and police dramas provide highly popular forms of entertainment, Bundy's story could be confused with fictional narratives like the hugely popular American drama series *Dexter*.[35] The long-running TV series, which achieved cult status, was based on the novel *Darkly Dreaming Dexter*, the central character of which was in turn reportedly modelled after Bundy.[36] In the field of high-profile crime, the difficulty of teasing apart myth and reality is also compounded by 'true crime' literature such as the book *The Stranger Beside Me* by the American author Ann Rule.[37] Rule grew close to Bundy whilst working on a telephone helpline in Seattle in the early 1970s. Based on his life, this intimate biography, written by a friend, seamlessly mixes fact and speculation, representing Bundy in very human terms. At the time he was first arrested, Rule, like many others who knew him, believed that 'the man I know couldn't be responsible for any of the things he is accused of'.[38]

After the first arrest, Bundy became a media celebrity whose image was made available to a mass audience through press and television reportage. Whilst narratives of deviance were repeatedly attached to him, his image could never be made to signify the presence of evil in the way that the photograph of Myra Hindley was. And yet he exemplifies the notion of the monster as one who 'introduces disorder into the legal system'.[39] Despite his appearance of normality, Bundy was a highly transgressive figure, not only on account of the monstrous acts he performed, but also as a result of the way in which he blurred the boundaries between monstrous 'other' and the norm. The moral uncertainty generated by the contradictions between Bundy's physical appearance, his apparently 'normal' behaviour and the narratives of deviance attached to him undermines any attempt to identify him as categorically 'other', completely different to 'us', normal people.

Theorizing the Relation between Self and Monstrous Other

In her 2001 essay 'Phenomenology and Serial Murder: Asking Different Questions', the psychologist and criminologist Candice Skrapec asks, 'Is there something about the serial killer that makes him categorically different from us?' or 'Is it essentially a matter of degree that separates us from those who . . . repeatedly kill?'[40] It seems that there is a universal need to believe that criminal monsters such as Bundy are categorically different, and yet in this case the evidence fails. When the suspect looks normal it is difficult to set a clear and tangible boundary between 'really' normal people and someone who has been identified as a criminal monster. If, as Georges Canguilhem maintained, nineteenth-century science uncoupled physical deformity from the monstrous by classifying and accounting for it, the attempts of disciplines such as psychiatry, psychology and psychoanalysis to give meaning to the invisible inner world of the psychopathic killer have not been so successful. The traditional notion of the monster as recognizably alien 'other', physiognomically marked by insanity or evil, and therefore clearly separable from the 'normal' subject is no longer relevant in the face of a figure such as Bundy. As Margrit Shildrick has observed, 'what lies beyond the unproblematic horror of the absolute other is the far more risky perception that the monstrous may not be recognised as such, for it is not so different after all'.[41] The invisible and unrepresented nature of Bundy's criminality is perhaps even more profoundly monstrous than the crimes he committed because it suggests that the violent and primitive urges beneath his veneer of normality may be lurking within any of us.

In order to find a new theoretical framework for this invisible monstrosity that resists categorical separation from self, and to understand better the complexity of our relationship to the criminal monster, it is perhaps useful to turn to Julia Kristeva's philosophical notion of the abject. Consistent with Foucault's 'real question of monstrosity' – that is, the transgression of natural limits or classifications – abjection is a human reaction to the collapse of meaning that arises when the distinction between subject and object, or self and other becomes blurred. In Kristeva's words, what causes abjection is that which '. . . disturbs identity, system, order. What does not respect borders, positions, rules. The in-between, the ambiguous, the composite'.[42] She goes on to list as abject characters 'the traitor, the liar, the criminal with a good conscience, the shameless rapist, the killer who claims he is a saviour . . . [and] any crime, because it draws attention to the fragility of the law'.[43] The types of abject individual listed by Kristeva are all apparently 'normal' human beings who, like serial killers, lack one significant human quality – the capacity for empathy with their victims.

In her book, *Powers of Horror*, Kristeva asks, 'How can I be without border?'[44] For her, the crisis of identity that underlies this question is produced by an encounter not with the absolute 'other', but with the abject – that which must be expelled from self, but which at the same time sustains identity and provides a boundary for the self. According to Kristeva, improper, unclean or taboo forces, ranging from excrement to incestuous desire and the violence of birth, are rejected by the human subject, but cannot really be left behind. These are the forces that disrupt identity and render it provisional, drawing attention to the impossibility of a coherent, stable and 'clean' self. The violent impulses and inappropriate desires of the criminal monster may be added to this list of abject forces that, for many people, trouble normal identity. Although most people would never feel compelled to act on these inappropriate desires and impulses, they cannot be categorically set apart from the psyche of the 'normal' individual 'norm'.

The concept of the abject as something that is unacceptable but never completely externalized provides a useful tool for thinking about the behaviour of criminal monsters in general, and of serial killers such as Bundy in particular. Whilst most people are unlikely ever to meet someone like Bundy face to face, the threat of an empty subjectivity which appears to mirror our own whilst in fact failing to do so fundamentally challenges the definition of what it is to be human. Like the abject, the serial killer is a part of 'us' – he or she appears to function as a 'normal' member of society, whilst at the same time being utterly alien. To return to Kristeva:

> There looms, within abjection, one of those violent, dark revolts of being, directed against a threat that seems to emanate from an exorbitant outside or inside, ejected beyond the scope of the possible, the tolerable, the thinkable. It lies there quite close, but it cannot be assimilated.[45]

Even if the criminal monster has a human face, his or her unassimilable behaviour must be visibly removed from society.

Whilst Bundy's execution was performed in front of just twelve witnesses, his death was very much in the public eye. It is reported that over three hundred reporters from around the world gathered across the street from Florida State Prison where he was executed, along with hundreds of spectators. At the moment an officer came out to pronounce Bundy dead, members of the crowd outside cheered, whilst others demonstrated against the barbarism of the death penalty. In Bundy's case, the spectacle of the actual death was closeted, available to only a select few. But the carnival outside the prison, coupled with the narrative of his execution, which was broadcast on television networks across America and throughout the world, are reminiscent of Foucault's image of the public execution of the eighteenth-century criminal Robert Damiens. The ritual of Bundy's death demonstrated the power of the State, which enacted punishment on his body in a final gesture designed to assert that the crimes of which he was accused really did take place.

Because Bundy's life ended when he was relatively young, his image remains, like that of Myra Hindley, frozen in time. For many people he continues to be the typical, young, successful, handsome, late twentieth-century American whose mediated narrative is as enthralling as any televised crime drama. The question of who Bundy really was remains unanswered in many ways. Whilst he blamed social factors such as exposure to violent pornography for his own compulsive actions, the only cause that has been reliably attached to Bundy's murders is a personal one. He was, apparently, traumatized after the break-up of his relationship with girlfriend Stephanie Brooks in 1968, and as a consequence compulsively murdered women who looked like her. If Bundy's personal anguish was what led him to carry out so many devastating murders, perhaps his monstrous actions can be read as a sign of the self-centred alienation of a late twentieth-century capitalist society. Bundy's answer when asked what it was like to murder someone is telling in this respect. He replied that murder is not about lust or violence, but possession. As an apparently ideal all-American boy obsessed with consumption and control, Ted Bundy seems to have embodied the values of his society, epitomizing Foucault's notion of the dangerous individual who refuses to answer the question, 'Who are you?'

Anders Behring Breivik

When seen in the context of human monstrosity, the more recent phenomenon of the Norwegian mass murderer Anders Behring Breivik reflects a different and perhaps more contemporary set of social issues. Like the Monster of Ravenna, whose mixed-up body acted as a symbol of social, moral and religious confusion in the early sixteenth century, the figure of Breivik points to a widespread but poorly articulated sense of threat, or perceived 'disorder', within early twenty-first-century Western society. On 22 July 2011 thirty-three-year-old Breivik bombed a government building in Oslo, killing eight people. On the same day he went on to kill sixty-nine young people in a mass shooting at a camp of the Workers' Youth League of the Norwegian Labour Party on the island of Utøya. He has admitted to killing all seventy-seven people but does not admit to murder, arguing that the deaths were 'cruel but necessary' to alert Norway to the threat of an Islamic takeover. In addition, Breivik declared war on members of the Norwegian Labour Party, whom he believed to be conducting a 'multicultural experiment' to promote the 'Muslim invasion' of Europe.

As the story unfolded during his trial, narratives of cause and origin were sought within Breivik's personal history in order to account for the crimes he committed. He is thought to have suffered a mental breakdown in 2006, after which he was increasingly reclusive, becoming obsessed with the politics of 'multiculturalism'. He subsequently spent a year playing the violent video game *World of Warcraft* for up to seventeen hours

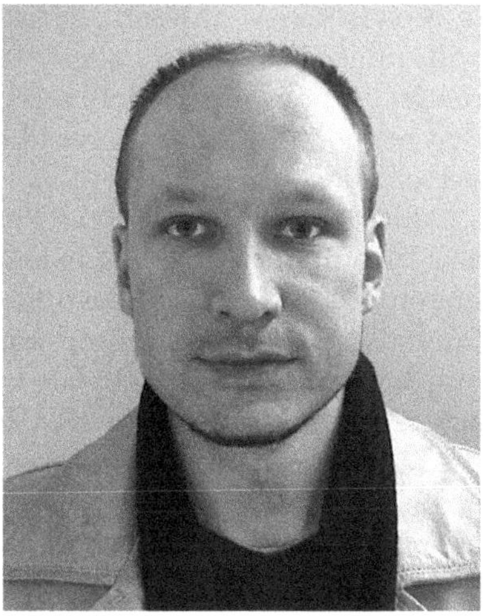

7.2: Anders Behring Breivik, passport photograph.

a day. During the early part of the trial Breivik claimed that this had helped him to train himself to kill. Whilst it is now clear that he spent years preparing himself both physically and mentally for the attacks that he carried out, it seems that he had no notable history of violent behaviour. Although there may be evidence to suggest that he was a difficult child with some emotional problems, there are, apparently, no specific personal experiences that can be made to explain his monstrous acts. As his passport photograph from 2009 (Figure 7.2) demonstrates, Breivik's outward appearance is equally unhelpful in the search for signs of a criminal character – he looks like a typical white, middle-class Norwegian man. But in the context of his attack against those he believed to be promoting 'multiculturalism' and the 'invasion of Europe' by Islam his looks are not entirely insignificant. His white skin and distinctly Nordic features align him with the nineteenth-century paradigm of a 'superior Aryan race' that was taken up by the Nazis, and with which he clearly identifies himself. If Breivik sees his appearance as a means of securing his own fragile identity, one feature in particular represents a tangible, corporeal inscription of his fears. In 1999, at the age of twenty, he had cosmetic surgery on his nose. According to his friends, Breivik underwent this surgery in an effort to appear 'more Aryan' in response to taunts that he had an 'Arabic' nose.[46] This detail, which emerged during the trial, shows how, in Breivik's view at least, physical appearance remains invested with political and ideological values. This reported attempt to render his appearance more acceptable to his peers also suggests that his political activities could have been motivated by a deep personal insecurity.[47]

Although, like Bundy, Breivik killed a large number of people and became the subject of extensive media coverage, there are important differences in the underlying motives for their crimes. Bundy's reasons for killing were apparently egocentric, the murders reinforcing his already inflated sense of power. Breivik's actions, which were informed by a significant ideology with broader social implications, seem to have been motivated by a profound sense of insecurity. Breivik's extreme behaviour, which has prompted comparisons to both Adolf Hitler and Osama bin Laden, reflects an anxiety about the relationship between self and cultural identity that is both personal to him and endemic in modern societies.

Aside from his own identity crisis, Breivik continued to maintain that he had an important political message to deliver. He repeatedly insisted that he was acting on behalf of a pan-European anti-Muslim militant group called the 'Knights Templar'. Although it is very unlikely that such a group existed, Breivik and his defence lawyers made every effort to maintain the credibility of his political message, and to ensure that his belief in the imminent threat of a 'Muslim invasion' of Norway was taken seriously. In order to try to demonstrate that his views are not unique, individuals of a similar persuasion were called to give evidence at Breivik's trial. One right-wing advocate, Arne Tumyr, the leader of an organization called 'Stop the Islamization of Norway', is reported to have called Islam 'a religion of violence, a religion of wars' that poses 'a threat to Norwegian society and values'.[48]

Whilst there is clear evidence that Breivik performed the actions he is accused of, the case against him is not straightforward. The main focus of the murder trial was to determine whether or not he should be diagnosed as 'insane'. An initial psychiatric evaluation conducted in November 2011 by two court-appointed psychiatrists found him to be a paranoid schizophrenic and therefore not responsible for his actions. In April 2012 a second evaluation concluded that he was sane and should be held to account.[49] Individuals such as Mr Tumyr were subsequently called to court in order to try to show that, because there are others who share his beliefs, Anders Breivik cannot be deemed insane.

Breivik seems to be emerging as a significant contemporary incarnation of the 'criminal monster', his actions drawing attention to a particularly contemporary kind of social and ideological instability. Creating unrest within one of the wealthiest and most secure countries in the world, the attacks carried out by Breivik provoked widespread political debate – in the Norwegian courtroom, in the international mass media as well as in more informal settings – around the notion of 'multiculturalism'. In this sense, Breivik is a truly modern monster. His unspeakably monstrous acts have given tangible form to that which currently challenges the established order of identities, systems, borders and rules – for him personally and for a whole range of different individuals and social and cultural groups. Symbolically, Breivik's role is similar to that of the Monster of Ravenna, whose bodily transgressions were seen as an emblem of evil for both Catholics and Protestants during the religious wars of the sixteenth century. Breivik's extensively documented trial provided a focus for the expression of divergent views on the relationship between Islam and the West, the influence of the far right on Western society, and notions of national identity. All of these are current and emotive concerns for people of all religious convictions and cultural backgrounds. The monstrous murders carried out by Breivik certainly act as a symbolic warning, although the nature of that warning remains open to interpretation.

In his rambling and contradictory 1,500-page manifesto entitled '2083: A European Declaration of Independence', Breivik presents himself as a right-wing nationalist with a strong hatred of Muslims, Marxists and those he labels 'multiculturalists'. Then he writes:

> I don't hate Muslims at all. I acknowledge that there are magnificent Muslim individuals in Europe. In fact, I have had several Muslim friends over the years, some of whom I still respect. This does not mean however that I will accept an Islamic presence in Europe. Muslim individuals who do not assimilate 100% by 2020 will be deported as soon as we manage to seize power. Although I do admit that I am disgusted by the current development, I would rather say I'm driven by my love for Europe, European culture and all Europeans. This does not mean that I oppose diversity. But appreciating diversity does not mean that you support genocide of your own culture and people by accepting for example Islamic Demographic Warfare.[50]

This statement is culturally significant because it draws out some of the confusion and tension that occur as the structure of society changes. Breivik argued that he was acting in the interests of political necessity. He has claimed that he killed seventy-seven people in order to broadcast his political message and save millions from impending Islamic colonization in the face of media censorship of his writings on the subject. Whilst his views and actions overtly reflect those of the modern far right, which sees Islam as its main enemy, they also indirectly reflect a much broader sense of unrest, highlighting some of the more general conflicts that exist around the concept of multiculturalism. At a time of economic strain, when certain political leaders were declaring a failure of multiculturalism in Europe, the details of Breivik's trial provoked widespread political debate about the ways in which European cultural identity may be understood. Some, like Breivik himself, believe in the threat of an 'Islamic colonization' of Europe, whilst others argue that minority cultures such as Islam should be protected from the ignorance and prejudice of mainstream Western culture. This unrest suggests that political extremism such as that brought to light by the Breivik case may be the most modern form of monstrousness to threaten the stability of individual and social identities.

During his trial Breivik was characterized in the media as 'rambling, repetitive, obsessive', 'fixated on a threat he never truly managed to articulate', 'profoundly abnormal' and suffering from 'underlying delusions of grandeur'.[51] Comments such as these offer a means of categorically setting this criminal character apart from the 'norm', identifying him as someone who cannot share the common reality of 'normal' people and who is not responsible for his own 'evil', inhuman actions. If Breivik's trial had concluded with a verdict of insanity, therefore, his right-wing views may have been considered the distorted product of a disturbed mind, and consequently of little account. But, in August 2012, the jury brought a unanimous verdict of sanity. Breivik was deemed to be responsible for his actions and a danger to society. A twenty-one-year sentence of 'preventive detention' was imposed on him. Since he has been officially deemed sane, the idea of Breivik as 'a monster made by multiculturalism', or 'a distinctively right-wing kind of monster' can act as another means of dismissing the kind of extremist ideology he upholds. If he is not 'mad', he must be a monster.

The appearance of modern 'monsters' such as Bundy and Breivik seems to support Foucault's argument that physical appearance can no longer be relied upon as a visible sign of monstrousness. But this does not mean that human monstrosity has disappeared from view. Even if monstrousness is no longer manifested in the physique of those we consider 'monsters', the international mass media continue to ensure that monstrosity remains an embodied phenomenon. Media coverage of high-profile figures like Bundy and Breivik guarantees that monstrousness can still be publicly attributed to an identifiable individual, who can then be tried by a court of law and must either be held to account, or deemed 'insane'.

Afterword

The project to investigate how and why human monstrosity exists was initially inspired by my practice as a visual artist. This book has, therefore, focused on the visual significance of human monstrosity. Inspired by the picture of the Monstrous Races discussed in Chapter 1, my investigation began with a desire to find a context for the idea that monstrosity is not an essential form of being. An unwieldy mass of interdisciplinary material soon began to accumulate around the visual images that led this research. It was only when I discovered Michel Foucault's series of lectures on the abnormal that I was able to imagine a coherent form for the work. In particular, his assertion that in the late eighteenth century somatic monstrosity gave way to 'something that really will be a monstrosity' – that is, monstrosity of character. Here Foucault implicitly raises the question of the visual significance of monsters, although he does not pursue it.

My understanding of the social function of human monsters has also been developed with Foucault's unconventional and anti-establishment approach to history in mind. His work seemed to give credibility to my impulse to bring together various different historical examples in a loosely chronological order, but with no intention of trying to assemble a history of monsters. In *The Archeology of Knowledge*, for example, Foucault explains that 'the problem [of history] is no longer one of tradition, of tracing a line, but one of division, of limits; it is no longer one of lasting foundations, but one of transformations that serve as new foundations'.[1] Here he seems to be describing history as a process in which monsters, as transformative figures, would play a vital role. In later work he goes on to characterize history as a genealogy that must look beyond a particular phenomenon for the social and cultural conditions of its possibility. This rationale has been central to my study of monsters. The significance both of the enduring values of ancient Greece and of the nineteenth century as a period of rapid transition became increasingly evident during the course of my research. Against a background of core values that have changed little since classical times, the interlinked processes of industrialization, increased social mobility, the development of modern medical and forensic sciences and the emergence of photography have radically altered what, in modern Western society, is considered a monstrosity.

Giving tangible presence to the terrible and unspeakable forces of monstrousness, monstrosity is both formed by, and at the same time instrumental in breaking down and re-forming, the cultural and social narratives that determine who and what we can be as 'civilized' humans. But, as Georges Canguilhem wrote in 'Monstrosity and the Monstrous', 'there is nothing monstrous about monstrosities'.[2] 'Real' human monsters and the monstrosities they exhibit are social constructs created in order to articulate monstrousness and, by bringing it into being, to 'domesticate' it. I have tried to show that, even though the monsters described in this book take different forms according to the context in which they are found, their social function remains consistent. In fact, each of the examples discussed here could be considered a marker of the social and cultural challenges of its time. Most obviously, the strange bodies of the ancient Monstrous Races reflect a sense of wonder at human diversity that, from a contemporary perspective, seems acutely naive. With hindsight we can also see the much more recent 'criminal monster' Ted Bundy as a personification of the bleak alienation at the heart of twentieth-century consumer capitalism.

I hope that collectively the examples presented here have demonstrated that monsters are always contingent, their existence dependent upon a viewing subject, from whose 'norm' the monstrous 'other' is seen to deviate. From the Monstrous Races – those strange creatures that were once believed to inhabit unknown territories at the farthest edges of the globe, to people such as Bundy and Breivik, who could pass as ordinary citizens until held to account for their inhuman acts, the 'monsters' that make up this study are found in increasingly close proximity to 'us', 'normal' people. Indeed, since the late nineteenth century, human 'monsters' have been attributed a subjectivity that calls for identification, empathy and fascination on the one hand, and elicits fear and rejection on the other. This modern form of monstrosity is exemplified in the figure of Bundy, whose performance of normality misled even those who thought they knew him well. Bundy seems to have transgressed and even obscured the boundaries between the normal and the unspeakably monstrous in an especially challenging way. In the end it was not his monstrous acts so much as his unknowability, the apparent absence of humanity beneath the public mask of normality, that made him such a fascinating, but also disturbing, example to study.

The various historical monsters discussed in the preceding chapters have been selected in order to show that there is an established tradition in Western culture of articulating narratives of self and other visually, in the form of strange bodies and unconventional behaviours. Most specifically, Chapter 6 aimed to show that the public acknowledgement of a particular individual as an 'icon of evil' depends on the circulation of recognizable visual images. As Margrit Shildrick has recently stated, visual images are reassuring because they 'provoke a familiar mode of response to otherness'.[3] Indeed, what other strategy do we have for ensuring that monstrous difference may be set apart from the norm? Without an identifiable visual image, how can we situate what is monstrous in the place of the 'other'? Looking at Bundy, for example, we might ask, 'If this is how a monster looks, how do I know that those closest to me are not like him or, worse still, how do I know that I myself will not become like him?' I have argued that monstrosity remains a visual phenomenon even if it has, as Foucault proposed, moved from the domain of somatic and natural disorder to that of criminality. At times of social and moral unrest in particular, the visible presence of a human monster offers an important form of reassurance that society has a means of dealing with the disruptive forces in play. But what happens if the process of visualization fails? Surely what is most disturbing, and thus most truly monstrous, in any particular situation is the 'evil' that can be neither articulated nor represented visually.

Perhaps a moment of reflection on our individual responses to those who emerge as the significant monsters of our time can help each of us to acknowledge our own subjective position in the face of the 'otherness' they manifest. If they exist to reinforce the norm, to reassure us about who and what we are by manifesting what we are not, what will happen if we discover that these 'others' are not so different from ourselves? Or worse, what if the trajectory followed by the monsters discussed in this book is completed and identity itself becomes unstable? How do we construct an acceptable image of self without an identifiable image of 'otherness'? Monsters call for change, but they also reveal fear of changes to the existing order of things, and perhaps most fundamentally a fear of the possibility that we might not be who we think we are. The moment that the monstrous 'other' becomes indistinguishable from the image we see in the mirror is the terrible moment when monstrosity fails.

Notes

Introduction

1 See: Cousins, Mark and Athar, Hussain, *Michel Foucault*, London: Macmillan Books, 1984, p. 3.

2 Foucault, Michel, *Les Anormaux: Cours au Collége de France 1974–5*, trans. as *Abnormal* by Graham Burchill, New York: Picador, 2003; and Foucault, Michel, 'The Dangerous Individual', in *Philosophy, Culture and Other Writings, 1977–1984*, trans. by Alan Sheridan, ed. by Lawrence Kritzman, New York: Routledge, 1988. This lecture was originally delivered at York University in Toronto in 1978.

3 Canguilhem, Georges, 'Monstrosity and the Monstrous', *Diogenes* 40, 1962, pp. 27–42.

4 Davidson, Arnold I., *Foucault and his Interlocutors*, London: University of Chicago Press, 1997, p. 21.

5 Canguilhem, Georges, *The Normal and the Pathological*, New York: Zone Books, 1991, p. 13.

6 Canguilhem, 'Monstrosity and the Monstrous', p. 30.

7 Ibid., p. 38.

8 Ibid. See also: Sharpe, Andrew, 'Structured Like a Monster: Understanding Human Difference Through a Legal Category', *Law and Critique* 18(2), 2007, p. 216.

9 Foucault, *Abnormal*, p. 73.

10 Ibid., p. 74.

11 Ibid., p. 57.

12 Canguilhem, 'Monstrosity and the Monstrous', p. 36.

13 Ibid., p. 63.

14 With regard to Fritzl, see, for example: 'I'm No Monster', *Daily Mirror*, 7 May 2008, p. 5; Flanagan, Padraic, 'I'm No Monster: I Could Have Killed Them', *Daily Express*, 8 May 2008, pp. 8–9; and 'Fritzl Lodger Set to Tell Police: I Saw the Cellar Monster's Wife Help Take Food to Sex Slave Dungeon', *Daily Mail*, 1 May 2008, available online at: www.dailymail.co.uk/news/article-563326/Fritzl-lodger-set-tell-police-I-saw-cellar-monsters-wife-help-food-sex-slave-dungeon.html. For reference to Huntley see: Troup, John, 'Monster Copied De Niro', *Sun*, 1 August 2002, available online at: www.thesun.

co.uk/sol/homepage/news/80693/monster-copied-de-niro.html (accessed 14 January 2013).

15 Shildrick, Margrit, *Embodying the Monster*, London: Sage, 2002, p. 17.

Chapter 1

1 The Arnstein Bible is now kept in the British Library.

2 From a conversation with Alixe Bovey, former curator of manuscripts at the British Library, 17 November 2008.

3 See: Williams, David, *Deformed Discourse: The Function of the Monster in Medieval Thought and Literature*, Exeter: Exeter University Press, 1996, p. 137. Conversely, creatures such as the centaur, in which a human head is combined with an animal body, symbolize a distortion of form that preserves reason.

4 In *Politics* Book I, chapter ii, 1253a 9–10 Aristotle states, 'man is the only animal who has the gift of speech', see: Aristotle, *Politics*, trans. by B. Jowett, in *The Complete Works of Aristotle*, ed. by Jonathan Barnes, Princeton: Princeton University Press, 1984, p. 1988. Also, Kate Soper discusses the legacy of Descartes' seventeenth-century argument that the use of language is exclusively human and offers a clear-cut standard for dividing animals from humans: Soper, Kate, *What Is Nature? Culture, Politics and the Non-human*, Oxford: Blackwell, 1995, pp. 52–70. Stephen Horigan identifies Descartes' understanding of language as 'the most important criterion used to distinguish between humans and animals' in Horigan, Stephen, *Nature and Culture in Western Discourses*, London: Routledge, 1988, p. 75.

5 See: Fudge, Erica, *Animal*, London: Reaktion Books, 2002, pp. 117–18.

6 Wittkower, Rudolf, 'Marvels of the East', in Rudolf Witkower, *Allegory and the Migration of Symbols*, London: Thames & Hudson, 1977.

7 Ibid., p. 50.

8 See: Wilson, Dudley, *Signs and Portents: Monstrous Births from the Middle Ages to the Enlightenment*, London: Routledge, 1993, p. 4.

9 Friedman, John Block, *The Monstrous Races in Medieval Art and Thought*, Cambridge, MA: Harvard University Press, 1981.

10 Ibid., pp. 24–5.

11 The origins of the Monstrous Races are unknown, but Ctesias' treatise is understood to be one of the earliest surviving accounts. See: Wittkower, 'Marvels of the East', p. 46 and McCrindle, J.W., *Ancient India as Described by Ctesias the Knidian*, Calcutta: Thacker, Spink & Co., 1882.

12 See, for example: Wittkower, 'Marvels of the East', p. 47, and McCrindle, *Ancient India*, p. 5.
13 Higgs Strickland, Debra, *Saracens, Demons, and Jews: Making Monsters in Medieval Art*, Princeton: Princeton University Press, 2003, pp. 11–12.
14 McCrindle, *Ancient India*, p. 5. See also: Wittkower, 'Marvels of the East', p. 48.
15 Ibid., p. 54.
16 Pliny the Elder, *Natural History*, trans. by H. Rackham, London: Loeb Classical Library, Harvard University Press, 1999, book VII, 23–5.
17 Ibid., book VII, 22.
18 Friedman, *The Monstrous Races*, p. 26.
19 Ibid., pp. 26–7.
20 See, for example: Shildrick, Margrit, *Embodying the Monster*, London: Sage, 2002, p. 16, and Velazco y Trianosky, Gregory, 'Savages, Wild Men, and Monstrous Races: The Social Construction of Race in the Early Modern Era', in Peggy Zeglin Brand (ed.), *Beauty Revisited*, Bloomington, IN: Indiana University Press, 2012, pp. 45–71.
21 Stallybrass, Peter, and White, Allon, *The Politics and Poetics of Transgression*, London: Methuen, 1986, p. 5.
22 Barnhart, Robert (ed.), *Chambers Dictionary of Etymology*, Edinburgh: Harrap, 2000, p. 1160.
23 Foucault, Michel, 'A Preface to Transgression,' in Michel Foucault, *Language, Counter-memory, Practice*, ed. by Donald F. Bouchard, trans. by Donald F. Bouchard and Sherry Simon, Ithaca, NY: Cornell University Press, 1977, p. 34.
24 This is the *Oxford English Dictionary* definition: Thompson, Della (ed.), *Concise Oxford English Dictionary*, Oxford: Clarendon Press, 1995.
25 Fabian, Johannes, *Time and the Work of Anthropology, Critical Essays, 1971–1991*, London: Routledge, 1991, p. 208.
26 Kearney, Richard, *Strangers, Gods and Monsters: Interpreting Otherness*, London: Routledge, 2003, p. 117.
27 Crick, Malcolm, *Explorations in Language and Meaning: Towards a Semantic Anthropology*, London: Malaby Press, 1976, p. 165.
28 Levinas, Emmanuel, 'The Trace of the Other', in William McNeill and Karen Feldman (eds), *Continental Philosophy: An Anthology*, Oxford: Blackwell, 1998, p. 177.
29 Said, Edward, *Orientalism*, London: Routledge and Kegan Paul, 1978.
30 Sontag, Susan, 'The Anthropologist as Hero', in Eugene Hayes (ed.), *Claude Lévi-Strauss: The Anthropologist as Hero*, Cambridge, MA: MIT Press, 1970, p. 185.

31 Foucault, Michel, *Les Anormaux: Cours au Collége de France 1974–5*, trans. as *Abnormal* by Graham Burchill, New York: Picador, 2003, p. 63.

32 Ibid., p. 65.

33 Ibid., p. 64.

34 See, for example: Horigan, *Nature and Culture*, p. 4, and White, Hayden, 'The Forms of Wildness', in E. Dudley and M. Novak (eds), *The Wild Man Within*, Pittsburgh: Pittsburgh University Press, 1972, p. 15.

35 On a conceptual level the boundary between humans and animals is less clearly defined in the contemporary context (see: Fudge, *Animal*). However, in the field of genetic science the taboos surrounding the mixture of human and animal material remain strong (see: Sharpe, Andrew, 'Structured Like a Monster: Understanding Human Difference Through a Legal Category', *Law and Critique* 18(2), 2007, pp. 221–6).

36 Paré, Ambroise, *Monstres et Prodiges; On Monsters and Marvels*, trans. by Janis Pallister, Chicago: University of Chicago Press, 1982, p. 67.

37 Canguilhem, 'Monstrosity and the Monstrous', pp. 30–1.

38 Foucault, *Abnormal*, p. 56.

39 Ibid.

40 Higden, Ranulph, *Polycronicon*, trans. by John Trevisa, London: William Caxton, 1482. Quoted with reference to the Monstrous Races in Park, Katherine, and Daston, Lorraine, *Wonders and the Order of Nature*, New York: Zone Books, 1998, p. 25. The Englishman Higden was in this case referring to Ireland as the edge of the world.

41 Park and Daston, *Wonders*. See also: Thrower, N.J.W., *Maps and Civilization: Cartography in Culture and Society*, Chicago: University of Chicago Press, 2007. pp. 42–6.

42 Ibid., p. 43.

43 Friedman, John Block, 'Cultural Conflicts in Medieval World Maps', in Stuart B. Schwartz (ed.), *Implicit Understandings: Observing, Reporting and Reflecting on the Encounters Between Europeans and Other People in the Early Modern Era*, Cambridge: Cambridge University Press, 1995, p. 69.

44 Wittkower, in 'Marvels of the East', and Park and Daston, in *Wonders*, indicate that myth still figured strongly in both Eastern and Western interpretations of the world during the Middle Ages.

45 Park and Daston, *Wonders*, p. 60.

46 Barthes, Roland, 'Myth Today', in *Selected Writings*, London: Fontana, 1982, p. 93.

47 Ibid., p. 132.

48 Ibid., p. 106.
49 Wittkower, 'Marvels of the East', pp. 61–9.
50 Barthes, 'Myth Today', pp. 93–4.
51 Ibid.
52 Ibid., pp. 102–3.
53 Wittkower, 'Marvels of the East', p. 72.
54 Ibid.
55 Baldo Ubaldi, quoted in Friedman, *Monstrous Races*, p. 180.

Chapter 2

1 Newton, Michael, *Savage Girls and Wild Boys: A History of Feral Children*, London: Faber & Faber, 2002, p. 236.
2 Miller, Fred, 'The State and the Community in Aristotle's *Politics*', *Reason Papers* 1, pp. 61–3, available online at: www.reasonpapers.com/pdf/01/rp_1_5.pdf (accessed 20 December 2012).
3 Aristotle, *Politics*, trans. by B. Jowett, in *The Complete Works of Aristotle*, ed. by Jonathan Barnes, Princeton: Princeton University Press, 1984, Book III, Chapter v, 1278a, 26–7, p. 2028.
4 Foucault, Michel, *Les Anormaux: Cours au Collége de France 1974–5*, trans. as *Abnormal* by Graham Burchill, New York: Picador, 2003, p. 56.
5 Williams, Raymond, *Keywords: A Vocabulary of Culture and Society*, London: Fontana, 1983, p. 219.
6 Soper, Kate, *What Is Nature? Culture, Politics and the Non-human*, Oxford: Blackwell, 1995, p. 73.
7 Ibid., p. 15.
8 Ibid., p. 155.
9 Ibid., p. 21.
10 Ibid., p. 156.
11 Ibid., p. 16.
12 Williams, *Keywords*, p. 87.
13 Ibid., pp. 76–82.
14 Williams shows that this meaning evolved in the eighteenth century: ibid., pp. 77–8.
15 Ibid., pp. 48–50.
16 Lovejoy, Arthur O., *The Great Chain of Being: A Study of the History of an Idea*, Cambridge, MA: Harvard University Press, 1936, pp. 58–9.
17 A scan of the original volume of the tenth edition of *Systema Natura* in Latin is available online at: www.biodiversitylibrary.org/item/10277 (accessed 20 December 2012).
18 Douthwaite, Julia, *The Wild Girl, Natural Man and the Monster: Dangerous Experiments in the Age of Enlightenment*, Chicago: University of Chicago Press, 2002, pp. 16–17.

19 See: Horigan, Stephen, *Nature and Culture in Western Discourses*, London: Routledge, 1988, p. 69.

20 Rousseau, Jean-Jacques, *A Discourse on the Origin and Foundation of the Inequality of Mankind*, London: R. & J. Dodsley, 1761, p. 17.

21 Comte de Buffon, Georges-Louis Leclerc, *Histoire Naturelle*, Amsterdam: J.H. Schneider, 1766.

22 The word 'savage' is of Latin origin. Derived from silva, meaning forest, it originally meant simply 'wild' or 'of the woods'. It was first used in English in the sense of 'uncivilized' around the fourteenth century (Barnhart, Robert (ed.), *Chambers Dictionary of Etymology*, Edinburgh: Harrap, 2000).

23 Cuvier, Georges, *The Animal Kingdom: Arranged in Conformity with its Organization*, trans. by H.M. Murtrie, New York: G. & C. & H. Carvill, 1831, vol. 1, p. 52.

24 Ibid.

25 Ibid.

26 Darwin, Charles, *On the Origin of Species by Means of Natural Selection; Or the Preservation of Favoured Races in the Struggle for Life*, London: John Murray, 1859; Darwin, Charles, *The Descent of Man and Selection in Relation to Sex*, New York: D. Appleton & Co., 1871; Huxley, Thomas, *Evidence as to Man's Place in Nature*, New York: D. Appleton & Co., 1863; Lyall, Charles, *Geological Evidences of the Antiquity of Man*, Philadelphia: George W. Childs, 1863.

27 Lyall, *Geological Evidences*, p. 501.

28 Huxley, *Evidence as to Man's Place in Nature*, p. 123.

29 See: Bernheimer, Richard, *Wild Men in the Middle Ages: A Study in Art, Sentiment, and Demonology*, Cambridge, MA: Harvard University Press, 1952, pp. 10 and 23, and Husband, Timothy, *The Wild Man, Medieval Myth and Symbolism*, New York: Museum of Metropolitan Art, 1980, p. 2.

30 Bernheimer, *Wild Men in the Middle Ages*, p. 1.

31 Husband, *The Wild Man*, p. 1.

32 White, Hayden, 'The Forms of Wildness', in E. Dudley and M. Novak (eds), *The Wild Man Within*, Pittsburgh: Pittsburgh University Press, 1972, p. 4.

33 Bernheimer, *Wild Men in the Middle Ages*, p. 8.

34 See: White, 'The Forms of Wildness', p. 28.

35 Husband, *The Wild Man*, p. 5.

36 Ibid., p. 13.

37 Hirst, P. and Woolley, P., *Social Relations and Human Attributes*, London: Tavistock, 1982, p. 46.

38 White, 'The Forms of Wildness', p. 7.

39 See: Bernheimer, *Wild Men in the Middle Ages*, pp. 33–5, and White, 'The Forms of Wildness', p. 22.

40 Bernheimer, *Wild Men in the Middle Ages*, p. 33.
41 Ibid.
42 See: Velazco y Trianosky, Gregory, 'Savages, Wild Men, and Monstrous Races: The Social Construction of Race in the Early Modern Era', in Peggy Zeglin Brand (ed.), *Beauty Revisited*, Bloomington, IN: Indiana University Press, 2012, p. 49.
43 See Chapter 4 for a discussion of freak shows.
44 For a thorough analysis of the cultural implications of the 'What Is It?', see: Cook, James W. Jr, 'Of Men, Missing Links and Nondescripts: The Strange Career of P.T. Barnham's "What Is It?" Exhibition', in Rosemarie Garland-Thomson (ed.), *Freakery, Cultural Spectacles of the Extraordinary Body*, New York: New York University Press, 1996, pp. 139–57.
45 Malson, Lucien, *Wolf Children*, London: New Left Books, 1972, pp. 80–2. This is one of many lists identified by Adriana Benzaquén in *Encounters with Wild Children: Temptation and Disappointment in the Study of Human Nature*, Montreal: McGill-Queen's University Press, 2006, pp. 271–80. Benzaquén notes that Malson's list has several errors.
46 Itard's account is reproduced in full in Malson, *Wolf Children*, pp. 95–178.
47 Ibid., p. 95.
48 Benzaquén, *Encounters with Wild Children*.
49 Ibid., pp. 244–50. Genie is a pseudonym.
50 Ibid., pp. 259–62.
51 *Jensen!*, RTL5, 23 April 2007, available online at: www.rtl.nl/components/shows/jensen/169_anamorf/miMedia/2007/week17/ma_gasten_23apr.avi_plain.xml (accessed 9 November 2012).
52 Dragonfly Film and Television Productions, *Feral Children*, episode 1, 'The Monkey Boy of Uganda', first shown in the UK on Animal Planet, 24 September 2012.
53 Benzaquén, *Encounters with Wild Children*, p. 259.
54 Hirst and Woolley, *Social Relations and Human Attributes*, p. 44.
55 From: Fry, Lyn, 'Oxana Malaya', unpublished article given to the author on 21 August 2012.
56 Scream Films, *Mindshock: Feral Children*, Channel 4 documentary, first shown in UK on 17 June 2006.
57 Interview with Ed Stagg, BBC Midland Radio, 21 September 2012, available online at: http://raisedwild.files.wordpress.com/2012/10/bbc-midlands-hud_discovery-feral-children.mp3 (accessed 9 November 2012).
58 Dragonfly Film and Television Productions, *Feral Children*, episode 2, 'The Dog-Girl of Ukraine', first shown in UK on Animal Planet, 1 October 2012.

59 Fry, 'Oxana Malaya'.
60 Ibid.
61 Dudley and Novak, *The Wild Man Within*, p. 35.
62 Grice, Elizabeth, 'Cry of an Enfant Sauvage', *Daily Telegraph*, 17 July 2006, available online at: www.telegraph.co.uk/culture/tvandradio/3653890/Cry-of-an-enfant-sauvage.html (accessed 20 December 2012).
63 Ibid.

Chapter 3

1 Bordo, Susan, *Unbearable Weight: Feminism, Western Culture, and the Body*, Berkeley: University of California Press, 1993, p. 165.
2 Kemp, Martin, 'The Art of Physiognomy', *Guardian*, 23 April 2007, published online at: http://blogs.guardian.co.uk/art/2007/04/the_art_of_physiognomy.html (accessed 15 August 2008).
3 Douglas, Mary, *Natural Symbols: Explorations in Cosmology*, London: Routledge, 1996, p. xxxviii.
4 Ibid., p. 78.
5 Ibid., pp. 72 and 91.
6 Foucault, Michel, *Les Anormaux: Cours au Collége de France 1974–5*, trans. as *Abnormal* by Graham Burchill, New York: Picador, 2003, p. 63.
7 Ibid., p. 57.
8 Plato, *Timaeus*; quoted in Barkan, Leonard, *Nature's Work of Art: The Human Body as Image of the World*, New Haven, CT: Yale University Press, 1975, p. 9.
9 Ibid., p. 8.
10 Ibid., p. 22. The oldest known astrological texts date back to the first half of the Babylonian Hammurabi dynasty, around the middle of the eighteenth century BC. By the fourth century BC astrology was important in Chinese, Indian, Native American and Western cultures.
11 Barkan, *Nature's Work of Art*, p. 23.
12 See: Davidson, Arnold I., 'The History of Horror, Abominations, Monsters and the Unnatural', in Arnold I. Davidson (ed.), *The Emergence of Sexuality: Historical Epistemology and the Formation of Concepts*, London: Harvard University Press 2002, p. 106.
13 Women were not thought to be fully human. See, for example: Aristotle, *Generation of Animals*, trans. by A.L. Peck, London: Heinemann, 1943, p. 401.
14 Garland, Robert, *The Eye of the Beholder: Deformity and Disability in the Graeco-Roman World*, London: Duckworth, 1995, p. 89.
15 Potts, Alex, *Flesh and the Ideal: Winklemann and the Origins of Art History*, New Haven, CT: Yale University Press, 1994, p. 145.
16 Gombrich, E.H., *The Story of Art*, London: Phaidon, 2003, p. 90.

17 There are several different marble, bronze and plaster copies of the lost original. In this one, held at the British Museum, the head is looking the wrong way – the figure should be looking towards the discus.
18 Foucault, *Abnormal*, p. 57.
19 Park, Katherine and Daston, Lorraine, *Wonders and the Order of Nature*, New York: Zone Books, 1998, pp. 177–80.
20 Barkan, *Nature's Work of Art*, p. 46.
21 Earlier versions of the Monster of Ravenna are modelled on another monster believed to have been born in Florence in 1506. See Park and Daston, p. 178. See also: Niccoli, Ottavia, *Prophecy and People in Renaissance Italy*, trans. by Lydia Cochrane, Chicago: University of Chicago Press, 1990, pp. 36–43, for a comprehensive genealogy of the monster and its political significance.
22 See: Gould, G.M., and Pyle, W.L., *Anomalies and Curiosities of Medicine*, Philadelphia: W.B. Saunders, 1897, p. 213.
23 See: Laplanche, Jean, 'The Unfinished Copernican Revolution', in Jean Laplanche, *Essays on Otherness*, ed. by John Fletcher, London: Routledge, 1988, p. 56.
24 Luca Landucci records the sacking of Ravenna in his diary entry of 29 March 1512: Landucci, Luca, *A Florentine Diary from 1450 to 1516 by Luca Landucci, Continued by an Anonymous Writer Until 1542, with Notes by Iodoco Del Badia*, trans. by Alice de Rosen Jervis, New York: Dutton, 1927, p. 250.
25 Roman Chronicler, Sebastiano di Branca Tedallini, quoted in Niccoli, *Prophecy and People in Renaissance Italy*, p. 35.
26 Lykke, Nina and Braidotti, Rosi (eds), *Between Monsters, Goddesses and Cyborgs: Feminist Confrontations with Science, Medicine and Cyberspace*, London: Zed Books, 1996, p. 150.
27 Quoted in Park and Daston, *Wonders*, pp. 181–2.
28 Boaistuau, Pierre, *Histoires prodigieuses*, trans. by Edward Fenton as *Certaine Secrete Wonders of Nature*, London: Henry Bynneman, 1569, p. 139.
29 Williams, David, *Deformed Discourse: The Function of the Monster in Medieval Thought and Literature*, Exeter: Exeter University Press, 1996, p. 197.
30 For example: Janis Pallister, in appendix to Paré, Ambroise, *On Monsters and Marvels*, Chicago: University of Chicago Press, 1982; Hamburger, Viktor, 'Monsters in Nature', *Ciba Symposia* 9, 1947, pp. 966–83; Walton, Michael, Fineman, Robert and Walton, Phyllis, 'Of Monsters and Prodigies: The Interpretation of Birth Defects in the Sixteenth Century', *American Journal of Medical Genetics* 47(1), 1993, p. 12.
31 Lycosthenes, Conrad, *Prodigiorum ac Ostentorum Chronicon*,

trans. by Stephen Bateman as *The Doome Calling All Men to the Judgement: Wherein Are Contayned for the Most Parte All the Straunge Prodigies Hapened In the Worlde*, London: Ralph Nubery, 1581, p. 285.

32 Wilson, Dudley, *Signs and Portents: Monstrous Births from the Middle Ages to the Enlightenment*, London: Routledge, 1993, p. 8.

33 See: Friedman, John Block, *The Monstrous Races in Medieval Art and Thought*, Cambridge, MA: Harvard University Press, 1981, pp. 108–11.

34 Wittkower, Rudolf, 'Marvels of the East', in *Allegory and the Migration of Symbols*, Thames & Hudson, 1977, p. 56.

35 *Oxford English Dictionary* definition: Thompson, Della (ed.), *Concise Oxford English Dictionary*, Oxford: Clarendon Press, 1995. The problem of evil is discussed in more detail in Chapter 6.

36 Landucci, *A Florentine Diary*, p. 249.

37 Park and Daston, *Wonders*, p. 182.

38 See: Hamilton, Peter, 'Policing the Face', in Peter Hamilton and Roger Hargreaves, *The Beautiful and the Damned: The Creation of Identity in Nineteenth Century Photography*, London: Lund Humphries and National Portrait Gallery, 2001, p. 63; also Higgs Strickland, Debra, *Saracens, Demons, and Jews: Making Monsters in Medieval Art*, Princeton: Princeton University Press, 2003, pp. 37–8. Higgs Strickland points out that this text is now attributed to a 'Pseudo-Aristotle'.

39 Pseudo-Aristotle, 814a, quoted in Evans, Elizabeth C., 'Physiognomics in the Ancient World', *Transactions of the American Philosophical Society*, New Series 59(5), 1969, p. 9.

40 See: Kwakkelstein, Michael, 'Leonardo da Vinci's Grotesque Heads and the Breaking of the Physiognomic Mould', *Journal of the Warburg and Courtauld Institutes* 54, 1991, p. 129–30.

41 Ibid., p. 133.

42 Della Porta, Giambattista, *De Humana Physiognomonia, Libri IIII*, Vici Æquensis: Apud J. Cacchium, 1586.

43 See: Ross, Stephanie, 'Painting the Passions: Charles LeBrun's Conference sur L'Expression', *Journal of the History of Ideas* 45(1), January–March 1984, pp. 25–47.

44 See: Hartley, Lucy, *Physiognomy and the Meaning of Expression in Nineteenth-Century Culture*, Cambridge: Cambridge University Press, 2001, pp. 21–6.

45 Le Brun's system divides 'man' into three general classes according to his passions: mild passions which do not alter the features, generous passions which leave a particular mark and blameworthy or vile passions which degrade the features.

46 Lavater, Johann Kaspar, *Physiognomische Fragmente: Essays on*

Physiognomy; for the Promotion of the Knowledge and the Love of Mankind, 4 vols, trans. by Thomas Holcroft, London: G.G.J. & J. Robinson, 1789.

47 Lavater, quoted in Garland, *The Eye of the Beholder*, p. 88.

48 Socrates posed a problem for physiognomists because he proved that humans could not be put into preconceived categories. He was profoundly ugly and yet highly intelligent and so disproved the Greek association of beauty with goodness and truth. See: Shortland, Michael, 'Skin Deep: Barthes, Lavater and the Legible Body', *Economy and Society* 14(3), August 1985, pp. 290–1.

49 Lavater, quoted in Berland, Kevin, 'Reading Character in the Face: Lavater, Socrates, and Physiognomy', *Word & Image* 9(3), July–September 1993, p. 263.

50 Ibid., p. 269.

51 See Chapter 2.

52 See: Davis, Lennard, 'Constructing Normalcy: The Bell Curve, the Novel and the Invention of the Disabled Body in the Nineteenth Century', in Lennard Davis (ed.), *The Disability Studies Reader*, London: CRC Press, 2006, pp. 14–15; and Green, David, 'Veins of Resemblance: Photography and Eugenics', *Oxford Art Journal* 7(2), 1984, pp. 8–9.

53 Ibid., p. 17.

54 Foucault, *Abnormal*, pp. 81–2.

55 Hamilton, 'Policing the Face', pp. 57–8.

56 Sekula, Allan, 'The Body and the Archive', in Richard Bolton (ed.), *Contest of Meaning*, London: MIT Press, 1996, p. 350.

57 Hamilton, 'Policing the Face', p. 62.

58 See Chapter 6.

59 Sekula, 'The Body and the Archive', p. 347

60 Galton, Francis, 'Composite Portraits, Made by Combining Those of Many Different Persons into a Single Resultant Figure', *Journal of the Anthropological Institute of Great Britain and Ireland* 8, 19 April 1878, p. 133.

61 See: Novak, Daniel, 'A Model Jew: Literary Photographs and the Jewish Body in Daniel Deronda', *Representations* 85, winter 2004, pp. 58–97.

62 Sekula, 'The Body and the Archive', p. 360.

63 Hamilton, 'Policing the Face', p. 67.

64 Hannavy, John, *Encyclopedia of Nineteenth-Century Photography*, London: Routledge, 2008, p. 151.

65 See: Hamilton, 'Policing the Face', p. 106.

66 Lombroso, Cesare, *Criminal Man*, trans. and ed. by Mary Gibson and Nicole Hahn Rafter, London: Duke University Press, 2006, p.48.

67 Franz Joseph Gall formalized the theory of phrenology in the late eighteenth century. Phrenology is based on the idea that particular mental faculties are linked to specific areas of the brain. Phrenologists believed that the physical size of an area of the brain corresponds to a particular mental capacity and that the topography of the skull follows the development of the brain. By this account an individual's personality traits could be determined by measuring his or her skull.

68 Lombroso, Cesare, *Criminal Man According to the Classification of Cesare Lombroso, Briefly Summarized by his Daughter Gina Lombroso Ferrero, with an Introduction by Cesare Lombroso*, London: G.P. Puttnams, 1911, pp. 5 and 11.

69 Ibid., p.14.

70 See: Hamilton, 'Policing the Face', p. 100.

71 Lombroso, *Criminal Man*, trans. and ed. by Gibson and Hahn Rafter, pp. 81–4.

72 Ibid., p. 343.

73 Morison, Sir Alexander, *The Physiognomy of Mental Diseases*, London: Longman & Co., 1843, p. 1.

74 Ibid., p. 17.

75 Bucknill, J.C., and Tuke, D.H., *A Manual of Psychological Medicine*, London, J. & A. Churchill, 1879, p. 418.

76 Ibid., p. 424.

77 Ibid., p. 421.

78 Ibid., p. 422.

79 Ibid., p. 423.

80 Connolly, John, 'The Physiognomy of Insanity', *Medical Times and Gazette* 16, January 1858, p. 3.

81 Ibid.

82 Ibid.

83 Hamilton, 'Policing the Face', p. 79.

84 Gilman, Sander, *Seeing the Insane: A Cultural History of Madness*, Chichester: Wiley & Sons, 1982, p. 167.

85 Ibid., pp. 236–40.

86 Foucault's characterization of nineteenth-century asylums has been contested. See, for example: Porter, Roy, 'Lunatic Ideas and the Truth about Asylums', *Times Higher Education*, 10 October 1997, available online at: www.timeshighereducation.co.uk/story.asp?storyCode=103990&sectioncode=26 (accessed 20 December 2012).

87 Foucault, Michel, *Madness and Civilization*, trans. by Richard Howard, London: Routledge, 2001, p. 128.

Chapter 4

1 Foucault, Michel, *Discipline and Punish: The Birth of the Prison*, trans. Alan Sheridan, London: Penguin Books, 1977, p. 184.
2 Davis, Lennard, 'Constructing Normalcy: The Bell Curve, the Novel and the Invention of the Disabled Body in the Nineteenth Century', in Lennard Davis (ed.), *The Disability Studies Reader*, London: CRC Press, 2006, p. 6.
3 Canguilhem, Georges, 'Monstrosity and the Monstrous' *Diogenes* 40, 1962, p. 38.
4 Foucault, Michel, *Les Anormaux: Cours au Collége de France 1974–5*, trans. as *Abnormal* by Graham Burchill, New York: Picador, 2003, p. 73.
5 Altick, Richard, *The Shows of London*, London: Harvard University Press, 1978, p. 35.
6 Ibid., pp. 34–49. See also: Wilson, Philip K., 'Eighteenth-Century "Monsters" and Nineteenth-Century "Freaks": Reading the Maternally Marked Child', *Literature and Medicine* 21(1), 2002, pp. 1–25, and Wilson, Dudley, *Signs and Portents: Monstrous Births from the Middle Ages to the Enlightenment*, London: Routledge, 1993, p. 179.
7 See: Fahy, Thomas, *Freak Shows and the Modern American Imagination*, Basingstoke: Palgrave Macmillan, 2006, p. 3.
8 'A monstrosity; an abnormally developed individual or thing; an abnormal or bizarre occurrence': Thompson, Della (ed.), *Concise Oxford English Dictionary*, Oxford: Clarendon Press, 1995.
9 Barnhart, Robert (ed.), *Chambers Dictionary of Etymology*, Edinburgh: Harrap, 2000.
10 Garland-Thomson, Rosemarie (ed.), *Freakery, Cultural Spectacles of the Extraordinary Body*, New York: New York University Press, 1996, p. 4.
11 Bogdan, Robert, *Freak Show: Presenting Human Oddities for Amusement and Profit*, London: University of Chicago Press, 1988, pp. 54–5.
12 See: Garland-Thomson, Rosemarie, *Extraordinary Bodies, Figuring Physical Disability in American Culture and Literature*, New York: Columbia University Press, 1997, p. 65.
13 Garland-Thomson, *Freakery*, p. 12.
14 Ibid. (un-paginated section between chapters 2 and 3).
15 Garland-Thomson, *Extraordinary Bodies*, p. 60.
16 Debord, Guy, *Society of the Spectacle and Other Films*, London: Rebel Press, 1992, p. 61.
17 Stallybrass, Peter and White, Allon, *The Politics and Poetics of Transgression*, London: Methuen, 1986, p. 4.
18 See: Bogdan, *Freak Show*, chapter 4, pp. 94–118.

19 Mitchell, Michael, *Monsters: Human Freaks in America's Gilded Age, the Photographs of Chas. Eisenmann*, Toronto: ECW Press, 2002, p. 50.
20 Ibid.
21 Barnum. P.T., *Struggles and Triumphs, or Forty Years' Recollections*, Buffalo: Warren, Johnson & Co., 1871, available online at: www.archive.org/details/strugglestriumph00barnrich (accessed 20 December 2012).
22 See Chapter 2.
23 The shape of Johnson's head has led some to believe that he suffered from microcephaly, a disorder in which the circumference of the head is smaller than normal because the brain has not developed properly or has stopped growing. However, it is unlikely that Johnson was microcephalic as his intellectual ability seems to have been normal.
24 Mitchell, *Monsters*, p. 94.
25 'The Leopard Boy', Royal Aquarium Playbills Box, 1876–84, Victoria & Albert Museum Theatre and Performance Archives.
26 Durbach, Nadja, *Spectacle of Deformity: Freak Shows and Modern British Culture*, London: University of California Press, 2010, p. 30.
27 Davis, 'Constructing Normalcy', p. 91
28 See Chapter 2.
29 See: Mitchell, *Monsters*, p. 94, and Bogdan, *Freak Show*, pp. 134–5.
30 Bogdan, *Freak Show*, p. 135; Fahy, *Freak Shows and the Modern American Imagination*, p. 22.
31 Fahy, *Freak Shows and the Modern American Imagination*, p. 55.
32 Bogdan, *Freak Show*, p. 134.
33 Cook, James W. Jr, 'Of Men, Missing Links and Nondescripts: The Strange Career of PT Barnham's "What Is It?" Exhibition', in Garland-Thomson (ed.), *Freakery*, p. 144.
34 Brown, Bill, *The Material Unconscious*, London: Harvard University Press, 1996, p. 217.
35 Adams, Rachel, *Sideshow U.S.A.: Freaks and the American Cultural Imagination*, Chicago: University of Chicago Press, 2001, p. 6.
36 For example, 'gaffs', who faked physical anomalies by pretending to have missing limbs.
37 Adams, *Sideshow U.S.A.*, p. 13.
38 Garland-Thomson, *Extraordinary Bodies*, p. 66.
39 Ibid. (unpaginated section between chapters 2 and 3).
40 Ibid.
41 See: Lemagny, Jean-Claude, and Rouillé, André (eds), *A History of Photography: Social and Cultural Perspectives*, trans. by Janet Lloyd, Cambridge: Cambridge University Press, 1987, p. 40.

42 Batchen, Geoffrey, 'Dreams of Everyday Life', in Martha Langford (ed.), *Image and Imagination*, Montreal: McGill-Queen's University Press, 2005, p. 72.
43 Lemagny and Rouillé, *A History of Photography*, p. 39.
44 Batchen, 'Dreams of Everyday Life', p. 64.
45 'Racial' freaks were usually photographed as outsiders, or exotic 'others', whilst Western freaks with physical deformities were depicted as aggrandized members of society.
46 See: Adams, *Sideshow U.S.A.*, p. 113.
47 Lemagny and Rouillé, *A History of Photography*, p. 40.
48 Bogdan, *Freak Show*, p. 108.
49 Ibid., p. 224.
50 See: Fahy, *Freak Shows and the Modern American Imagination*, p. 65.
51 Durbach, *Spectacle of Deformity*, p. 107.
52 O'Connor, Erin, *Raw Material: Producing Pathology in Victorian Culture*, Durham, NC: Duke University Press, 2001, p. 195.
53 Durbach, *Spectacle of Deformity*, p. 47.
54 Fahy, *Freak Shows and the Modern American Imagination*, p. 2.
55 Davis, 'Constructing Normalcy', p. 9.
56 Ibid.
57 Ibid., pp. 3–16. See also: Garland-Thomson, *Freakery*, p. 12.
58 Davis, 'Constructing Normalcy', p. 10. See also: Sekula, Allan 'The Body and the Archive', in Richard Bolton (ed.), *Contest of Meaning*, London: MIT Press, 1996, pp. 353–4.
59 Edwards, Martha, 'Constructions of Physical Disability in the Ancient Greek World: The Community Concept', in David Mitchell and Sharon Snyder (eds), *The Body and Physical Difference: Discourses of Disability*, Ann Arbor, MI: University of Michigan Press, 2000, p. 44.
60 Davis, 'Constructing Normalcy', p. 4.
61 Garland, Robert, *The Eye of the Beholder: Deformity and Disability in the Graeco-Roman World*, London: Duckworth, 1995, p. 14.
62 Aristotle, *Politics*, Book VII, Chapter xvi, 1335b, 20–1, p. 2119.
63 Garland, *The Eye of the Beholder*, p. 24.
64 Quoted in Friedman, John Block, *The Monstrous Races in Medieval Art and Thought*, Cambridge, MA: Harvard University Press, 1981, p. 179.
65 Foucault, *Abnormal*, p. 63.
66 Ibid., p. 64.
67 Canguilhem, 'Monstrosity and the Monstrous', p. 38.
68 On a practical level, the disabled body has conventionally been seen to signify a lack of ability to work, which – in a capitalist context – denotes a subjectivity that is less valuable than that of a 'normally' embodied person See: Edwards, Claire and Imrie,

Rob, 'Disability and Bodies as Bearers of Value', *Sociology* 37, 2003, pp. 239–56. For a theoretical context see: Foucault, Michel, *Language, Counter Memory, Practice*, ed. by Donald F. Bouchard, trans. by Donald F. Bouchard and Sherry Simon, Ithaca, NY: Cornell University Press, 1977, p. 148.

69 Garland, *The Eye of the Beholder*, p. 5.

70 Landucci, Luca, *A Florentine Diary from 1450 to 1516 by Luca Landucci, Continued by an Anonymous Writer Until 1542 with Notes by Iodoco Del Badia*, trans. by Alice de Rosen Jervis, New York: Dutton, 1927.

71 Durbach, *Spectacle of Deformity*, pp. 176–7.

Chapter 5

1 Foucault, Michel, *Les Anormaux: Cours au Collége de France 1974–5*, trans. as *Abnormal* by Graham Burchill, New York: Picador, 2003, p. 74.

2 His birth date has been disputed: in Merrick's autobiography it is recorded as 5 August 1860 and Ashley Montagu records it as 21 April 1864. The date given here comes from Howell and Ford, who identified Merrick from his birth certificate: Howell, Michael, and Ford, Peter, *The True History of the Elephant Man*, London: Allison & Busby, 1980, p. 32.

3 Joseph Merrick's autobiography is reproduced in: Howell and Ford, *True History*, appendix 1, pp. 173–5.

4 For documentation of Merrick's early life see: Howell and Ford, *True History*; Graham, P. and Oehlshlaeger, F.H., *Articulating the Elephant Man*, London: Johns Hopkins University Press, 1992, and Montague, Ashley, *The Elephant Man: A Study in Human Dignity*, London: Allison & Busby, 1972. For an emotive primary account, see: Treves, Frederick, *The Elephant Man and Other Reminiscences*, London: Cassell & Co., 1923.

5 See: Huet, Marie-Hélène, *Monstrous Imagination*, London: Harvard University Press, 1993, and Shildrick, Margrit, *Embodying the Monster*, London: Sage, 2002, pp. 36–47.

6 Howell and Ford, *True History*, appendix 1, pp. 173–5.

7 Ibid., pp. 4–5.

8 Evans, Jonathan, *Treves and the Elephant Man*, London: Royal London Hospital, 2003, p. 9.

9 Ibid., p. 10.

10 Ibid., p. 9.

11 From: Norman, Tom, 'Somewhat Different: Unusual as Usual', undated unpublished manuscript held at National Fairground Archive, University of Sheffield. See also: Howell and Ford, *True History*, p. 77, and Norman, Tom, *The Penny Showman:*

Memoirs of Tom Norman 'Silver King', ed. by George Barnum Norman-Noakes, London: Norman-Noakes, 1985.

12 Evans, *Treves and the Elephant Man*, p. 11.

13 Durbach, Nadja, *Spectacle of Deformity: Freak Shows and Modern British Culture*, London: University of California Press, 2010, p. 34.

14 Howell and Ford, *True History*, pp. 88–90.

15 Ibid., pp. 74–8. However, Treves' story is supported in a pamphlet published by Jonathan Evans, archivist at the Royal London Hospital, who has written: 'Although many modern day readers may feel that it presents a romanticised and patronising picture of Merrick during his four year stay at the London Hospital, the story told by Treves does not need to be factually altered until the time of Joseph's death' (Evans, *Treves and the Elephant Man*, p. 52).

16 Ibid., pp. 15–18.

17 Treves, *Reminiscences*, p. 20.

18 Montagu, *The Elephant Man*, p. 28.

19 Shelley, Mary, *Frankenstein; Or the Modern Prometheus*, London: Lackington, Hughes, Harding, 1818; Hugo, Victor, *The Hunchback of Notre Dame*, ed. and trans. by Robin Waterfield, London: Puffin, 1996.

20 Howell and Ford, *True History*, pp. 150–1, and Evans, *Treves and the Elephant Man*, pp. 53–4.

21 Evans, *Treves and the Elephant Man*, p. 47, and Norman, 'Somewhat Different'.

22 Durbach, *Spectacle of Deformity*, p. 56.

23 Canguilhem, Georges, *The Normal and the Pathological*, New York: Zone Books, 1991, pp. 42, 131–5, 142 and 210; Canguilhem, Georges, 'Monstrosity and the Monstrous', *Diogenes* 40, 1962, pp. 37–40.

24 Canguilhem, 'Monstrosity and the Monstrous', pp. 36–7.

25 Geoffroy de St Hilaire, Etienne, *Philosophie anatomique: des monstruosités humaines, ouvrage contenant une classification des monstres . . .*, 2 vols, Paris: Auteur, 1818–22.

26 Foucault, *Abnormal*, p. 131.

27 Geoffroy de St Hilaire, Isidore, *Histoire générale et particulière des anomalies . . .*, Paris: J.B. Baillière, 1832, vol. 1, p. 18.

28 Ibid., p. xii.

29 Ibid.

30 Canguilhem, 'Monstrosity and the Monstrous', p. 38.

31 Ibid., p. 41.

32 Ibid., p. 37.

33 See, for example: Evans, *Treves and the Elephant Man*, pp. 54–5.

34 See, for example: Ablon, Joan, '"The Elephant Man" as "Self"

and "Other": The Psycho-Social Costs of a Misdiagnosis', *Social Science and Medicine* 40(11), June 1995, pp. 1481–9.

35 Evans, *Treves and the Elephant Man*, pp. 54–5.

36 Foucault, *Abnormal*, p. 73.

37 Canguilhem, 'Monstrosity and the Monstrous', p. 40.

38 Foucault, *Abnormal*, p. 131.

39 Excerpt from Joseph Merrick's autobiography, reproduced in Howell and Ford, *True History*, pp. 173–5.

40 Most sources agree that this text is unlikely to have been written by Merrick himself, but of interest here is what the text says about the public perception of Merrick, not its authenticity.

41 This was written some forty years after the event took place.

42 Treves, *Reminiscences*, pp. 1–2.

43 Darwin, Charles, *On the Origin of Species by Means of Natural Selection; Or the Preservation of Favoured Races in the Struggle for Life*, London: John Murray, 1859.

44 *The Times*, 4 December 1886, p. 6.

45 *The Times*, 16 April 1890, p. 6.

46 Evans, *Treves and the Elephant Man*, p. 39.

47 Ibid., p. 46.

48 Statement made by Jonathan Evans, archivist at the Royal London Hospital, in conversation with the author, 1 June 2005.

49 Kemp, Martin, '"A Perfect and Faithful Record": Mind and Body in Medical Photography before 1900', in Ann Thomas (ed.), *Beauty of Another Order: Photography in Science*, London: Yale University Press, 1997, p. 149.

50 Gilman, Sander, *Seeing the Insane*, London: Wiley & Sons, 1982, p. 226.

51 Ibid., p. 120.

52 Kemp, 'A Perfect and Faithful Record', p. 148.

53 The original prints are available for viewing by appointment at the Royal London Hospital Archives.

54 Hannavy, John, *Encyclopedia of Nineteenth-Century Photography*, London: Routledge, 2008, p. 277.

55 Lalvani, Suren, *Photography, Vision and the Production of Modern Bodies*, New York: SUNY Press, 1996, p. 191.

56 Sekula, Allan, 'The Body and the Archive', in Richard Bolton (ed.), *Contest of Meaning*, London: MIT Press, 1996, p. 345.

57 Graham and Oehlshlaeger, *Articulating the Elephant Man*, p. 18.

58 I refer here to the written account of Merrick's disabilities in Carr Gomm's earlier letter to *The Times* (see note 44 above).

59 Evans, *Treves and the Elephant Man*, p. 42.

60 Graham and Oehlshlaeger, *Articulating the Elephant Man*, p. 58.

61 Evans, *Treves and the Elephant Man*, p. 41.

62 Ibid., pp. 41–2.

63 Ibid., pp. 8–9.
64 Halsted, D.G., *A Doctor in the Nineties*, London: Christopher Johnson, 1959, p. 39.
65 From an (undated) account published in the *British Medical Journal*, reproduced as an appendix in Howell and Ford, *True History*, p. 178.
66 Montagu, *The Elephant Man*, p. 49.

Chapter 6

1 Jordanova, Ludmilla, 'Reading Faces in the Nineteenth Century', *Art History* 13(4), December 1990, p. 571.
2 See, for example: Douglas, John E., Ressler, R., et al., 'Criminal Profiling from Crime Scene Analysis', *Behavioral Sciences and the Law* 4(4), 1986, pp. 401–21.
3 Holmes, Ronald and Holmes, Stephen, *Profiling Violent Crimes: An Investigative Tool*, London: Sage, 2008, p. 4.
4 See, for example: Douglas, John E., et al. (eds), *Crime Classification Manual: A Standard System for Investigating and Classifying Violent Crimes*, Oxford: Maxwell Macmillan International, 1992.
5 Schmid, David, *Natural Born Celebrities: Serial Killers in American Culture*, London: University of Chicago Press, 2005, pp. 177 and 207.
6 Tithecott, Richard, *Of Men and Monsters: Jeffrey Dahmer and the Construction of the Serial Killer*, Madison, WI: University of Wisconsin Press, 1997, p. 34.
7 Ibid., p. 6.
8 See: White, Hayden, *The Content of the Form: Narrative Discourse and Historical Representation*, London: Johns Hopkins University Press, 1987, p. 36.
9 Sutcliffe's victims who were not prostitutes included a sixteen-year-old shop assistant, Jayne McDonald, whom he killed in 1977; Josephine Whitaker, a nineteen-year-old bank clerk killed in 1979; and students Barbara Leach (also in 1979) and Jacqueline Hill (in 1980).
10 Barthes, Roland, 'Introduction to the Structural Analysis of Narratives', in *Selected Writings*, Glasgow: Fontana, 1989, p. 294.
11 The etymology of the word 'spectacle' is derived from the Latin roots *spectare*, 'to view or watch', and *specere*, 'to look at'.
12 'Dangerous outsiders' is a term borrowed from Philip Jenkins: Jenkins, Philip, 'Catch Me Before I Kill More: Seriality as Modern Monstrosity', *Cultural Analysis* 2, 2002, p. 5. See also: Jenkins, Philip, *Intimate Enemies: Moral Panics in Contemporary Great Britain*, Hawthorne, NY: Aldine de Gruyter, 1992, and Jenkins, Philip, *Using Murder: The Social Construction of Serial Homicide*, Hawthorne, NY: Aldine de Gruyter, 1994.

13 For example, the former US President George W. Bush popularized notions of a 'war against terrorism and evil' and of an 'axis of evil' between countries whose policies were completely foreign to his own.
14 Kekes, John, 'Understanding Evil', *American Philosophical Quarterly* 25(1), January 1988, p. 13.
15 Robert Ressler, co-founder of the FBI Behavioral Science Unit, claims to have first coined the term 'serial killer' in the mid-1970s (see: Seltzer, Mark, *Serial Killers: Death and Life in America's Wound Culture*, London: Routledge, 1998, p. 16, and Biressi, Anita, *Crime, Fear and the Law in True Crime Stories*, Basingstoke: Palgrave, 2001, p. 166), although this has been disputed (see: Jenkins, 'Catch Me Before I Kill More', p. 15). For a longer discussion of the relationship between serial killing and the FBI, see: Schmid, *Natural Born Celebrities*, pp. 77–83.
16 Jenkins, 'Catch Me Before I Kill More', pp. 2–3.
17 Ibid.
18 Norris, Joel, *Serial Killers: The Growing Menace*, New York: Doubleday, 1988, p. 19.
19 Cameron D., and Frazer, E., *The Lust to Kill: A Feminist Investigation of Sexual Murder*, New York: New York University Press, 1987, p. 27; Tithecott, *Of Men and Monsters*, p. 4.
20 Norris, *Serial Killers*, p. 19.
21 'News from Whitechapel', *Daily Telegraph*, 1 October 1888, p. 143.
22 Although it was never confirmed that the murders were the work of one person, the most popular suspects were Aaron Kosminski, a Polish Jew; Severin Klosowski, another Pole; Francis Tumblety, an Irish-American physician; Michael Ostrog, a supposed Russian doctor, and John Druitt, a middle-class British teacher.
23 Poe, Edgar Allan, *The Murders in the Rue Morgue: The Dupin Tales*, ed. by Matthew Pearl, London: Vintage Books, 2006; Conan Doyle, Arthur, *The Complete Sherlock Holmes*, Feltham: Hamlyn, 1984. True crime is a literary genre in which an actual crime and real people are used as a basis for a narrative that mixes factual information with fictionalized account. In the context of the true crime narrative monstrous acts are removed from the everyday and turned into a form of entertainment.
24 Oldridge, Darren, 'Casting the Spell of Terror: The Press and the Early Whitechapel Murders', in A. Warwick and M. Willis (eds), *Jack the Ripper: Media, Culture, History*, Manchester: Manchester University Press, 2007, p. 47.
25 *Jack the Ripper's Face 'Revealed'*, documentary first shown on Channel 5, 21 November 2006.

26 Statement recorded in the Channel 5 documentary, also quoted at: BBC News Online, 20 November 2006, available online at: http://news.bbc.co.uk/1/hi/uk/6164544.stm (accessed 20 December 2012).
27 *BBC News*, Monday 20 November 2006, available online at: http://news.bbc.co.uk/1/hi/uk/6164544.stm (accessed 20 December 2012).
28 Curtis Jr, L. Perry, *Jack the Ripper and the London Press*, London: Yale University Press, 2001, p. 41.
29 Smith, Joan, *Misogynies*, London: Faber & Faber, 1989, p. 117.
30 Philip Jacobson, quoted in Cameron and Frazer, *The Lust to Kill*, p. 27. Feminist studies of serial murder include: Smith, *Misogynies*; Holloway, Wendy, '"I Just Wanted to Kill a Woman" Why? The Ripper and Male Sexuality', *New Feminist Review* 9, 1981, pp. 33–40; Walkowitz, Judith, 'Jack the Ripper and the Myth of Male Violence', *Feminist Studies* 8, 1982, pp. 543–74.
31 Caputi, Jane, 'The New Founding Fathers: The Lore and Lure of the Serial Killer in Contemporary Culture', in Jane Caputi, *Goddesses and Monsters*, London: University of Wisconsin Press, 2004, p. 121.
32 Ibid., p. 10.
33 Jenkins, 'Catch Me Before I Kill More', p. 4.
34 Schmid, *Natural Born Celebrities*, p. 229.
35 See, for example: *Daily Mirror*, 11 December 1965, p. 1.
36 Ibid.
37 Reported on *BBC News*, 15 November 2002, available online at: http://news.bbc.co.uk/1/hi/uk/581580.stm (accessed 20 December 2012). Also quoted in Stanford, Peter, 'Myra Hindley: Notorious Child Murderer Whose Protestations of Repentance Failed to Assuage Public Revulsion', *Guardian*, 15 November 2002. A version of this article is available online at: www.guardian.co.uk/obituaries/story/0,3604,841049,00.html (accessed 20 December 2012).
38 Brady has repeatedly been refused the right to be moved from Ashworth, where he is subject to force-feeding, to a prison. The prison service has no right to force-feed inmates.
39 Jones, David, 'He Should Be Condemned to Live', *Daily Mail*, 16 March 2012, available online at: www.dailymail.co.uk/news/article–2116178/Ian-Brady-Furious-reaction-Moors-murderers-victims-decision-allow-public-hearing-battle-starve-death.html (accessed 20 December 2012).
40 Jewkes, Yvonne, *Media and Crime*, London: Sage, 2004, p. 128.
41 It is significant that the death penalty for murder was abolished in Britain in 1965, during the time that Hindley and Brady were

awaiting trial. If they had been sentenced to death, perhaps the moral transgressions attributed to Hindley and Brady would have been symbolically removed from society and they would have faded from view.

42 Birch, Helen, 'If Looks Could Kill: Myra Hindley and the Iconography of Evil', in Helen Birch (ed.), *Moving Targets: Women, Murder and Representation*, Berkeley: University of California Press, 1994, p. 32.

43 Ibid., pp. 48–9.

44 Ibid., p. 53.

45 Bertillon's technique, first published under the title *La Photographie judiciaire* (1890), still remains valid. It demands that an individual should be photographed full face and in profile, with the face well lit and the ear should be clearly visible in the profile image.

46 Available online at: www.telegraph.co.uk/news/2105864/Myra-Hindley-Victim's-mother's-desperate-plea.html (accessed 20 December 2012).

47 See, for example, an article inviting comment by Lord Longford (who was a supporter of Hindley) and Ann West, the mother of victim Lesley Ann Downey, who was vehemently against Hindley's release: 'Should Myra Hindley Ever Be Freed? Opinion', *Sun*, 30 October 1997.

48 The original photograph seems to be attributed a mythical power, by both the police and the media. For example, in trying to gain access to the original police print, I was treated with suspicion by the *Manchester Evening News*. When I finally located the print in a 'deep store' facility at the Cheshire Police Headquarters I was granted access to it only after submitting several letters of justification. Eventually permission was withdrawn. The case had been reopened and the photograph was deemed 'too sensitive' to be moved to a place where I could view it. I was sent a scan of the picture instead.

49 See: Young, Alison, *Judging the Image: Art, Value, Law*, London: Routledge, 2005, p. 34; also: Thorpe, Vanessa, 'Hindley Picture Is a Sensation Too Far for Artist Ayres', *Independent*, 21 September 1997, available online at: www.independent.co.uk/news/hindley-picture-is-a-sensation-too-far-for-artist-ayres-1240388.html (accessed 20 December 2012).

50 See, for example: *Daily Express*, 17 December 1986, pp. 2–3. Hindley herself was not physically attacked. She died in prison on 15 November 2002 at the age of sixty. She was Britain's longest-serving female prisoner.

51 See, for example: an article entitled 'Icon of Evil', *Daily Star*, 16 November 2002, pp. 8–9.

52 Documented online at: http://news.bbc.co.uk/1/hi/uk/7580261.stm (accessed 20 December 2012).
53 Hattenstone, Simon, 'Myra, Margaret and Me', *Guardian* Weekend, 21 February 2009, p. 29.
54 Tithecott, *Of Men and Monsters*, p. 6.
55 Barthes, Roland, 'The Photographic Message', in *Selected Writings*, Glasgow, Fontana, 1989, p. 194.
56 Ibid., p. 204.
57 Ibid., p. 205.
58 See: Halberstam, Judith, *Skin Shows, Gothic Horror and the Technology of Monsters*, London: Duke University Press, 1995, p. 3.

Chapter 7

1 Foucault, Michel, *Discipline and Punish*, London: Penguin, 1977, pp. 3–5. Foucault also describes a similarly brutal execution in his 'Abnormal' lecture of 29 January 1975: Foucault, Michel, *Les Anormaux: Cours au Collége de France 1974–5*, trans. as *Abnormal* by Graham Burchill, New York: Picador, 2003, pp. 84–5.
2 Lecture given on 22 January 1975, in ibid., pp. 55–79.
3 Foucault, Michel, 'The Dangerous Individual', in Michel Foucault, *Philosophy, Culture and Other Writings, 1977–1984*, ed. by Lawrence Kritzman, trans. by Alan Sheridan, New York: Routledge, 1988, p. 144.
4 Ibid.
5 Ibid., p. 128.
6 Ibid., p. 131.
7 Ibid., p. 134.
8 Canguilhem, Georges, 'Monstrosity and the Monstrous', *Diogenes* 40, 1962, p. 38. See also Foucault's discussion of psychiatry in his 'Seminar of 19th March, 1975', in Foucault, *Abnormal*, pp. 291–321.
9 Foucault, 'The Dangerous Individual', pp. 125–6.
10 Ibid., p. 127.
11 Masters, Brian, *Killing for Company: The Case of Dennis Nilsen*, London: Arrow Books, 1995.
12 Tithecott, Richard, *Of Men and Monsters: Jeffrey Dahmer and the Construction of the Serial Killer*, Madison, WI: University of Wisconsin Press, 1997, p. 53.
13 Seltzer, Mark, *Serial Killers: Death and Life in America's Wound Culture*, London: Routledge, 1998, p. 12.
14 See, for example: Michaud, Stephen and Aynesworth, Hugh, *Ted Bundy: Conversations with a Killer*, New York: Signet, 1989, p. xi; and Michaud, Stephen and Aynesworth, Hugh, *The Only Living Witness: The True Story of Serial Sex Killer, Ted Bundy*, Irving,

TX: Authorlink, 1999, p. i. See also A&E Biography Channel documentary about Ted Bundy currently (January 2013) available online at: www.youtube.com/watch?v=sdq6ViwYHLA. Audio documentation of the confessions is available online at: www.kirotv.com/news/4182402/detail.html (accessed 20 December 2012).

15 Extract from an anonymous confessional letter published in an Ohio newspaper, quoted in Seltzer, *Serial Killers*, p. 9.

16 It is thought that Bundy may have murdered as many as one hundred women.

17 For a discussion of Bundy's status as a psychopath see: Caputi, Jane, *The Age of Sex Crime*, Bowling Green, OH: Bowling Green State University Popular Press, 1987, p. 109. The term 'moral insanity' was coined by the physician, J.C. Pritchard, in 1835. He defined it as: 'a morbid perversion of the natural feelings, affections, inclinations, temper, habits, moral dispositions and natural impulses, without any remarkable disorder or defect of the intellect or knowing and reasoning faculties, and particularly without any insane illusion or hallucination': Prichard, J.C., *A Treatise on Insanity and Other Disorders Affecting the Mind*, New York: Arno, 1837, p. 16.

18 See, for example: Cleckley, H., *The Mask of Sanity*, St Louis, MO: C.V. Mosby, 1941, pp. 198–9; Hare, Robert, *Without Conscience: The Disturbing World of the Psychopaths Among Us*, New York: Guilford Press, 1999, and Hare, Robert, 'Psychopathy: A Clinical Construct whose Time Has Come', *Criminal Justice and Behavior* 23(1), 1996, pp. 25–54.

19 Halberstam, Judith, 'Skinflick: Posthuman Gender in Jonathan Demme's *The Silence of the Lambs*', *Camera Obscura* 27, September 1991, p. 37.

20 Dr James Dobson's company, Focus on the Family, refused to grant permission to publish a still from the documentation of this interview because, 'as per our contract with Mr. Bundy, we are not allowed to use or license the footage from his interview for any purpose except for fighting pornography'. The interview footage is, however, available on YouTube. An 'official' version, with contextual introduction is also available online at: www.pureintimacy.org/piArticles/A000000433.cfm (accessed 20 December 2012).

21 Quoted in: Rule, Ann, *The Stranger Beside Me*, London: Warner, 1994, p. 394.

22 Bremner, Charles, 'String of Confessions Fails to Stay Killer's Execution; Ted Bundy', *The Times*, 24 January 1989, and 'Bundy Interview Seen After Execution', *The Times*, 26 January 1989;

Stewart, Helen, 'Ted Bundy: Natural Porn Killer', *Sunday Times*, 13 August 2006.

23 For example: 'Death of the Devil', *Daily Express*, 25 January 1989, p. 3.

24 A&E Biography Channel documentary.

25 See, for example: Schmid, David, *Natural Born Celebrities: Serial Killers in American Culture*, London: University of Chicago Press, 2005, pp. 211–12.

26 All the quotes in this section are from the documentation of Bundy's final interview.

27 Seltzer, *Serial Killers*, p. 42.

28 A& E Biography Channel documentary.

29 From US TV news article, available online at: www.youtube.com/watch?v=eJHrcLzttHY&feature=relmfu (accessed 20 December 2012).

30 Jenkins, Philip, *Using Murder: The Social Construction of Serial Homicide*, Hawthorne, NY: Aldine de Gruyter, 1994, p. 53.

31 Jackson, Rosemary, *Fantasy: The Literature of Subversion*, London: Routledge, 1988, p. 45.

32 Quoted in Tucker, Carol, 'Constructing Images of Serial Killers', *University of Southern California Chronicle*, 10 November 1997, p. 6.

33 Seltzer, *Serial Killers*, p. 115.

34 Dietz, Mary Lorenz, 'Killing Sequentially: Expanding the Parameters of the Conceptualization of Serial and Mass Murder', in Thomas O'Reilly Fleming (ed.), *Serial and Mass Murder*, Toronto: Canadian Scholar's Press, 1996, p. 111.

35 The first episode was shown on Showtime (US TV) on 1 October 2006.

36 Lindsay, Jeff, *Darkly Dreaming Dexter*, London: Orion Books, 2004.

37 Rule, *The Stranger Beside Me*.

38 Ibid., p. 147.

39 Foucault, *Abnormal*, p. 324.

40 Skrapec, Candice, 'Phenomenology and Serial Murder: Asking Different Questions', *Homicide Studies* 5, 2001, p. 47.

41 Shildrick, Margrit, *Embodying the Monster*, London: Sage, 2002, p. 45.

42 Kristeva, Julia, *Powers of Horror*, New York: Columbia University Press, 1982, p. 4.

43 Douard, John, 'Loathing the Sinner, Medicalizing the Sin: Why Sexually Violent Predator Statutes Are Unjust', *International Journal of Law and Psychiatry* 30(1), 2007, p. 45.

44 Kristeva, *Powers of Horror*, p. 4.

45 Ibid., p. 1.

46 'Breivik "Cut Contact with Friends" in Run-up to Attacks', BBC Europe Online, 29 May 2012, available online at: www.bbc.co.uk/news/world-europe–18248116 (accessed 20 December 2012).

47 Breivik himself said that the surgery to his nose was necessary after a fight with a Pakistani man, which represents an equivalent statement.

48 'Norwegian Far Right Defend Breivik's Views on Islam', BBC News Online, 5 June 2012, available online at: www.bbc.co.uk/news/world-europe-18332442 (accessed 4 January 2013).

49 See: 'Norway's Mass Killer Breivik Declared Sane', BBC News Online, 10 April 2012, available online at: www.bbc.co.uk/news/world-europe-17663958 (accessed 4 January 2013).

50 Breivik, Anders, '2083: A European Declaration of Independence', translation available online at: www.breiviksmanifesto.com.

51 Pidd, Helen, 'Remorseless and Baffling, Breivik's Testimony Leaves Norway No Wiser', *Guardian*, 17 April 2012, available online at: www.guardian.co.uk/world/2012/apr/17/breivik-court-boasts-killing-utoya; Beaumont, Peter, 'Anders Breivik Was Challenging and Aggressive Child, Court Hears', *Guardian*, 14 June 2012, available online at: www.guardian.co.uk/world/2012/jun/14/anders-breivik-challenging-aggressive-child?INTCMP=ILCNETTXT3487, and 'Anders Breivik and the Trouble with Defining Sanity', *Guardian*, 18 June 2012, available online at: www.guardian.co.uk/commentisfree/2012/jun/18/anders-breivik-defining-sanity (all accessed 4 January 2013).

Afterword

1 Foucault, Michel, *The Archeology of Knowledge*, New York: Pantheon Books, 1972, p. 5.

2 Canguilhem, Georges, 'Monstrosity and the Monstrous', *Diogenes* 40, 1962, p. 41.

3 Shildrick, Margrit, 'On Longing for the Monstrous, Some Precautionary Observations', unpublished keynote lecture given at Sensualising Deformity conference, University of Edinburgh, 15 June 2012.

Bibliography and Further Reading

Books and Journal Articles

Ablon, Joan, '"The Elephant Man" as "Self" and "Other": The Psycho-Social Costs of a Misdiagnosis', *Social Science and Medicine* 40(11), June 1995, pp. 1481–9.

Adams, Rachel, *Sideshow U.S.A.: Freaks and the American Cultural Imagination*, Chicago: University of Chicago Press, 2001.

Aldrovandi, Ulysses, *Monstrorum Historia*, Bologna: N. Tebaldinus, 1642.

Altick, Richard, *The Shows of London*, London: Harvard University Press, 1978.

Aristotle, *Generation of Animals*, trans. by A.L. Peck, London: Heinemann, 1943.

—— *Politics*, trans. by B. Jowett, in *The Complete Works of Aristotle*, ed. by Jonathan Barnes, Princeton: Princeton University Press, 1984.

St Augustine, *City of God*, trans. by J.W.C. Wand, London: Oxford University Press, 1963.

Baltrusaitis, Jurgis, *Aberrations*, trans. by Richard Miller, London: Oktober Books, MIT Press, 1989.

Bann, Stephen, *Frankenstein: Creation and Monstrosity*, London: Reaktion Books, 1994.

Barkan, Leonard, *Nature's Work of Art: The Human Body as Image of the World*, New Haven, CT: Yale University Press, 1975.

Barnhart, Robert (ed.), *Chambers Dictionary of Etymology*, Edinburgh: Harrap, 2000.

Barnum, P.T., *Struggles and Triumphs, or Forty Years' Recollections*, Buffalo, NY: Warren, Johnson & Co., 1871.

Barthes, Roland, *Selected Writings*, London: Fontana Press, 1982.

—— and Duisit, Lionel, 'An Introduction to the Structural Analysis of Narrative', *New Literary History* 6(2), Winter 1975, pp. 237–72.

Bartra, Roger, *The Artificial Savage: Modern Myths of the Wild Man*, Ann Arbor, MI: University of Michigan Press, 1997.

—— *Wild Men in the Looking Glass: The Mythic Origins of European Otherness*, Ann Arbor, MI: University of Michigan Press, 1994.

Batchen, Geoffrey, 'Dreams of Everyday Life', in Martha Langford (ed.), *Image and Imagination*, Montreal: McGill-Queen's University Press, 2005.

Belsay, Catherine, *Culture and the Real*, London: Routledge, 2005.

Benzaquén, Adriana, *Encounters with Wild Children: Temptation and Disappointment in the Study of Human Nature*, Montreal, McGill-Queen's University Press, 2006.

Berland, Kevin, 'Reading Character in the Face: Lavater, Socrates, and Physiognomy', *Word & Image* 9(3), July–September 1993, pp. 252–69.

Bernheimer, Richard, *Wild Men in the Middle Ages: A Study in Art, Sentiment, and Demonology*, Cambridge, MA: Harvard University Press, 1952.

Birch, Helen, 'If Looks Could Kill: Myra Hindley and the Iconography of Evil', in Helen Birch (ed.), *Moving Targets: Women, Murder and Representation*, Berkeley: University of California Press, 1994.

Biressi, Anita, *Crime, Fear and the Law in True Crime Stories*, Basingstoke: Palgrave, 2001.

Boaistuau, Pierre, *Histoires prodigieuses* (first published in French 1560), trans. by Edward Fenton as *Certaine Secrete Wonders of Nature*, London: Henry Bynneman, 1569.

Bogdan, Robert, *Freak Show: Presenting Human Oddities for Amusement and Profit*, London: University of Chicago Press, 1988.

Bordo, Susan, *Unbearable Weight: Feminism, Western Culture, and the Body*, Berkeley: University of California Press, 1993.

Braidotti, Rosie, *Metamorphoses: Towards a Materialist Theory of Becoming*, Cambridge: Polity Press, 2002.

—— *Nomadic Subjects*, New York: Columbia University Press, 1994.

Breton, David le, 'Dualism and Rennaisance: Sources for a Modern Representation of the Body', trans. by R. Scott Walker, *Diogenes* 36(142), 1988, pp. 47–69.

Brown, Bill, *The Material Unconscious*, London: Harvard University Press, 1996.

Bucknill, J.C. and Tuke, D.H., *A Manual of Psychological Medicine*, London: J. & A. Churchill, 1879 (facsimile of the 1858 edition, with an introduction by Francis J. Braceland).

Buffon, Georges-Louis Leclerc, Comte de, *Histoire Naturelle*, Amsterdam: J.H. Schneider, 1766.

Bulwer, John, *Anthropometamorphosis*, London: William Hunt, 1653.

Burrows, Adrienne and Schumacher, Iwan, *Portraits of the Insane: The Case of Dr. Diamond*, London: Quartet Books, 1990.

Butler, Judith, *Bodies that Matter: On the Discursive Limits of Sex*, London: Routledge, 1993.

Cameron, D. and Frazer, E., *The Lust to Kill: A Feminist Investigation of Sexual Murder*, New York: New York University Press, 1987.

Canguilhem, Georges, 'Monstrosity and the Monstrous', *Diogenes* 40, 1962, pp. 27–42.

—— *The Normal and the Pathological*, New York: Zone Books, 1991.

Caputi, Jane, *The Age of Sex Crime*, Bowling Green, OH: Bowling Green State University Popular Press, 1987.

—— 'The New Founding Fathers: The Lore and Lure of the Serial Killer in Contemporary Culture', in Jane Caputi, *Goddesses and Monsters*, London: University of Wisconsin Press, 2004.

Céard, Jean, *La Nature et les prodiges: l'insolite au XVIe siècle, en France*, Geneva: Librairie Droz, 1977.

Chomsky, Noam, *Language and Mind*, Cambridge: Cambridge University Press, 2006.

Chrisman, Miriam, *Lay Culture, Learned Culture: Books and Social Change in Strasbourg, 1480–1599*, New Haven, CT: Yale University Press, 1982.

Cleckley, H. *The Mask of Sanity*, St Louis, MO: C.V. Mosby, 1941.

Coffey, John, *Life After the Death of God: Michel Foucault and Postmodern Atheism*, Cambridge Papers Toward a Biblical Mind, vol. 5, no. 4, Cambridge: Cambridge University Press, 1996.

Cohen, J.J., *Monster Theory: Reading Culture*, London: University of Minneapolis Press, 1996.

Conan Doyle, Arthur, *The Complete Sherlock Holmes*, Feltham: Hamlyn, 1984.

Connolly, John, 'The Physiognomy of Insanity', *Medical Times and Gazette* 16, 1858, pp. 2–4 and 56–8.

Cousins, Mark, 'Disabling Beauty', *Portfolio Magazine* 30, December 1999, pp. 52–3.

—— and Athar, Hussain, *Michel Foucault*, London: Macmillan, 1984.

Crick, Malcolm, *Explorations in Language and Meaning: Towards a Semantic Anthropology*, London: Malaby Press, 1976.

Curtis Jr, L. Perry, *Jack the Ripper and the London Press*, London: Yale University Press, 2001.

Curtiss, Susan, *Genie: A Psycholinguistic Study of a Modern Day Wild Child*, London: Academic Press, 1977.

Cuvier, Georges,*Tableau élémentaire de l'histoire naturelle des animaux*, Paris: Baudouin, 1798 (trans. by H.M. Murtrie as *The Animal Kingdom: Arranged in Conformity with its Organization*, New York: G. & C. & H. Carvill, 1831).

da Vinci, Leonardo, 'Of the Order to be Observed in Study', in Edward MacCurdy (ed.), *The Notebooks of Leonardo da Vinci*, New York: George Brazilier, 1958.

Darwin, Charles, *The Descent of Man and Selection in Relation to Sex*, New York: D. Appleton & Co., 1871.

—— *On the Origin of Species by Means of Natural Selection; Or the Preservation of Favoured Races in the Struggle for Life*, London: John Murray, 1859.

Davidson, Arnold I., *Foucault and his Interlocutors*, London: University of Chicago Press, 1997.

— 'The History of Horror, Abominations, Monsters and the Unnatural', in Arnold I. Davidson (ed.), *The Emergence of Sexuality: Historical Epistemology and the Formation of Concepts*, London: Harvard University Press, 2002.

Davis, Lennard, 'Constructing Normalcy: The Bell Curve, the Novel and the Invention of the Disabled Body in the Nineteenth Century', in Lennard Davis (ed.), *The Disability Studies Reader*, London: CRC Press, 2006.

Debord, Guy, *Society of the Spectacle and Other Films*, London: Rebel Press, 1992.

della Porta, Giambattista, *De Humana Physiognomonia, Libri IIII*, Vici Æquensis: Apud J. Cacchium, 1586.

Dietz, Mary Lorenz, 'Killing Sequentially: Expanding the Parameters of the Conceptualization of Serial and Mass Murder', in Thomas O'Reilly Fleming (ed.), *Serial and Mass Murder*, Toronto: Canadian Scholar's Press, 1996.

Dorrian, Mark, 'Monstrosity Today', *Artifice* 5, 1996, pp. 48–59.

— 'On the Monstrous and the Grotesque', *Word & Image* 16(3), 2000, pp. 310–17.

Douard, John, 'Loathing the Sinner, Medicalizing the Sin: Why Sexually Violent Predator Statutes are Unjust', *International Journal of Law and Psychiatry* 30(1), 2007, pp. 36–48.

Douglas, John E., Ressler, R. et al., 'Criminal Profiling from Crime Scene Analysis', *Behavioral Sciences and the Law* 4(4), 1986, pp. 401–21.

— et al. (eds), *Crime Classification Manual: A Standard System for Investigating and Classifying Violent Crimes*, Oxford: Maxwell Macmillan International, 1992.

Douglas, Mary, *Natural Symbols: Explorations in Cosmology*, London: Routledge, 1996.

— *Purity and Danger*, London: Routledge, 1966.

Douthwaite, Julia, *The Wild Girl, Natural Man and the Monster: Dangerous Experiments in the Age of Enlightenment*, Chicago: University of Chicago Press, 2002.

Dudley, E. and Novak, M., *The Wild Man Within*, Pittsburgh: Pittsburgh University Press, 1972.

Durbach, Naja, *Spectacle of Deformity: Freak Shows and Modern British Culture*, London: University of California Press, 2010.

Ebert, Thomas G., *A Social History of the Asylum: Mental Illness and its Treatment in the Late 19th and Early 20th Century*, Bristol, IN: Wyndham Hall Press, 1999.

Edwards, Claire and Imrie, Rob, 'Disability and Bodies as Bearers of Value', *Sociology* 37, 2003, pp. 239–56.

Edwards, Elizabeth (ed.), *Anthropology and Photography: 1860–1920*,

London: Yale University Press in association with the Royal Anthropological Institute, 1992.

Edwards, Martha, 'Constructions of Physical Disability in the Ancient Greek World: The Community Concept', in David Mitchell and Sharon Snyder (eds), *The Body and Physical Difference: Discourses of Disability*, Ann Arbor, MI: University of Michigan Press, 2000.

Evans, Elizabeth C., 'Physiognomics in the Ancient World', *Transactions of the American Philosophical Society*, New Series 59(5), 1969, pp. 1–101.

Evans, Jonathan, *Treves and the Elephant Man*, London: Royal London Hospital, 2003.

Fabian, Johannes, *Time and the Work of Anthropology: Critical Essays, 1971–1991*, London: Routledge, 1991.

Fahy, Thomas, *Freak Shows and the Modern American Imagination*, Basingstoke: Palgrave Macmillan, 2006.

Fielder, Lesley, *Freaks: Myths and Images of the Secret Self*, London: Penguin, 1978.

Foucault, Michel, *Les Anormaux, cours au Collége de France 1974–5*, trans. by Graham Burchill as *Abnormal*, New York: Picador, 2003.

—— *The Archeology of Knowledge*, New York: Pantheon Books, 1972.

—— *The Birth of the Clinic*, London: Routledge, 1989.

—— 'The Dangerous Individual', in Michel Foucault, *Philosophy, Culture and Other Writings, 1977–1984*, ed. by Lawrence Kritzman, trans. by Alan Sheridan, New York: Routledge, 1988.

—— *Discipline and Punish: The Birth of the Prison*, trans. by Alan Sheridan, London: Penguin Books, 1977.

—— *Foucault Live, Interviews 1961–1984*, ed. by Sylvere Lotringer, trans. by Lysa Hochroth and John Johnston, New York: Semiotext(e), 1989.

—— *Madness and Civilization*, trans. by Richard Howard, London: Routledge, 2001.

—— *The Order of Things*, London: Routledge, 1989.

—— 'A Preface to Transgression,' in Michel Foucault, *Language, Counter-memory, Practice*, ed. by Donald F. Bouchard, trans. by Donald F. Bouchard and Sherry Simon, Ithaca, NY: Cornell University Press, 1977.

Freedburg, David, *The Power of Images: Studies in the History and Theory of Response*, Chicago: University of Chicago Press, 1989.

Friedman, John Block, 'Cultural Conflicts in Medieval World Maps', in Stuart B. Schwartz (ed.), *Implicit Understandings: Observing, Reporting and Reflecting on the Encounters between Europeans and Other People in the Early Modern Era*, Cambridge: Cambridge University Press, 1995.

—— *The Monstrous Races in Medieval Art and Thought*, Cambridge, MA: Harvard University Press, 1981.

Fudge, Erica, *Animal*, London: Reaktion Books, 2002.

Fuss, Diana, 'Monsters of Perversion: Jeffrey Dahmer and the Silence of the Lambs', in Marjorie Garber, Jann Matlock and Rebecca L. Walkowitz (eds), *Media Spectacles*, London: Routledge, 1993.

Galton, Francis, 'Composite Portraits, Made by Combining Those of Many Different Persons into a Single Resultant Figure,' *Journal of the Anthropological Institute of Great Britain and Ireland* 8, 19 April 1878, pp. 132–44.

—— *Inquiries into Human Faculty*, London: Eugenics Society, 1883.

Garland, Robert, *The Eye of the Beholder: Deformity and Disability in the Graeco-Roman World*, London: Duckworth, 1995.

Garland-Thomson, Rosemarie, *Extraordinary Bodies, Figuring Physical Disability in American Culture and Literature*, New York: Columbia University Press, 1997.

—— (ed.), *Freakery: Cultural Spectacles of the Extraordinary Body*, New York: New York University Press, 1996.

Geoffroy de St Hilaire, Etienne, *Philosophie anatomique: des monstruosités humaines, ouvrage contenant une classification des monstres . . .*, Paris: Auteur, 2 vols, 1818–22.

Geoffroy de St Hilaire, Isidore, *Histoire générale et particulière des anomalies de l'organisation chez l'homme et les animaux*, vol. 1, Paris: J.B. Baillière, 1832.

—— *Traité de tératologie*, vol. 1, Paris: J.B. Bailliere,1836.

Gilman, Sander, *Difference and Pathlogy: Stereotypes of Sexuality, Race and Madness*, London: Cornell University Press, 1985.

—— *The Face of Madness: Hugh W. Diamond and the Origin of Psychiatric Photography*, London: Routledge, 1982.

—— *Seeing the Insane: A Cultural History of Madness*, Chichester: Wiley, 1985.

Glacken, Terence, *Traces on the Rhodean Shore: Nature and Culture in Western Thought from Ancient Times to the End of the Eighteenth Century*, Berkeley: University of California Press, 1967.

Gombrich, E.H., *The Story of Art*, London: Phaidon, 2003.

Gomel, Elana, 'Written in Blood: Serial Killing and Narratives of Identity', *Post-Identity* 2(1), 1999, pp. 24–71.

Gould, G.M. and Pyle, W.L., *Anomalies and Curiosities of Medicine*, Philadelphia: W.B. Saunders, 1897.

Graham, P. and Oehlshlaeger, F.H., *Articulating the Elephant Man*, London: Johns Hopkins University Press, 1992.

Green, David, 'On Foucault: Disciplinary Power and Photography', in Jessica Evans (ed.), *The Camerawork Essays: Context and Meaning In Photography*, London: Rivers Oram, 1997.

— 'Veins of Resemblance: Photography and Eugenics', *Oxford Art Journal* 7(2), 1984, pp. 3–16.

Halberstam, Judith, *Skin Shows: Gothic Horror and the Technology of Monsters*, London: Duke University Press, 1995.

— 'Skinflick: Posthuman Gender in Jonathan Demme's The Silence of the Lambs', *Camera Obscura* 27, September 1991, pp. 37–52.

Halsted, D.G., *A Doctor in the Nineties*, London: Christopher Johnson, 1959.

Hamburger, Viktor, 'Monsters in Nature', *Ciba Symposia* 9, 1947, pp. 966–83.

Hamilton, Peter and Hargreaves, Roger, *The Beautiful and the Damned: The Creation of Identity in Nineteenth Century Photography*, London: Lund Humphries and National Portrait Gallery, 2001.

Hannavy, John, *Encyclopedia of Nineteenth-Century Photography*, London: Routledge, 2008.

Hare, Robert, 'Psychopathy: A Clinical Construct whose Time Has Come', *Criminal Justice and Behavior* 23(1), 1996, pp. 25–54.

— *Without Conscience: The Disturbing World of the Psychopaths Among Us*, New York: Guilford Press, 1999.

Hartley, Lucy, *Physiognomy and the Meaning of Expression in Nineteenth-Century Culture*, Cambridge: Cambridge University Press, 2001.

Higden, Ranulph, *Polycronicon*, trans. by John Trevisa, London: William Caxton, 1482.

Higgs Strickland, Debra, *Saracens, Demons, and Jews: Making Monsters in Medieval Art*, Princeton: Princeton University Press, 2003.

Hirst, P. and Woolley, P. *Social Relations and Human Attributes*, London: Tavistock, 1982.

Holloway, Wendy, '"I Just Wanted to Kill a Woman" Why? The Ripper and Male Sexuality', *New Feminist Review* 9, 1981, pp. 33–40.

Holmes, Ronald and Holmes, Stephen, *Profiling Violent Crimes: An Investigative Tool*, London: Sage, 2008.

Horigan, Stephen, *Nature and Culture in Western Discourses*, London: Routledge, 1988.

Horn, David, *The Criminal Body: Lombroso and the Anatomy of Deviance*, London: Routledge, 2003.

Horton, David M. and Rich, Katherine E., *The Criminal Anthropological Articles of Cesare Lombroso Published in the English Language Periodical Literature During the Late 19th and Early 20th Centuries*, New York: Edwin Mellen Press, 2004.

Howell, Michael and Ford, Peter, *The True History of the Elephant Man*, London: Allison & Busby, 1980.

Huet, Marie-Hélène, *Monstrous Imagination*, London: Harvard University Press, 1993.

Hugo, Victor, *The Hunchback of Notre Dame*, ed. and trans. by Robin Waterfield, London: Puffin, 1996.
Husband, Timothy, *The Wild Man, Medieval Myth and Symbolism*, New York: Museum of Metropolitan Art, 1980.
Huxley, Thomas Henry, *Evidence as to Man's Place in Nature*, New York: D. Appleton & Co., 1863.
Isidore of Seville, 'The Medical Writings', trans. by W.D. Sharpe, in *Transactions of the American Philosophical Society* 54(2), 1964, pp. 1–75.
Jackson, Rosemary, *Fantasy: The Literature of Subversion*, London: Routledge, 1988.
Jenkins, Philip, 'Catch Me Before I Kill More: Seriality as Modern Monstrosity', *Cultural Analysis* 2, 2002, pp. 1–17.
— *Intimate Enemies: Moral Panics in Contemporary Great Britain*, Hawthorne, NY: Aldine de Gruyter, 1992.
— *Using Murder: The Social Construction of Serial Homicide*, Hawthorne, NY: Aldine de Gruyter, 1994.
Jewkes, Yvonne, *Media and Crime*, London: Sage, 2004.
Jordanova, Ludmilla, 'Reading Faces in the Nineteenth Century', *Art History* 13(4), December 1990, pp. 570–5.
Kearney, Richard, *Strangers, Gods and Monsters: Interpreting Otherness*, London: Routledge, 2003.
Kekes, John, 'Understanding Evil', *American Philosophical Quarterly* 25(1), January 1988, pp. 13–24.
Kemp, Martin, '"A Perfect and Faithful Record": Mind and Body in Medical Photography before 1900', in Ann Thomas (ed.), *Beauty of Another Order: Photography in Science*, London: Yale University Press, 1997.
Kristeva, Julia, *Powers of Horror*, New York: Columbia University Press, 1982.
— *Strangers to Ourselves*, New York: Columbia University Press, 1991.
Kwakkelstein, Michael W., 'Leonardo da Vinci's Grotesque Heads and the Breaking of the Physiognomic Mould', *Journal of the Warburg and Courtauld Institutes* 54, 1991, pp. 127–36.
Lacan, Jacques, *Écrits*, Paris: Seuil, 1966.
— *Écrits: A Selection*, trans. by Alan Sheridan, London: Tavistock, 1977.
Lalvani, Suren, *Photography, Vision and the Production of Modern Bodies*, New York: SUNY Press, 1996.
Landucci, Luca, *A Florentine Diary from 1450 to 1516 by Luca Landucci, Continued by an Anonymous Writer Until 1542, With Notes by Iodoco Del Badia*, trans. by Alice de Rosen Jervis, New York: Dutton, 1927.
Laplanche, Jean, 'The Unfinished Copernican Revolution', in Jean

Laplanche, *Essays on Otherness*, ed. by John Fletcher, London: Routledge, 1988.

Lavater, Johann Kaspar, *Physiognomische Fragmente: Essays on Physiognomy; for the Promotion of the Knowledge and the Love of Mankind*, trans by Thomas Holcroft, London: G.G.J. & J. Robinson, 4 vols, 1789.

Lemagny, Jean-Claude and Rouillé, André (eds), *A History of Photography: Social and Cultural Perspectives*, trans. by Janet Lloyd, Cambridge: Cambridge University Press, 1987.

Lenneberg, E.H., *Biological Foundations of Language*, London: Wiley, 1967.

Lévi-Strauss, Claude, *The Elementary Structures of Kinship*, London: Eyre and Spottiswoode, 1969.

Levinas, Emmanuel, 'The Trace of the Other', in William McNeill and Karen Feldman (eds), *Continental Philosophy: An Anthology*, Oxford: Blackwell, 1998.

Lindsay, Jeff, *Darkly Dreaming Dexter*, London: Orion Books, 2004.

Linneaus, Caroleus, *Systema Naturae*, trans. by M.S.J. Engel-Ledeboer and H. Engel, Niewwkoop: B de Graaf, 1964 (facsimile of the first edition, 1735).

Lombroso, Cesare, *Criminal Man*, trans. and ed. by Mary Gibson and Nicole Hahn Rafter, London: Duke University Press, 2006.

— *Criminal Man According to the Classification of Cesare Lombroso. Briefly Summarised by his Daughter Gina Lombroso Ferrero. With an Introduction by Cesare Lombroso*, London: G.P. Puttnams, 1911.

Lovejoy, Arthur O., *The Great Chain of Being: A Study of the History of an Idea*, Cambridge, MA: Harvard University Press, 1936.

Lyall, Charles, *Geological Evidences of the Antiquity of Man*, Philadelphia: George W. Childs, 1863.

Lycosthenes, Conrad, *Prodigiorum ac Ostentorum Chronicon* (first published 1557), trans. by Stephen Bateman as *The Doome Calling All Men to the Judgement: Wherein Are Contayned For the Most Parte All the Straunge Prodigies Hapened In the Worlde*, London: Ralph Nubery, 1581.

Lykke, Nina and Braidotti, Rosi (eds), *Between Monsters, Goddesses and Cyborgs: Feminist Confrontations with Science, Medicine and Cyberspace*, London: Zed Books, 1996.

McCrindle, J.W., *Ancient India as Described by Ctesias the Knidian*, Calcutta: Thacker, Spink & Co., 1882.

McGrath, Roberta, 'Medical Police', *10:8* 14, 1984, pp. 13–18.

Malik, Kenan, *The Meaning of Race: Race, History and Culture in Western Society*, New York: New York University Press, 1996.

Malson, Lucien, *Wolf Children*, London: New Left Books, 1972.

Masters, Brian, *Killing for Company: The Case of Dennis Nilsen*, London: Arrow Books, 1995.

Michaud, Stephen and Aynesworth, Hugh, *The Only Living Witness: The True Story of Serial Sex Killer, Ted Bundy*, Irving, TX: Authorlink, 1999.
— and Aynesworth, Hugh, *Ted Bundy: Conversations with a Killer*, New York: Signet, 1989.
Miller, Fred, 'The State and the Community in Aristotle's *Politics*', *Reason Papers* 1, 1974, pp. 61–3, available online at: www.reasonpapers.com/pdf/01/rp_1_5.pdf (accessed 20 December 2012).
Mitchell, Michael, *Monsters: Human Freaks in America's Gilded Age, the Photographs of Chas. Eisenmann*, Toronto: ECW Press, 2002.
Montague, Ashley, *The Elephant Man: A Study in Human Dignity*, London: Allison & Busby, 1972.
Morison, Sir Alexander, *The Physiognomy of Mental Diseases*, London: published for the author, 1840.
Newton, Michael, *Savage Girls and Wild Boys: A History of Feral Children*, London: Faber & Faber, 2002.
Niccoli, Ottavia, *Prophecy and People in Renaissance Italy*, trans. by Lydia Cochrane, Chicago: University of Chicago Press, 1990.
Norman, Tom, *The Penny Showman: Memoirs of Tom Norman 'Silver King'*, ed. by George Barnum Norman-Noakes, London: Norman-Noakes, 1985.
Norris, Joel, *Serial Killers: The Growing Menace*, New York: Doubleday, 1988.
Novak, Daniel, 'A Model Jew: Literary Photographs and the Jewish Body in *Daniel Deronda*', *Representations* 85, Winter 2004, pp. 58–97.
O'Connor, Erin, *Raw Material: Producing Pathology in Victorian Culture*, Durham, NC: Duke University Press, 2001.
Packard, F.R., *The Life and Times of Ambroise Paré*, Oxford: Oxford University Press, 1921.
Paré, Ambroise, *Monstres et Prodiges; On Monsters and Marvels*, trans. by Janis Pallister, Chicago: University of Chicago Press, 1982.
Park, Katherine and Daston, Lorraine, *Wonders and the Order of Nature*, New York: Zone Books, 1998.
Paton, W.R., *The Greek Anthology*, book 9, vol. 3, London: Loeb Classical Library, Heinemann, 1917.
Pinel, Philippe, *A Treatise on Insanity*, trans. by D.D. Davis, London: Cadell & Davies, 1806.
Pliny the Elder, *Natural History*, trans. by H. Rackham, London: Loeb Classical Library, Harvard University Press, 1999.
Poe, Edgar Allan, *The Murders in the Rue Morgue: The Dupin Tales*, ed. by Matthew Pearl, London: Vintage Books, 2006.
Porter, Roy, 'History of the Body', in Peter Burke (ed.), *New Perspectives on Historical Writing*, Cambridge: Polity Press, 1991.

Potts, Alex, *Flesh and the Ideal: Winklemann and the Origins of Art History*, New Haven, CT: Yale University Press, 1994.
Prichard, J.C., *A Treatise on Insanity and Other Disorders Affecting the Mind*, New York: Arno, 1837.
Purcell, Rosamund, *Special Cases*, San Francisco: Chronicle Books, 1997.
Rawlinson, H.G., *Intercourse between India and the Western World from the Earliest Times to the Fall of Rome*, Cambridge: Cambridge University Press, 1916.
Ritvo, Harriett, *The Platypus and the Mermaid and Other Figments of the Classifying Imagination*, Cambridge, MA: Harvard University Press, 1997.
Rose, Gillian, *Visual Methodologies*, London: Sage, 2001.
Ross, Stephanie, 'Painting the Passions: Charles LeBrun's Conference Sur L'Expression', *Journal of the History of Ideas* 45(1), January–March 1984, pp. 25–47.
Rousseau, Jean-Jacques, *A Discourse upon the Origin and Foundation of the Inequality among Mankind*, London: R. & J. Dodsley, 1761.
Rule, Ann, *The Stranger Beside Me*, London: Warner, 1994.
Said, Edward, *Orientalism*, London: Routledge and Kegan Paul, 1978.
Schmid, David, *Natural Born Celebrities: Serial Killers in American Culture*, London: University of Chicago Press, 2005.
Sekula, Alan, 'The Body and the Archive', in Richard Bolton (ed.), *Contest of Meaning*, London: MIT Press, 1996.
Seltzer, Mark, *Serial Killers: Death and Life in America's Wound Culture*, London: Routledge, 1998.
Sharpe, Andrew, 'Structured Like a Monster: Understanding Human Difference Through a Legal Category', *Law and Critique* 18(2), 2007, pp. 207–28.
Shaviro, Steven, *The Cinematic Body*, Minneapolis: University of Minnesota Press, 1993.
Sheehan, James and Sosna, Morton (eds), *The Boundaries of Humanity: Humans, Animals, Machines*, Berkeley: University of California Press, 1991.
Shelley, Mary, *Frankenstein; or, The Modern Prometheus*, London: Lackington, Hughes, Harding, 1818.
Sheridan, Alan, *Michel Foucault: The Will to Truth*, London: Tavistock Publications, 1980.
Shildrick, Margrit, *Embodying the Monster*, London: Sage, 2002.
Shortland, Michael, 'Skin Deep: Barthes, Lavater and the Legible Body', *Economy and Society* 14(3), August 1985, pp. 290–1.
Skrapec, Candice A. 'Phenomenology and Serial Murder', *Homicide Studies* 5(1), 2001, pp. 46–63.
Smith, Joan, *Misogynies*, London: Faber & Faber, 1989.
Sontag, Susan, 'The Anthropologist as Hero', in Eugene Hayes (ed.),

Claude Lévi-Strauss: The Anthropologist as Hero, Cambridge, MA: MIT Press, 1970.

Soper, Kate, *What Is Nature? Culture, Politics and the Non-human*, Oxford: Blackwell, 1995.

Stallybrass, Peter and White, Allon, *The Politics and Poetics of Transgression*, London: Methuen, 1986.

Tagg, John, *The Burden of Representation: Essays on Photographies and Histories*, Basingstoke: Macmillan, 1988.

—— 'Power and Photography – A Means of Surveillance: the Photograph as Evidence in Law', in Tony Bennett, Graham Martin et al. (eds), *Culture, Ideology and Social Process: A Reader*, London: Batsford Academic and Educational in association with Open University Press, 1981.

Thompson, Della (ed.), *Concise Oxford English Dictionary*, Oxford: Clarendon Press, 1995.

Thrower, N.J.W., *Maps and Civilization: Cartography in Culture and Society*, Chicago: University of Chicago Press, 2007.

Tithecott, Richard, *Of Men and Monsters: Jeffrey Dahmer and the Construction of the Serial Killer*, Madison, WI: University of Wisconsin Press, 1997.

Treves, Frederick, *The Elephant Man and Other Reminiscences*, London: Cassell & Co., 1923.

Twine, Richard, 'Physiognomy, Phrenology and the Temporality of the Body', *Body and Society* 8(1), March 2002, pp. 67–88.

Velazco y Trianosky, Gregory, 'Savages, Wild Men, and Monstrous Races: The Social Construction of Race in the Early Modern Era', in Peggy Zeglin Brand (ed.), *Beauty Revisited*, Bloomington, IN: Indiana University Press, 2012.

Walkowitz, Judith, 'Jack the Ripper and the Myth of Male Violence', *Feminist Studies* 8, 1982, pp. 543–74.

Walton, Michael, Fineman, Robert and Walton, Phyllis, 'Of Monsters and Prodigies: The Interpretation of Birth Defects in the Sixteenth Century', *American Journal of Medical Genetics* 47(1), 1993, pp. 7–13.

Warwick, A. and Willis, M. (eds), *Jack the Ripper: Media, Culture, History*, Manchester: Manchester University Press, 2007.

White, Hayden, *The Content of the Form: Narrative Discourse and Historical Representation*, London: Johns Hopkins University Press, 1987.

—— 'The Forms of Wildness', in E. Dudley and M. Novak (eds), *The Wild Man Within*, Pittsburgh: Pittsburgh University Press, 1972.

Williams, David, *Deformed Discourse: The Function of the Monster in Medieval Thought and Literature*, Exeter: Exeter University Press, 1996.

Williams, Raymond, *Keywords: A Vocabulary of Culture and Society*, London: Fontana, 1983.
Wilson, Dudley, *Signs and Portents: Monstrous Births from the Middle Ages to the Enlightenment*, London: Routledge, 1993.
Wilson, Philip K., 'Eighteenth-Century "Monsters" and Nineteenth-Century "Freaks": Reading the Maternally Marked Child', *Literature and Medicine* 21(1), 2002, pp. 1–25.
Wittkower, Rudolf, 'Marvels of the East', in Rudolf Wittkower, *Allegory and the Migration of Symbols*, London: Thames & Hudson, 1977.
Young, Alison, *Imagining Crime*, London: Sage Publications, 1996.
— *Judging the Image: Art, Value, Law*, London: Routledge, 2005.

Newspaper and Magazine Articles

On Joseph Merrick

Carr Gomm, F.C., letters to *The Times*: 4 December 1886; 16 April 1890.

On Jack the Ripper

'News from Whitechapel', *Daily Telegraph*, 1 October 1888.

On Myra Hindley

Blanchard, Tamsin, 'Sensation as Ink and Egg are Thrown at Hindley Portrait', *Independent*, 17 September 1997, available online at: www.independent.co.uk/news/arts-sensation-as-ink-and-egg-are-thrown-at-hindley-portrait-1239892.html (accessed 4 January 2013).
Hattenstone, Simon, 'Myra, Margaret and Me', *Guardian* Weekend, 21 February 2009, p. 29.
'Icon of Evil', *Daily Star*, 16 November 2002, p. 8.
Kent, Sarah, 'Rogue's Gallery', *Time Out*, 1414, 1997, pp. 16–17.
'My Bid to Kill Moors Murderer', *Daily Mirror*, 9 January 1978, p. 5.
'Myra: Inside the Mind of a Monster', *Sun*, 18 November 2002.
'Myra May Go Free', *Daily Star*, 28 October 2002, p. 30.
'Should Myra Hindley Ever Be Freed? Opinion', *Sun*, 30 October 1997.
Stanford, Peter, 'Myra Hindley: Notorious Child Murderer Whose Protestations of Repentance Failed to Assuage Public Revulsion', *Guardian*, 15 November 2002, available online at: www.guardian.co.uk/obituaries/story/0,3604,841049,00.html (accessed 4 January 2013).
— 'Obituary: Myra Hindley: Notorious Child Murderer whose Protestations of Repentance Failed to Assuage Public Revulsion', *Guardian*, 16 November 2002, available online at: www.guardian.co.uk/news/2002/nov/16/guardianobituaries.ukcrime (accessed 4 January 2013).

Teichmann, Esther, 'Myra, Margaret and Me, *Guardian Weekend*, 21 February 2009.

Thorpe, Vanessa, 'Hindley Picture is a Sensation Too Far for Artist Ayres', *Independent*, 21 September 1997, available online at: www.independent.co.uk/news/hindley-picture-is-a-sensation-too-far-for-artist-ayres-1240388.html (accessed 4 January 2013).

Tucker, Carol, 'Constructing Images of Serial Killers', *University of Southern California Chronicle*, 10 November 1997.

'Victim's Mother's Desperate Plea', *Telegraph*, 10 June 2008, available online at: www.telegraph.co.uk/news/2105864/Myra-Hindley-Victim's-mother's-desperate-plea.html (accessed 20 December 2012).

Walker, John A., 'Marcus Harvey's Sick Disgusting Painting of Myra Hindley: A Semiotic Analysis', *Tate* 14, 1998, pp. 56–7.

Ted Bundy

Bremner, Charles, 'String of Confessions Fails to Stay Killer's Execution; Ted Bundy', *The Times*, 24 January 1989.

'Bundy Interview Seen After Execution', *The Times*, 26 January 1989.

'Death of the Devil', *Daily Express*, 25 January 1989.

Lamar, Jacob, 'I Deserve Punishment', *Time Magazine*, 6 February 1989.

Schwarz, Jerry, 'Cheers as Bundy Goes to his Death', *Independent*, 25 January 1989.

Stewart, Helen, 'Ted Bundy: Natural Porn Killer', *Sunday Times*, 13 August 2006.

Other

Edgar, David, 'Seeing Isn't Believing', *Sunday Times*, 22 August 1993.

Flanagan, Padraic, 'I'm No Monster: I Could Have Killed Them', *Daily Express*, 8 May 2008, pp. 8–9.

'Fritzl Lodger Set to Tell Police: I Saw the Cellar Monster's Wife Help Take Food to Sex Slave Dungeon', *Daily Mail*, 1 May 2008, available online at: www.dailymail.co.uk/news/article-563326/Fritzl-lodger-set-tell-police-I-saw-cellar-monsters-wife-help-food-sex-slave-dungeon.html (accessed 4 January 2013).

Grice, Elizabeth, 'Cry of an Enfant Sauvage', *Daily Telegraph*, 17 July 2006, available online at: www.telegraph.co.uk/culture/tvandradio/3653890/Cry-of-an-enfant-sauvage.html (accessed 20 December 2012).

'I'm No Monster', *Daily Mirror*, 7 May 2008, p. 5.

Jones, David, 'He Should Be Condemned to Live', *Daily Mail*, 16 March 2012, available online at: www.dailymail.co.uk/news/article–2116178/Ian-Brady-Furious-reaction-Moors-murderers-

victims-decision-allow-public-hearing-battle-starve-death.html (accessed 20 December 2012).
Kemp, Martin, 'The Art of Physiognomy', *Guardian*, 23 April 2007, available online at: http://blogs.guardian.co.uk/art/2007/04/the_art_of_physiognomy.html (accessed 15 August 2008).
Morrison, Helen, 'Partners in Savagery', *The Times*, 7 May 2004.
Porter, Roy, 'Lunatic Ideas and the Truth about Asylums', *Times Higher Education*, 10 October 1997, available online at: www.timeshighereducation.co.uk/story.asp?storyCode=103990&sectioncode=26 (accessed 20 December 2012).
Smith, Joan, 'The Fear and the Fantasy', *Guardian*, 18 June 1993.
Troup, John, 'Monster Copied de Niro', *Sun*, 1 August 2002, available online at: www.thesun.co.uk/sol/homepage/news/80693/monster-copied-De-Niro.html (accessed 14 January 2013).

Film and Television

'2012 Hindley Image Use Condemned', BBC News, 25 August 2008, available online at: http://news.bbc.co.uk/1/hi/uk/7580261.stm.
A & E Biography Channel, 'Biography of Ted Bundy', part 1 available online at: http://www.youtube.com/watch?v=sdq6ViwYHLA (accessed 4 January 2013).
Bodyshock television documentary series, Mentorn/Channel 4, episodes: 'I Am the Elephant Man', 7 April 2008; 'Born With Two Heads', 20 February 2006; 'Riddle of the Elephant Man', 5 January 2004; 'Wild Child', 15 December 2003.
Born to Kill television documentary series, Sky three television, episodes: 'Harold Shipman', 31 March 2009; 'Fred West', 19 March 2009; 'Myra Hindley', 2 April 2009; 'Jeffrey Dahmer', 9 April 2009.
'Breivik "Cut Contact with Friends" in Run-up to Attacks', BBC Europe online, 29 May 2012, available online at: www.bbc.co.uk/news/world-europe–18248116 (accessed 20 December 2012).
'Bundy Confession Tapes Revealed for the First Time', kirovtv.com, 9 February 2005, available online at: www.kirotv.com/news/4182402/detail.html.
The Elephant Man, dir. David Lynch, EMI Films, 1980, 118 min.
Extraordinary People, 'The Woman with Giant Legs', *Centini*, first broadcast on Channel 5, 21 August 2008.
Feral Children, Dragonfly Film and Television Productions, first shown in the UK on Animal Planet: episode 1, 'The Monkey Boy of Uganda', 24 September 2012, and episode 2, 'The Dog-Girl of Ukraine', 1 October 2012.
Freaks, dir. Tod Browning, Metro Goldwyn Mayer, 1932.
Fred and Rose – the West Murders, three-part documentary series

produced by Creative Consortium in association with United Productions. Broadcast on Channel 5, 2–4 October 2001.

Interview with Ed Stagg, BBC Midland Radio, 21 September 2012, available online at: http://raisedwild.files.wordpress.com/2012/10/bbc-midlands-hud_discovery-feral-children.mp3 (accessed 9 November 2012).

Jack the Ripper's Face 'Revealed', television documentary, Channel 5, 21 November 2006.

'Jack the Ripper's Face Revealed', BBC News, 20 November 2006, available online at: http://news.bbc.co.uk/1/hi/uk/6164544.stm.

Jensen!, RTL5, 23 April 2007, available online at: www.rtl.nl/components/shows/jensen/169_anamorf/miMedia/2007/week17/ma_gasten_23apr.avi_plain.xml (accessed 9 November 2012).

Mind of a Murderer, three-part documentary, BBC television, 4, 11 and 18 September 2001.

Mindshock: Feral Children, television documentary, Channel 4, 17 June 2006.

'Myra Hindley: A Hate Figure', BBC News Online, 15 November 2012, available online at: http://news.bbc.co.uk/1/hi/uk/581580.stm (accessed 4 January 2013).

'Norway's Mass Killer Breivik Declared Sane', BBC News Online, 10 April 2012, available online at: www.bbc.co.uk/news/world-europe-17663958 (accessed 4 January 2013).

'Norwegian Far Right Defend Breivik's Views on Islam', BBC News Online, 5 June 2012, available online at: www.bbc.co.uk/news/world-europe-18332442 (accessed 4 January 2013).

'On this Day 1966: Moors Murderers Jailed for Life', BBC News Online (television report, first broadcast 6 May 1966), available online at: http://news.bbc.co.uk/onthisday/hi/dates/stories/may/6/newsid_2512000/2512119.stm (accessed 4 January 2013).

The True Story of the Elephant Man, QED, BBC1, 28 May 1997.

Index

abject, the/abjection 156–7
abnormality/abnormal 54, 68, 78, 79, 80, 83, 86, 100, 108, 120, 121, 139, 147, 162
Abnormal, The (Foucault) 3, 28, 48, 79, 164
Adams, Rachel 89, 90
Alexander the Great 12, 36, 37
alien/alienation 18, 28, 91, 148, 153, 155, 157, 158, 165
Alien (Ridley Scott) 5
Altick, Richard 80
appearance 1, 3, 6, 13, 15, 35, 51, 61, 64, 67, 70–1, 73, 74, 75, 78, 79–82, 85, 98, 99, 107, 112–14, 118, 120, 123, 125, 126, 131, 133, 139, 143–4, 145, 148, 149, 151, 152–5, 159–60, 162–3
Aristotle 28, 31, 32, 61, 100
Arnstein Bible *8*, 9–11, 21
astrology 5, 47–9, 61, 125
Augustine, Saint 14

Barkan, Leonard 49
Barnum, P.T. 81, 82, 85, 86, 88, 97
Barthes, Roland 25, 92, 127–8, 142
Batchen, Geoffrey 93
bearded lady 81, 82, 85, *95*, *96*, 97
Benjamin, Ashbury 86–9, *88*
Benzaquén, Adriana 42–3
Bernheimer, Richard 35, 39
Bertillon, Alphonse 70, 137
Birch, Helen 136
Blemmaye 12, 16
body, the 1, 6, 10, 25, 26, 47–50, 52, 59, 60, 61, 62, 63, 65, 67, 68, 70, 73, 89, 99, 100–2, 104, 112, 114, 116, 125, 128, 145; of the monster 5, 9, 11, 17, 18, 51, 54–8, 60, 61, 81, 90, 140, 144, 158
Bogdan, Robert 83, 87, 94
boundary 5, 11, 20, 26, 27, 28, 29, 31, 39, 40, 41, 43, 46, 48, 78, 82, 155, 156
Brady, Ian 130, 135–6, *137*
Breivik, Anders 2, 7, 128, 145, 146, 158–63, 165
Bucknill, John Charles, Sir 74–5
Bundy, Ted 7, 145, 148–58, 160, 162, 163, 165, 166

Canguilhem, Georges 3, 4, 5, 20, 79, 80, 101, 110, 111, 112, 147, 155, 165
Caputi, Jane 134
Carr Gomm, F.C. 105, 114, 115, 124
carte de visite 80, 89, 92–4, 99, 118, 119, 120, 122, 124
celebrity 93, 94, 153, 155
Chain of Being, the 31–2
character 6, 26, 36, 47, 49, 61, 62–3, 65, 68, 70, 80, 95, 96, 101, 104, 105, 107, 109, 112, 114, 115, 120–2, 124, 147, 149, 153, 159; monstrosity of 4, 79, 112, 126, 144, 145, 148, 164
Christians 5, 12, 17, 19, 22, 60, 150
civilization/civilized 1, 5, 9, 11,

16, 21, 27, 28, 31, 33–7, 40, 43, 49, 67, 74, 78, 83, 120, 131, 165
classification/classify 18, 31–4, 48, 49, 63, 67, 70, 75, 78, 79, 81, 111, 112, 155, 156
criminality/criminal 6, 28, 47, 61, 67–8, 70–3, 75, 104, 107, 125, 126–8, 129, 130, 131, 133, 136, 137, 141, 144, 145–8, 152, 154–7, 159, 161, 162, 165, 166
Ctesias 12, 14, 15
culture 2, 5, 9, 10, 11, 13–21, 24, 26, 27–31, 34, 38, 40, 43, 47, 52, 61, 62, 67, 78, 81, 82, 90, 92, 108, 109, 125, 128, 134, 135, 142, 149, 154, 161, 162, 166
customs 1, 11, 15, 16
Cuvier, Georges 33, 34, 41, 67
cynocephali 11, 13, 16

da Vinci, Leonardo 49, *50*, 62, *63*, 67
Damiens, Robert 145, 157
'The Dangerous Individual' 3, 146, 147, 158
Darwin, Charles 33, 40, 41, 67, 71, 86, 114
Daston, Lorraine 24
Davis, Lennard 79, 86, 87, 99, 100, 101
deformity/deformed 4, 5, 6, 10, 18, 20, 48, 50, 54, 55, 58, 59, 60, 61, 62, 65, 79, 80, 83, 84, 91, 99, 100–2, 103, 104, 105, 107, 108, 109, 111–12, 114–15, 118–24, 137, 155
Descartes, René 64, 73
Devere, Jane (Madame Devere) 85, 94–7
deviant/deviance 17, 21, 48, 51, 61, 67, 68, 79, 81, 83, 89, 96–7, 116, 137, 147, 151, 155
difference 1, 11, 15, 17, 18, 24, 26, 34, 58, 70, 79, 80, 82, 83, 84, 85, 89–92, 93, 99, 100, 101, 102, 105, 110, 116, 127, 160, 166
disability/disabled 5, 6, 18, 79, 82, 86–7, 90, 99–102, 106
'Discobolus' ('Discus Thrower') 52, *53*
disorder 5, 16, 28, 48, 49, 60, 61, 74, 90, 101, 104, 111, 112, 116, 132, 145, 149, 155, 158, 166
Dobson, James 150–2
dogs 11, 44, 45, 46, 59, 81; dog-faced/dog-headed 1, 10, 13, 14, 35, *84*, 85
Douglas, Mary 47
Durbach, Nadja 86, 97, 102, 108, 109

Eisenmann, Charles *84*, 86, 93, *95*, *96*, *98*
'Elephant Man', the *see* Merrick, Joseph
Evans, Jonathan 111–12
evil 18, 20, 60, 68, 71, 125, 128–9, 132, 135, 136, 137, 139, 140, 144, 145, 149, 150, 151, 155, 161, 162, 166
Extraordinary People 102–3

female 6, 16, 39, 48, 57, 58, 59, 68, 85, 94, 95, 96, 135, 139, 149, 150
feral children 5, 26, 27, 28, 29, 31, 32, 41–6
Foucault, Michel 2, 3, 4, 17, 19, 21, 28, 48, 54, 67, 78, 79, 80, 100, 103, 104, 105, 110, 112, 124, 125, 127, 145, 146, 147, 148, 156, 157, 158, 162, 164, 166
freak/freak show 5, 6, 41, 79–87, 89–94, 96, 97, 99, 102–3, 104, 105, 107, 108, 109, 110, 112, 113, 114, 115, 116, 120, 122, 123, 127, 145

Friedman, John Block 12, 15, 24

Galton, Francis 67, 68, *69*
Garland-Thomson, Rosmarie 81, 82, 83, 90
Geoffroy de St Hilaire, Etienne and Isidore 79, 110, 111, 112
Gilman, Sander 116
Greece/Greek 11, 13, 14, 15, 16, 18, 26, 27–8, 47, 51–3, 61, 65, 87, 100, 164

hierarchy/hierarchical 18, 27, 31, 32, 33, 34, 35, 47, 92, 121
Higgs Strickland, Debra 12
Hindley, Myra 6, 125, 129, 130, 135–44, 145, 151, 155, 157
Hirst, Paul 37–8, 43
Homer 16
horror 21, 114, 122, 123, 155, 156
human/animal 5, 9, 10, 11, 16, 19, 20, 21, 23, 26, 27, 28, 29, 31–5, 39, 40, 41, 43, 46, 58, 62, 64, 65, 67, 71, 83, 85, 86, 87, 97, 113, 114
human monster 1, 2, 5, 6, 9, 10, 12, 16, 17, 19, 24, 25, 27, 28, 31, 44, 49, 54, 79, 89, 90, 101, 104, 111, 127, 130, 146, 164, 165, 166
Husband, Timothy 35, 37
hybrid 9, 16, 19, 20, 40, 97, 112, 114

identity 1, 2, 3, 6, 19, 20, 26, 30, 54, 56, 65, 70, 82, 83, 89, 90, 105, 125, 126, 130, 131, 144, 147, 156, 159, 160, 161, 162, 166
insanity/insane 34, 67, 68, 70, 71, 73, 74, 75, 78, 126, 136, 146, 147, 149, 155, 160, 162, 163

Jack the Ripper 6, 125, 127, 129, 130, 131–4, 151
Jackson, Rosemary 154
Jeftichew, Fyodor *84*, 85, 94
Jenkins, Philip 129, 135, 153
Johnson, William Henry 85–7, *88*, 94
'JoJo, the Russian Dog-faced Boy' *see* Jeftichew, Fyodor

Kemp, Martin 47, 116
Kristeva, Julia 156–7

Lalvani, Suren 120
Landucci, Luca 59–60, 101
Lavater, Johann Kaspar 65–7, 71, 73
law, the/legal, 2, 3, 4, 17, 19–21, 26, 28, 30, 48, 49, 52, 71, 79, 87, 100, 104, 110, 111, 112, 125, 126, 128, 141, 145, 147, 152, 153, 155, 156, 163
Le Brun, Charles 63–5, 71, 73
'Leopard Boy', the *see* Benjamin, Ashbury
Levinas, Emmanuel 18
Linnaeus, Carolus 32–3
Lombroso, Cesare 70–3
London Hospital 105, 107, 108, 109, 110, 111, 116, *117*, 122
Lyall, Charles 34
Lycosthenes, Conrad 59

McCrindle, J.W. 12, 15
Malaya, Oxana 44–6
Malson, Lucien 41
Mappa Mundi 21, *22*, *23*
Masters, Brian 148
Merrick, Joseph 6, 104–24
Middle Ages/medieval 1, 5, 9, 10, 11, 12, 14, 19, 21, 22, 24, 25, 26, 27, 28, 31, 33, 34, 35, 36, 39, 48, 59, 73, 144
modernity 4, 6, 15, 24, 25, 28, 29, 32, 42, 47, 51, 54, 58, 59, 61, 65, 67, 68, 70, 71, 73, 78, 79, 80, 82, 83, 87, 97, 99, 108, 110, 112,

modernity *cont.* 116, 120, 125, 126, 128, 130, 132, 134, 135, 137, 141, 144, 145, 146, 147, 149, 151, 160, 161, 162, 165
Monster of Ravenna *see* Ravenna, Monster of
Monstrous Races 1–2, 4, *8*, 9–16, 18, 20, 21, 23, 24, 25, 26, 35, 54, 60, 81, 144, 145, 164, 165
multiculturalism 158–9, 161–2
murder/murderer 2, 7, 59, 125, 127, 129, 130–6, 139, 140, 146–50, 152–5, 158, 160, 161
Muslims 158, 160, 161
Myron 52, *53*
myth/mythological 4, 13, 15, 24, 25, 27, 34, 35, 39, 41, 43, 59, 81, 85, 86, 91, 92, 104, 105, 107, 111, 129, 130, 132, 133, 135, 139, 140, 144, 154

narrative 3, 10, 11, 21, 25, 40, 43, 65, 81, 83, 85, 86, 90, 91, 93, 94, 104, 105, 106, 109, 112, 115, 120, 121, 124, 125, 126, 127–8, 130, 131, 135, 137, 139, 141, 151, 154, 155, 157, 158, 165, 166
nature 1, 5, 6, 9, 10, 14, 15, 18, 19, 21, 27, 28, 29–31, 32, 34, 35, 36, 37, 39, 40, 43, 45, 58, 81, 99, 101, 104, 111, 112, 128
newspaper 46, 105, 130–1
Nilsen, Dennis 130, 147–8
norm/normal/normality 2, 3, 5, 6, 7, 15, 16, 17, 18, 26, 29, 35, 42, 46, 48, 49–50, 52, 54, 67, 68, 71, 78, 79, 81, 82, 83, 84, 87, 89, 90, 91, 93, 94, 96–7, 99–102, 103, 108, 109, 110, 111, 114, 115, 116, 118, 120, 121, 122, 123, 124, 127, 128, 129, 135, 136, 141, 143, 144, 145, 147, 148, 149, 151, 152, 153, 155, 156, 157, 162, 165, 166
Norman, Tom 107, 108, 109
Norris, Joel 129–30

Ochota, Mary-Ann 43, 44, 45
other/otherness 1, 3, 6, 7, 10, 12, 15, 16, 17–19, 22, 24, 27, 30, 33, 34, 35, 67, 68, 74, 75, 86, 89, 99, 112, 120, 122, 125, 147, 155–6, 165, 166; racial 83, 85, 87, 88
outsider 5, 6, 14, 15, 16, 26, 27–8, 29, 46, 84, 94, 121, 128

Panotii 12, *13*
Park, Katherine 24
photograph/photography/ photographic 6, 43, 47, 60, 61, 67–8, 70, 75, *76*, *77*, 78, 80, 86, 88, 89, 91, 92–4, 95, 97, 99, 100, 103, 104, 105, 115–22, 124, 125, 126, 130, 136–44, 145, 151, 155, 159, 165
physiognomy/physiognomic system 5, 47, 48, 61–78, 79, 80, 95, 100, 116, 120, 125, 137, 147, 155
Pinel, Philippe 41, 75, 147
Pliny the Elder 11, 14, 15, 16
police 6, 70, 108, 125, 126, 127, 130, 131–4, 136, 137, 138, 139, 140, 142, 143, 145, 154
primitiveness 10, 20, 27, 28, 36, 41, 71, 83, 86, 87, 97, 156
print 60, 82, 92, 118, 130, 144
psychiatry/psychiatrist 41, 71, 73, 74, 75, 76, 77, 78, 146, 147, 155, 160
psychologist/psychology/ psychological 2, 17, 44, 65, 73, 74, 78, 107, 112, 126, 129, 133, 146–7, 149, 150, 155
Pygmies 14, 15, 16

race/racial 11, 14, 15, 18, 20, 24, 33–4, 35, 40, 67, 71, 81, 82, 83,

85, 86, 87, 88, 90, 94, 99, 100, 159
Ravenna, Monster of 5, 26, 47, 48, *55*, *56*, 57–61, 81, 144, 145, 158, 161
religion/religious 11, 14, 19, 36, 52, 54, 56, 57, 58, 60, 61, 75, *76*, 79, 81, 125, 128, 158, 160, 161
Renaissance 49, 56, 59, 60, 61, 80, 82
romanticism 37, 42, 104, 109, 123
Rome/Roman 11, 26, 41, 42, 49, *52*, 53, 55, 59, 100
Rousseau, Jean-Jacques 32, 33, 43
Rule, Ann 154

savageness 20, 27, 31, 33, 34, 36, 37, 38, 43, 83, 132
Schmid, David 135
Sekula, Allan 68
self 2, 6, 10, 15, 17, 52, 68, 89, 160; and other 18, 27, 85, 155–8, 166
Selzer, Mark 152
serial killer 6, 7, 125, 127, 128, 129–30, 133, 134–5, 141, 145, 148, 154, 155, 156, 157
Shelley, Mary 109
Shildrick, Margrit 7, 155, 166
Sontag, Susan 18
Soper, Kate 29–30
spectacle/spectacular 21, 79, 80, 81, 83, 85, 89, 90, 101, 102, 107, 108, 110, 118, 122, 127, 128, 129, 145, 157
Ssebunya, John 42–3
Stallybrass, Peter 16, 83
subjectivity 61, 83, 103, 108, 157, 165
symbol/symbolic/symbolism 1, 4, 10, 11, 16, 21, 24, 25, 28, 32, 34, 36, 37, 39, 40, 46, 47, 48, 52, 54, 57, 58, 79, 83, 101, 103, 136, 145, 146, 158, 161

tabloids 44, 61, 130, 131, 135, 140, 143
Tithecott, Richard 126, 127, 129, 141, 148, 154
transgression/transgressive 1, 5, 10, 16, 17, 19, 20, 21, 28, 31, 38, 46, 48, 58, 60, 61, 81, 82, 83, 85, 112, 114, 136, 151, 155, 156, 161, 165
Treves, Frederick 105, 107, 108, 109, 110, 113, 114, 115, 116, 118, 121, 123, 124
Tripp, Charles 85, 90, 94, 97–9, 103

uncivilized people 20, 28, 33, 35, 41, 74, 87
unknown, the/unknowable 10, 16, 21, 42, 54, 121, 126, 132, 133, 165

Victorians 6, 93, 94, 97, 114, 125, 127, 132, 133
violence/violent 126, 133, 134, 135, 149, 151, 152, 153, 156, 157, 158, 159, 160
visual image 6, 12, 47, 48, 57, 66, 67, 78, 91, 103, 113, 125, 131, 135, 144, 164, 166
visual significance 2, 61, 104, 164
Volterra, Monster of 59

Welch Diamond, Hugh 75, *76*
White, Allon, 16, 83
White, Hayden 35, 39
Whitechapel 107, 113, 115, 130, 131, 132
wild man/wild woman 5, 26, 27, 28, 29, 32, 33, 34–41, 81, 85, 86, 87
Williams, Raymond 29–31
Wilson, Dudley 59

Wittkower, Rudolf 11, 13, 26
woman/women 28, 35, 36, 39, 46, 73, 75, 76, 80, 81, 82, 94, 95, 96, 97, 102, 107, 109, 114, 123, 125, 127, 129, 134, 135, 136, 139, 140, 148, 151, 153, 158
Woolley, Penny 38, 43

'Zip the Pinhead' *see* Johnson, William Henry

www.ingramcontent.com/pod-product-compliance
Ingram Content Group UK Ltd.
Pitfield, Milton Keynes, MK11 3LW, UK
UKHW021033150926
475561UK00003B/89

9 781780 763361

Advancing Multimodal and Critical Discourse Studies

Interdisciplinary Research Inspired by Theo van Leeuwen's Social Semiotics

Edited by Sumin Zhao, Emilia Djonov, Anders Björkvall, and Morten Boeriis

Routledge
Taylor & Francis Group
LONDON AND NEW YORK

First published 2018
by Routledge

2 Park Square, Milton Park, Abingdon, Oxfordshire OX14 4RN
52 Vanderbilt Avenue, New York, NY 10017

Routledge is an imprint of the Taylor & Francis Group, an informa business

First issued in paperback 2019

Library of Congress Cataloging-in-Publication Data
A catalog record for this book has been requested

ISBN: 978-1-138-69763-8 (hbk)
ISBN: 978-0-367-36639-1 (pbk)

Typeset in Sabon
by Apex CoVantage, LLC

Contents

List of Figures vii
List of Tables ix
Preface xi
Author Bios xv

1 Social Semiotics: A Theorist and a Theory in Retrospect and Prospect 1
EMILIA DJONOV AND SUMIN ZHAO

2 Changing Academic Common Sense: A Personal Recollection of Collaborative Work 19
GUNTHER KRESS

3 "Strangers in Europe": A Discourse-Historical Approach to the Legitimation of Immigration Control 2015/16 31
RUTH WODAK

4 The Limits of Semiotics—Epistemology and the Concept of 'Race' 51
PHILIP BELL

5 Can a Sign Reveal Its Meaning?: On the Question of Interpretation and Epistemic Contexts 67
STAFFAN SELANDER

6 Towards a Multimodal Social Semiotic Agenda for Touch 79
CAREY JEWITT

7 Reading That Which Should Not Be Signified: Community Currency in the UK 95
ANNABELLE MOONEY

8 A Sound Semiotic Investigation of How Subjective Experiences Are Signified in *Ex Machina* (2014) 115
GILBERT GABRIEL

9 Unravelling the Myth of Multiple Endings and the Narrative Labyrinth in *Mr. Nobody* (2010) 131
CHIAO-I TSENG

10 New Codifications, New Practices: The Multimodal Communication of CrossFit 147
PER LEDIN AND DAVID MACHIN

11 The 'Semiotics of Value' in Upcycling 165
ARLENE ARCHER AND ANDERS BJÖRKVALL

12 Multimodal Recontextualisations of Images in Violent Extremist Discourse 181
KAY L. O'HALLORAN, SABINE TAN, PETER WIGNELL, AND REBECCA LANGE

Revisiting the Family Silver: A Visual Essay on the Grammar of Visual Design 203
MORTEN BOERIIS

Index 217

Figures

3.1 The 'border fence' and related euphemisms (frequency by month 2015/16) 41
4.1 Beauty and the East—'race' 53
4.2 'Eurasian' Michelle Lee—she's got the look and science can prove it 54
4.3 Manipulated photograph—Barack Obama 59
4.4 Assimilation—photographic 'evidence' #1 61
4.5 Assimilation—photographic 'evidence' #2 62
4.6 'Face value'—art, not science, as coding orientation 64
7.1 Examples of community currencies analysed 98
9.1 Meaning strata—a multi-level meaning structure of text 133
9.2 Three analytical tools used in this section 136
9.3 Overall schematic structures of *Mr. Nobody* with five stages 137
9.4 Three examples of the hook: cohesive mechanisms of scene transitions and intercuts across different narrative strands 140
9.5 Goal plan and event progression of Nemo's choices and outcomes (en = enabling, psy = psychologically trigger, phy = physical trigger, mot = motivating) 143
10.1 The workout area shot from above 153
10.2 Warm up with bumper plates against the rough concrete wall in the workout area 155
10.3 Looking into the equipment area from the workout area 156
10.4 The WOD noted on the whiteboard, and above it, the digital clock 157
10.5 Exhausted man after the WOD wearing a Tee-shirt with writing 159
10.6 During the WOD 160
10.7 During the WOD 161
11.1 Upcycled tin aeroplane 166
11.2 Coasters 172
11.3 Plastic curtain 174
11.4 Wire bowls 177

12.1	A mixed-methods approach to the multimodal analysis of big data (O'Halloran, Tan, Pham, Bateman, & Vande Moere, 2016)	182
12.2	Examples of image-article type combinations in *Dabiq*, Issues 1–14	188
12.3a	Comparison of image-article type distribution in *Dabiq* Issue 1 (top) and Issue 12 (bottom)	193
12.3b	Image-article type frequency analysis for image category 'Near Enemy' and article type 'Near Enemy Issues', *Dabiq* Issues 1–14	194
12.3c	Comparison of image-article type connections for the image categories and sub-categories of Far and Near Enemies in *Dabiq* Issue 1 (top) and 12 (bottom) (Note: Near Enemy sub-categories are represented by blue arcs, Far Enemy sub-categories by red arcs.)	195
12.3d	Total number of image-article type connections in *Dabiq* Issues 1–14	196
12.3e	Reserve image search results for 'The Flood' in *Dabiq* Issue 2	197
12.3f	Images which have been recontextualised in *Dabiq*, e.g., Apocalyptic Event (Issue 2, left), and images which have been recontextualised elsewhere after appearing in *Dabiq*, e.g., ISIS Hero (Issue 8, right).	198
12.3g	Word cloud of URLs of websites with the same or similar images categorised as 'Far Enemy' in *Dabiq* Issue 1	199
VE.1	Process fusion	205
VE.2	Frontal planes	206
VE.3	Vertical viewpoint	207
VE.4	Horizontal viewpoint	208
VE.5	Horizontal viewpoint 2	209
VE.6	Viewpoint distance	210
VE.7	Grids as meaning	211
VE.8	Framing 1	212
VE.9	Framing 2	213
VE.10	Ideational information value 1	214
VE.11	Ideational information value 2	215

Tables

3.1 Selected list of content-related topoi in discriminatory discourses about immigration (adopted from Reisigl & Wodak, 2001, p. 74–80) 33
3.2 Periodisation in the debate about borders: July 2015—February 2016 38
3.3 Taxonomy: Legitimation Strategies (extrapolated from Van Leeuwen, 2008) 42
5.1 Knowledge-oriented context 75
7.1 Denominations and size 103
7.2 Security features 104
7.3 Paper feel 105
8.1 Transcription: Ava Session 1 121
8.2 Transcription: The subjective modality of intoxication 123
8.3 Transcription: The subjective modality of terror 126
12.1 Image classifications and explanations of key terms 186
12.2 Article types in *Dabiq* 187

Preface

In this Festschrift, we celebrate the illustrious academic career of Theo van Leeuwen, a social semiotician, a seasoned jazz pianist, and a founder of the research field of multimodality. Born in the Netherlands in 1947, Van Leeuwen's career in semiotics spans four decades and two continents.

Van Leeuwen first developed the desire to study semiotics in the late 1960s, as a student at the Dutch National Film Academy in Amsterdam, where engagement with theory was seen as a deterrent to creativity and discouraged. In 1972, after obtaining a BA in film direction and scriptwriting, he started working as a film/TV writer, editor, and producer. In 1973, he embarked on a journey to Australia and eventually to a career in academia. Over the following two decades, Van Leeuwen worked at Macquarie University in Sydney, designing and teaching courses in scriptwriting, film and television production, and film and media theory. He was also actively involved in establishing the Australian Film, Television and Radio School.

The 1980s is a defining period for Van Leeuwen's academic career. The decade began with a stint at the Centre for Interdisciplinary Studies in Semiotics, Anthropology and Sociology (Paris), where he studied cinema semiotics under the French film theorist Christian Metz. He went on to complete his first major piece of academic research in 1982 at Macquarie University—*Professional speech: Accentual and junctural style in radio announcing*, for which he was awarded an MA with honours. Several themes explored in his MA dissertation will be revisited, renewed, and developed throughout his research career, such as voices, sounds, listening, and the relation between theory and professional practices. In the mid 1980s, through the Newtown Semiotic Circle – whose members also included key figures in social semiotics, discourse analysis and cultural and media studies Bob Hodge, James R. Martin, Paul J. Thibault, Anne Cranny-Francis, and others – Van Leeuwen developed one of his most productive and enduring research partnerships—with Gunther Kress. In the Sydney suburb of Newtown, Kress and Van Leeuwen took their first steps towards building a social semiotic framework for the analysis of visual design.

The year 1990 saw the publication of an early edition of *Reading Images* by Deakin University Press, Australia. Two further editions of the book would be published by Routledge in 1996 and 2006. *Reading Images* laid the foundations for multimodality as a field of research with significant impact in design, education, communication, and media studies, as well as many other research fields and professional practices. In 1993, Van Leeuwen was awarded his PhD in linguistics from the University of Sydney. His doctoral thesis presented an innovative model for studying how written texts represent social practices. The model was based on Halliday's (1978) theory of language as a social semiotic, systemic functional linguistics (SFL), and Basil Bernstein's sociology of education, and was at the same time informed by key ideas from anthropology, philosophy, and sociology, including, among others, those of Pierre Bourdieu, Michel Foucault, Erving Goffman, Jürgen Habermas, and Claude Lévi-Strauss.

Van Leeuwen has since held several academic positions in Europe and Australia. In 1993, Van Leeuwen returned to Europe and began work as a principal lecturer and since 1996 as a professor at the London College of Printing (now London College of Communications). From 1999 to 2005, he held a professorship at the Centre for Language and Communication Research, Cardiff University, and served as the director of the centre between 2001 and 2005. Van Leeuwen returned to Australia in 2005 to take on the role of Dean of the Faculty of Arts and Social Sciences at the University of Technology Sydney, where he is now Emeritus Professor in Media and Communication. Since 2013, Van Leeuwen is a Professor at the Institute of Languages and Communication, University of Southern Denmark.

Van Leeuwen has published widely in multimodality, social semiotics, and critical discourse analysis, with many of his books and articles explicitly oriented to building bridges to domains such as journalism, art and design, education, and business. His books include: *The Media Interview: Confession, Contest, Conversation* (1994, with Philip Bell); *Reading Images: The Grammar of Visual Design* (2006 [1996]) and *Multimodal Discourse: The Modes and Media of Contemporary Communication* (2001), both with co-author Gunther Kress; *Speech, Music, Sound* (1999); *Introducing Social Semiotics* (2005); *Global Media Discourse* (2007, with David Machin); *Discourse and Social Practice: New Tools for Critical Discourse Analysis* (2008); *The Language of New Media Design* (2009, with Radan Martinec); and *The Language of Colour* (2011). He is one of the founding editors of the influential, international peer-reviewed journals *Social Semiotics* and *Visual Communication* (with Carey Jewitt) and a fellow of the Australian Academy of the Humanities.

This volume is envisaged as a celebration for Theo van Leeuwen's 70th birthday in 2017. Our aim with the festschrift is not simply to honour his towering achievements but also to capture the breadth of his theoretical outlook, his openness to dialogue, and his intellectual vigour and imaginative original vision. For the editors, and many others, Van Leeuwen is first and foremost a generous and inspiring mentor. Whereas a good mentor supports the research career of emerging scholars, a truly great mentor like Theo has made pursuing our own research agendas and visions possible.

We are grateful for the support we have received from our editor Alexandra Simmons at Routledge and all the contributors. We would also like to acknowledge many colleagues (and personal friends) of Theo van Leeuwen who have not been able to be involved directly in this project for various reasons: Professor Adam Jaworski, Professor Teal Triggs, Professor Carmen Caldas-Coulthard, Dr Radan Martinec, colleagues from the Centre for Multimodal Communication and Centre for Human Interactivity at University of Southern Denmark, the Multimodality Group at the University of New South Wales, the Learning Science Institute at the Australian Catholic University, and many others.

Author Bios

Arlene Archer is the director of the Writing Centre at the University of Cape Town, South Africa. She has co-edited three books on multimodality and has directed numerous research projects focusing on multimodal texts and pedagogies. Her research draws on popular culture and multimodal pedagogies to enable student access to writing and to higher education.

Philip Bell is an Emeritus Professor at the University of New South Wales. He has taught Media and Communications at Macquarie University and UTS and has spent sabbatical leaves or fellowships at the Slade School, UCL, the Institute of Education, Roskilde University, and the University of Southern Denmark. He retired in 2007, having served as a Foundation Professor of Media and Communication at UNSW since 1998.

Anders Björkvall is a Professor of Scandinavian languages at Örebro University, Sweden. He has directed research projects on technology in education, literacy, and multimodality. Anders also has an interest in the semiotics and ethnographies of artefacts.

Emilia Djonov is a lecturer in early childhood literacies at Macquarie University, Sydney, Australia. Her research interests are in the areas of (critical) multimodal and hypermedia discourse analysis, social semiotics, visual communication, multimodal learning, and multiliteracies education. She has published in journals such as *Visual Communication*, *Social Semiotics*, *Semiotica*, *Text & Talk*, *TESOL Quarterly*, *Children's Literature in Education*, and *Information Design Journal*.

Gilbert Gabriel is a professional musician and academic. He studied piano and film composition at several institutions, including Dartington College of Arts. He also studied piano with John Tilbury and music composition with the minimalist composer Howard Skempton. His work has been featured around the world on TV, film, and radio. He received an Ivor Novello nomination for his song "Sunchyme" in 1998 as well as industry awards for the radio play and sales of his music. He was an in-house composer at the London Film School and received a scholarship for a Master's in Film and TV Orchestration at Berklee Music College. He also studied film studies at Westminster University and obtained a PhD at Cardiff University in 2012, with a thesis exploring the semiotic power of film soundtracks called "Altered States, Altered Sounds," which uses sound semiotics to investigate how characters' subjective experiences are signified in a range of film soundtracks.

Carey Jewitt is a Professor of Technology and Learning at University College London, Institute of Education. She and colleagues have conducted research in a range of learning environments, notably school classrooms and museum galleries, with particular attention to how the digital re-mediates meaning-making and communication. This has included studies on the resources and use of interactive whiteboards, online learning, and mobile and tangible technologies for meaning-making and learning. Carey has led a number of projects that have contributed to the development of multimodal theory and methods, most recently the MODE project (*MODE.ioe.ac.uk*), with Bezemer, Price, and colleagues, and the MIDAS project (*MIDAS.ioe.ac.uk*), which explored the potential synergies between the social sciences and the arts. She has authored/edited a number of books on multimodality including: *Introducing Multimodality* (2016) with Jeff Bezemer and Kay O'Halloran; *The Routledge Handbook of Multimodal Analysis* (2009/2014); *Technology, Literacy and Learning: A multimodal Approach* (2008); *Urban English Classrooms: Multimodal teaching and learning* (2005), with Gunther Kress and colleagues; and *The Rhetorics of the Science Classroom: A multimodal approach* (2001), with Gunther Kress and colleagues.

Gunther Kress is a Professor of Semiotics and Education at the UCL Institute of Education, University of London. His interests are in communication and meaning (-making) in contemporary environments. His broad aims are to continue developing a social semiotic theory of (multimodal) communication, and, in that, to develop a theory in which communication, learning, identity are entirely interconnected. One part of that agenda is to develop apt tools for the 'recognition' and 'valuation' of learning. Some books along the road are: *Language as Ideology*; *Social Semiotics* (both with Bob Hodge); *Before Writing: Rethinking the paths to literacy*; *Reading Images: The grammar of visual design*; *Multimodal Discourse: The modes and media of contemporary communication* (both with Theo van Leeuwen); and *Literacy in the New Media Age*; *Multimodality: A social semiotic approach to contemporary communication*. Published by Routledge in 2016, his latest book is *Multimodality, Learning and Communication: A social semiotic frame* (with Jeff Bezemer).

Rebecca Lange is a computational specialist at the Curtin Institute for Computation at Curtin University. She has extensive programming, data analysis, and visualisation experience in astronomy and scientific imaging for heritage science. She is particularly interested in applying her technical skills to support and train researchers in the digital humanities.

Per Ledin is a Professor of Culture and Education at Södertörn University Sweden. He has published widely in different areas of discourse studies, including writing development, multimodality, and critical linguistics. His recent publications include papers on the assessment of writing tests and the semiotics of lists and tables.

David Machin is a Professor of Media and Communication at Örebro University, Sweden. His publications include *Visual Journalism* (Palgrave, 2015); *The Language of War Monuments* (Bloomsbury, 2013); and *The Language of Crime and Deviance* (Bloomsbury, 2012). He has published over 80 journal papers and book chapters and is the editor of two international peer-reviewed journals: *Social Semiotics* and the *Journal of Language and Politics*.

Annabelle Mooney is a Reader in Sociolinguistics at the University of Roehampton. Her most recent publications include: *Human Rights and the Body: Hidden in Plain Sight* (Ashgate, 2014), *Language and Law* (Palgrave, 2014) and *Language, Society and Power* (4th edition, Routledge, 2015, with Betsy Evans). Having worked on human rights, religion, and gender, she is now researching the language of money.

Morten Boeriis is working with Theo van Leeuwen at the University of Southern Denmark, cooperating on several projects such as, e.g., lighting as a semiotic resource and revising the grammar of visual design. He has edited the Routledledge book *Social Semiotics—key figures, new directions* (2015) (with Andersen, Maagerø, and Tønnessen) and the book *Nordisk Socialsemiotik—pædagogiske, multimodale og sprogvidenskabelige landvindinger* (2012) (with Andersen, published by Syddansk Universitetsforlag). He has written several articles and presented papers around the world on topics concerning audiovisual social semiotics and multimodality. Morten Boeriis teaches a variety of courses on visual analysis in business communication studies and film and media studies at the University of Southern Denmark. He has worked and continues to be involved in TV production and freelance photography.

Kay O'Halloran is a Professor in the School of Education, Faculty of Humanities at Curtin University. Her areas of research include multimodal analysis, social semiotics, mathematics discourse, and the development of interactive digital media technologies and visualisation techniques for multimodal and sociocultural analytics.

Staffan Selander is a Professor in Education and head of the unit IDEAL—Interaction Design and Learning, at the Department of Computer and Systems Sciences, Stockholm University. He has organised three international "Designs for Learning" conferences in Stockholm in 2008 and 2010 and 2014. He is the chief editor of the e-journal *Designs for Learning*, which, from now on, will be published as an online, open-access journal in cooperation with Stockholm University Press. Selander's research focuses on designs for learning, technology enhanced learning, self-regulated learning, multimodal texts and knowledge representations, games for learning and simulations, as well as rhetoric and interpretation theories/hermeneutics.

Sabine Tan is a Research Fellow in the School of Education, Faculty of Humanities at Curtin University. Her research interests include critical multimodal discourse analysis, social semiotics, and visual communication. She is particularly interested in the application of multidisciplinary perspectives within social semiotic theory to the analysis of institutional discourses involving traditional and new media.

Ruth Wodak is a Distinguished Professor of Discourse Studies at Lancaster University, UK, while she has remained affiliated with the University of Vienna (as a full professor of applied linguistics). Besides many other prizes, she was awarded the Wittgenstein Prize for Elite Researchers in 1996. In 2008, she was awarded the Kerstin Hesselgren Chair of the Swedish Parliament and an Honorary Doctorate from University of Örebro in Sweden in 2010. In 2011, she was awarded the Grand Decoration in Silver for Services for the Austrian Republic. She is a past president of the Societas Linguistica Europea and a member of the British Academy of Social Sciences and the Academia Europea. Her recent book publications include *The Politics of Fear. What Right-wing Populist Discourses Mean* (Sage, 2015); *The Discourse of Politics in Action: 'Politics as Usual'* (Palgrave, 2011); *Migration, Identity and Belonging* (with G. Delanty and P. Jones, LUP, 2011); *The Discursive Construction of History. Remembering the Wehrmacht's War of Annihilation* (with H. Heer, W. Manoschek, and A. Pollak, Palgrave, 2008), *Gedenken im Gedankenjahr* (with R. de Cillia, Studienverlag, 2009); *The SAGE Handbook of Sociolinguistics* (with B. Johnstone and P. Kerswill; Sage, 2010); *Critical Discourse Analysis* (four volumes, Sage Major Works, 2013); and *Analysing Fascism: Fascism in talk and text* (with J. Richardson, Routledge, 2013).

Peter Wignell is a Research Fellow in the School of Education, Faculty of Humanities at Curtin University. Peter's current research interests are in systemic functional linguistics, especially in its application to the analysis of multimodal texts. His research has also focused on the role of language in the construction of specialised knowledge.

Sumin Zhao is currently a Carlsberg Distinguished Postdoctoral Fellow at the University of Southern Denmark. Her research explores how young children learn to make meaning in different languages, mixing various semiotic modes, and across different technological platforms. She is also interested in the textual and visual practices of 'indie' culture, focusing on lifestyle magazines and social media. She publishes in the areas of critical multimodal discourse analysis, social semiotics, and early literacy. She was previously a Chancellor's Postdoctoral Fellow at the University of Technology Sydney.

1 Social Semiotics

A Theorist and a Theory in Retrospect and Prospect

Emilia Djonov and Sumin Zhao

1. Theo Van Leeuwen's Social Semiotics

When we look back at the body of work produced by Theo van Leeuwen, we cannot help but be struck by its breadth and evolving nature, its range in subjects and perspectives, and its transdisciplinary reach. For almost four decades, Van Leeuwen has examined phenomena as diverse as film (Van Leeuwen, 1985, 1991a, 2014; Van Leeuwen & Boeriis, 2017) and children's toys (Caldas-Coulthard & Van Leeuwen, 2001, 2002, 2003; Van Leeuwen, 2009b), music (Van Leeuwen, 1991b, 1999) and school textbooks (Van Leeuwen, 1992, 2000; Van Leeuwen & Humphrey, 1996; Van Leeuwen & Kress, 1995), women's magazines (Machin & Van Leeuwen, 2003, 2007) and kinetic art (Van Leeuwen, 2015a), news journalism (Van Leeuwen, 2006b; Van Leeuwen & Jaworski, 2002) and semiotic software such as PowerPoint (Djonov & Van Leeuwen, 2012, 2013; Van Leeuwen & Djonov, 2013; Zhao, Djonov, & Van Leeuwen, 2014; Zhao & Van Leeuwen, 2014). Van Leeuwen's work also gives voice to wide-ranging theories and perspectives, as he draws inspiration from the Paris and Prague schools of semiotics, especially the work of Roland Barthes and Roman Jakobson; Foucault's theory of discourse; the Bauhaus art and design movement; Rudolf Arnheim's psychology of visual perception; Raymond Murray Schafer's studies of music and sound; John Gage's theory of colour; and the anthropologist Erving Goffmann, to name just a few. This richness has enabled Van Leeuwen's own theories of legitimation in discourse (Van Leeuwen, 2007; see also Chapter 3 in this volume), the role of discourse in recontextualising social practice (Van Leeuwen, 2008a; see also Chapters 11 & 12 in this volume), new writing (Van Leeuwen, 2008b; see also Chapter 10 in this volume), and semiotic technologies (Djonov & Van Leeuwen, in press; Van Leeuwen, 2010; Zhao et al., 2014) to provide tools for understanding the seismic social, cultural, and political changes in the past two decades and thereby have influence beyond semiotics, communication studies, and applied linguistics, in fields such as education, arts, design, media, cultural, and management studies.

While diverse in scope and perspectives, Van Leeuwen's work is grounded in social semiotic theory. Van Leeuwen's key theoretical contributions to social semiotics are captured in his book *Introducing Social Semiotics* (Van Leeuwen, 2005), written in his staple accessible yet intellectually rich style, with intriguing examples from a wide array of semiotic practices. For Van Leeuwen, social semiotics is "not 'pure' theory, not a self-contained field" but "a form of enquiry" that "comes into its own when it is applied to specific instances and specific problems" (Van Leeuwen, 2005, p. 1). It is thus a theory that is both an 'appliable' (Halliday, 1985) and necessarily agile and interdisciplinary. Social semiotic enquiries pursue three central goals:

1. collect, document and systematically catalogue semiotic resources—including their history
2. investigate how these resources are used in specific historical, cultural and institutional contexts, and how people talk about them in these contexts—plan them, teach them, justify them, critique them, etc.
3. contribute to the discovery and development of new semiotic resources and new uses of existing semiotic resources. (Van Leeuwen, 2005, p. 3)

Central to Van Leeuwen's theory of social semiotics is the notion of 'semiotic resource', which reflects Halliday's (1978) model of language as a social semiotic resource whose meaning-making potential is dynamic, simultaneously shaped by and shaping the social contexts in which it is employed:

> Semiotic resources have a meaning potential, based on their past uses, and a set of affordances based on their possible uses, and these will be actualised in concrete social contexts where their use is subject to some form of semiotic regime.
>
> (Van Leeuwen, 2005, p. 285)

It also integrates a strong focus on materiality through Gibson's (1979) concept of 'affordances', the perceptible, physical qualities of objects that, together with the needs and interests of users, define their possible uses.

> Semiotic resources have a meaning potential, based on their past uses, and a set of affordances based on their possible uses, and these will be actualized in concrete social contexts where their use is subject to some form of semiotic regime.
>
> (Van Leeuwen, 2005, p. 285)

Studying semiotic resources for Van Leeuwen entails examining their roles in specific social practices and cultural-historical contexts. The origin of such an approach can be traced back to Malinowski's (1923) conceptualisation of 'context of situation' and 'context of culture'. Van Leeuwen's work also responds to Hodge and Kress's (1988) pan semiotic ambition that "texts and contexts, agents and objects of meaning, social structures and forces and their complex interrelationships together constitute the minimal and irreducible object of semiotic analysis" (p. viii). In particular, he draws on ethnographic approaches in the social sciences and considers not only how people use semiotic resources in specific socio-historical contexts but also the ways in which they talk about and legitimate (aspects of) these practices. This approach underpins Van Leeuwen's (2005, p. 47–68) inventory of semiotic regimes that govern people's meaning-making. The inventory includes (i) rules of personal authority, such as those developed by observing and conforming to trends, emulating role models, and drawing on the opinion of experts as well as rules imposed by people in power, and (ii) rules of impersonal authority, which are imposed through writing (the law, religion, etc.), tradition, and the design of technologies (e.g., PowerPoint) and objects (e.g., furniture) used in communication. Awareness of the emergence and changes in such norms is key to understanding and contributing to semiotic change.

As Van Leeuwen's work focuses on the relationship between meaning-making or semiotic resources, the interests/agency of meaning-makers, and the ways in which specific institutional and broader social contexts govern the use of semiotic resources, it has left enduring legacy in two strands of discourse studies—multimodal and critical discourse studies, and ultimately served as a catalyst for their merger (Djonov & Zhao, 2014; Machin & Mayr, 2012; Machin & Van Leeuwen, 2016; Van Leeuwen, 2013), as reflected in special issues on 'Critical Analysis of Musical Discourse' (2012) and 'Multimodal Critical Discourse Studies' (2013) of the journal *Critical Discourse Studies*; on 'Multimodality, Politics and Ideology' (2016) in *Journal of Language and Politics;* and on 'Gender and Multimodality' (2016) in *Gender and Language.*

2. Multimodality and Multimodal Discourse Studies

Van Leeuwen's most ground-breaking contribution consists in co-founding, alongside Gunther Kress, multimodality as a transdisciplinary field of research concerned with the meaning-making potential, use, and development of different semiotic resources. In two seminal publications, *Reading Images: The Grammar of Visual Design* (2006 [1996]) and *Multimodal Discourse: The Modes and Media of Contemporary Communication* (2001), Kress and Van Leeuwen have laid the groundwork for the two main directions in multimodal studies:

1. exploring the use and mapping the meaning-making potential of individual semiotic resources,
2. studying how choices from various semiotic resources interact to create meaning multimodally.

Reading Images incorporates insights from iconography, structural semiotics, Gestalt psychology, film, and the fine arts and explores a rich variety of Western-culture visual texts from different historical periods (advertising and news images, maps and technical diagrams, pages from magazines, picture books, and textbooks, three-dimensional objects such as sculptures and toys, and web pages). The book presents an analytical framework based on two central tenets of Halliday's systemic functional linguistics (Halliday & Matthiessen, 2004). The first is that every act of communication simultaneously constructs three broad types of meaning, or 'metafunctions':

- *ideational/representational*—representing patterns of experience (as configurations of processes, participants and circumstances) and the logico-semantic relations between them
- *interpersonal/interactional*—enacting social interactions, relations, attitudes, and values
- *textual/compositional*—interweaving ideational and interpersonal meanings into cohesive and coherent units, i.e. texts.

The second tenet is that the meaning potential of semiotic modes can be modelled as systems of interrelated choices, paradigmatically, where each option has a distinctive structural realisation.

While describing SFL as "a good source for thinking about all modes of representation" (Kress & Van Leeuwen, 2006 [1996], p. 20), *Reading Images* adds two interrelated caveats. The first is that although different modes may have the potential to make the same general types of meaning, their affordances and formal organisational principles differ (e.g., temporal organisation in spoken language vs. spatial organisation in images and spatio-temporal organisation in dance). To illustrate, as modelled in Halliday's system of 'modality' for English grammar (Halliday & Matthiessen, 2004, p. 143–150), linguistic resources for representing different versions of reality and truth values for different communities include modal verbs and modal adjuncts that construct degrees of probability and obligation between the polarity values of 'yes' and 'no'. In visual representations, as Kress and Van Leeuwen (2006 [1996]) show, modality relies on several cues such as colour saturation, colour differentiation, brightness, and detail, and their interaction may lead viewers to 'read' a picture as more or less naturalistic, abstract, sensory, or technical. The second is that the use of the term 'grammar' in the book's title is not intended to suggest that the visual mode has organisational or grammatical structures similar to those found in language, but to emphasise the need for visual analysis to move beyond interpreting the meaning of individual elements (e.g., a particular colour or shape) and represented objects, beyond what Kress and Van Leeuwen see as analogous to 'lexis' in language, and to examine the structures such elements form within a visual composition such as a photograph or a webpage.

In contrast to *Reading Images*, which focuses on visual design as a distinct mode, Kress and Van Leeuwen's *Multimodal Discourse* (2001, p. 2) presents "a view of multimodality in which common semiotic principles operate in and across different modes". Their key argument for adopting this type of multimodal perspective is that shifts in the semiotic landscape, and particularly advances in digital technologies, mean that non-specialists are increasingly able to select from and combine semiotic resources (e.g., typography, sound, layout) previously associated with discrete and highly specialised domains and professions. Studying contemporary communication thus requires "a unified and unifying semiotics" (ibid., p. 2).

Multimodal Discourse presents several fundamental principles for a unified theory of multimodality. The first is that the study of multimodal communication should focus on identifying broad semiotic principles that apply across different semiotic resources (in accordance with their unique affordances) and semiotic practices. These principles can then be built into frameworks for analysing multimodal interaction. Modality is one such principle, as not only language and images, but sound, too, can represent different degrees and kinds of truth depending on the extent to which it appears authentic or manipulated with technologies (Van Leeuwen, 1999, see also Chapter 8 in this volume).

The second key idea is that multimodal analysis must always consider semiotic resources in relation to specific, situated social practices, and should engage with each of four layers, or strata, of communication:

1. **Discourse,** "socially constructed knowledge(s) of (some aspects of) reality" (p. 4);
2. **Design,** blueprints or conceptualisations of the ways one or more discourses can be materialised and embedded in particular interactions through semiotic objects or events that involve certain combinations of semiotic resources;
3. **Production,** the material articulation of a semiotic object or event;
4. **Distribution,** "the technical 're-coding' of semiotic products and events, for purposes of recording [. . .] and/or distribution" (p. 21).

The stratum of discourse invites investigation into the relationship between epistemology (see also Chapters 4 & 5 in this volume), social roles and meaning-making. Kress and Van Leeuwen (2001) also emphasise the fluid boundaries between the strata of design and production, pointing out that "at any moment the implementer of a design can become a designer in respect to a particular facet of the productive process" (p. 56), as in jazz improvisation. The concepts of production and distribution, on the other hand, draw attention to the role of materiality and technologies for producing/recording and distributing semiotic products and events in specific communicative practices.

One of Van Leeuwen's distinctive contributions to multimodality lies in developing frameworks for studying material resources such as colour, texture, sound and (kinetic) typography, thereby drawing attention to semiotic resources that have generally been marginalised in linguistics, semiotics, and discourse analysis and providing tools for explicitly teaching and discussing them in semiotic theory as well as semiotic practice.

A strong focus on materiality in semiosis underpins Van Leeuwen's unified framework for analysing sound. Presented in *Speech, Music, Sound* (1999), it reflects his background in film production (where speech, music and sound can all be part of a soundtrack), jazz music practice, and his earlier research (Van Leeuwen, 1982) on intonation and rhythm (rhythm is a key organising principle for time-based modes and media such as radio). The framework incorporates principles from phonology, musicology, the psychology of perception, and conceptual metaphor theory.

As in *Reading Images*, in *Speech, Music, Sound*, tools from systemic functional linguistics such as the metafunctions provide a springboard for examining sound. For Van Leeuwen, sound is better equipped for realising interpersonal and textual rather than ideational meanings. He also argues that a 'bottom-up' approach (see also Chapter 8 in this volume), starting from material qualities (e.g., timbre, tempo), rather than larger structures, is more suitable for mapping the meaning potential of sound and other material semiotic resources, because compared to language they construct meaning "quite differently, on the basis either of an *experiential meaning potential*, hence grounded [. . .] in our bodily experience of [their] materiality, and/or *provenance*, hence grounded in intertextuality" (Van Leeuwen, 1999, p. 192). Experiential meaning is based on our ability to extend prior physical experiences metaphorically into knowledge, as Lakoff and Johnson (1980) have argued for linguistic metaphors (e.g., 'things are looking up').

In an earlier paper titled 'Taste in the Framework of a Semiotics of Materiality', for instance, Van Leeuwen (1998, p. 149) explains that such semiotics "must be placed in the still broader context of a semiotics of action, as it is only in our physical experience of materials, that the qualifies of those materials can be perceived". For taste, he would begin by inventorising the physical actions involved in tasting—touching, linking, sucking, biting, and chewing—and then the perception of various qualities (e.g., softness, temperature) that they afford in terms of the cultural values these qualities are assigned in specific contexts (e.g., does softness mean 'gentleness' or 'lack of discipline'). Provenance relies on familiarity with the origin of a signifier and related associations. The 'saltiness' and 'hardness' of Dutch liquorice for Van Leeuwen signifies the moral values of delayed gratification, restraint, and frugality upheld in the Dutch Calvinist tradition.

To model the experiential meaning potential of material resources, Van Leeuwen (2009a) develops what he calls 'parametric systems'. A parametric system presents those physical qualities, or affordances, of a given resource which people have taken up in communication. These qualities are always gradable and together define the meaning potential of a given signifier such as a certain type of voice, texture, or colour. A particular voice, for example, can be described as a combination of degrees of each of several parameters: tension, roughness, breathiness, loudness, vibrato, and nasality (Van Leeuwen, 1999, 2009a).

Van Leeuwen's notion of 'parametric system' is inspired by Jakobson and Halle's (1956) distinctive feature theory. That is, a phoneme can be described using a small number of distinctive features and identifying each feature as either present or absent, which allows one phoneme to be differentiated from another (e.g., the alveolar fricative consonants /z/ and /s/ have the same place and manner of articulation but differ in respectively presence vs. absence of voice). Unlike distinctive features, however, the parameters in Van Leeuwen's parametric systems are not simply absent or present (not binary choices) but gradable and not only allow one signifier to be differentiated from another but add layers of meaning to it.

In addition to sound and taste, Van Leeuwen has used the concepts of provenance and experiential meaning to tap into the semiotic potential of resources such as kinetic design (Van Leeuwen, 2015a; Van Leeuwen & Caldas-Coulthard, 2004), colour (Van Leeuwen, 2011a), (kinetic) typography (Van Leeuwen, 2006a; Van Leeuwen & Djonov, 2015), tactile and visual texture (Djonov & Van Leeuwen, 2011; see also Chapter 7 in this volume), and film lighting (Van Leeuwen & Boeriis, 2017). Most recently, Van Leeuwen (2017) has identified common qualities, including energy, brightness, regularity, among others, and examined the extent to which they are shared across different material resources such as colour, graphic shapes, timbre, and texture. This exploration concludes with a proposal for a social semiotic theory of synaesthesia which:

> should, on the one hand, be grounded in a solid knowledge of the material qualities of the semiotic resources we use, and the physical and physiological aspects of articulation and interpretation [. . .] On the other hand social semiotics must continue to focus on the way changing social practices of meaning making and interpretation create changing semiotic resources[,] for creating ever new expressions of individuality, authenticity, brightness, energy, expansiveness and so on.
>
> (Van Leeuwen, 2017, p. 118)

Van Leeuwen has also contributed significantly to establishing principles for understanding the interaction of various semiotic resources in a range of multimodal texts and events, following the direction set in Kress and Van Leeuwen (2001). In addition to modality, he has demonstrated the value of genre, style, framing, salience, rhythm, and conjunctive relations, for analysing both intra- and inter-semiotic interaction through a wide variety of examples (e.g., magazines, textbooks, three-dimensional objects, film, architectural space, soundtracks, and hypermedia) (e.g., Martinec & Van Leeuwen, 2009; Van Leeuwen, 1991a, 2003, 2005, 2011b; see also Chapter 9 in this volume).

Van Leeuwen's analyses of multimodal interaction are based on a keen focus on the role of socio-cultural and political factors in semiotic practices and the assumption that analysis and interpretation are themselves meaning-making processes driven by individual and institutional interests. This socio-political orientation has arguably contributed to the influence of his research beyond social semiotics, in areas such as literacy, media, and cultural studies. To illustrate, Van Leeuwen (2011c, 2015b) explains that although decoration is commonly viewed as purely a matter of form, by creating a sense of style and identity and drawing attention to itself, it serves important functions in promotional discourse and corporate branding. And precisely because aesthetic principles are not employed for representing specific ideas but instead carry meaning in covert ways, through vague reference to cultural values, Van Leeuwen (2015b) argues that 'aesthetic literacy' can no longer remain the province of design professionals.

3. Critical Discourse Studies

While all of Van Leeuwen's work on multimodality is underscored by an acute awareness of the ways social, historical, cultural, and political circumstances shape and are shaped by meaning-making practices, his direct contribution to critical discourse studies is best captured in *Discourse and Practice: New Tools for Critical Discourse Analysis* (2008a). The book presents a social semiotic framework for critical discourse analysis that is informed by a range of ideas from anthropology, sociology and philosophy, including, among others, those of Pierre Bourdieu, Michel Foucault, Erving Goffman, Jürgen Habermas, and Claude Lévi-Strauss. At its core is the idea that there is a distinction between social practices and their representation in texts, or discourses. Van Leeuwen defines a social practice as a sequence of physical and/or semiotic activities that includes the following elements: social actors, their activities and reactions to these activities or to other elements of the social practice; the location(s)and time(s) of the practice; and prescribed or freely chosen grooming, dress, tools, and materials.

The framework extends educational sociologist Basil Bernstein's (1990) theory of recontextualisation, which is concerned with the semantic shifts involved in transferring knowledge from the contexts of production to contexts of distribution and reproduction through pedagogic discourse, and the role of these shifts in maintaining the existing social order. Van Leeuwen (2008a, p. vii) argues that not only pedagogic discourse but "all discourses recontextualise [or change the meaning of] social practices"(vii) (see also Chapters 11 & 12 in this volume), which is why the same social practice may be subject to different representations, or attract "a plurality of discourses" (p. 6). He proposes relating social practices to discourses about them as a method for achieving the central goal of critical discourse analysis (CDA)—to reveal how discourses help perpetuate or expose and challenge social boundaries, oppression and inequality. This method involves two key steps: (1) analyse the semiotic practice into its components and then (2) identify how it has been transformed in discourse through the use of verbal and/or non-verbal resources. Such transformations may involve *substitution, deletion*, and *rearrangement* of the elements of a social practice and/or *addition* of evaluations, purposes, or legitimations. Van Leeuwen (2008a, p. 17–18) demonstrates, for instance, how in a text about the first day of school the use of a nominalisation ("the separation from families") transforms the action of a teacher separating children from their parents by representing it as a phenomenon ('the separation'), and deletes the teacher, who is a central actor in this activity, while substituting individual children and parents (e.g., Mary and her mother) with aggregate nouns ('families').

Like Norman Fairclough and many other critical discourse analysts, Van Leeuwen employs Halliday's systemic functional linguistic tools for analysing the role of language in recontextualising social practices. A distinguishing feature of his approach to CDA, however, is that it also explores the role non-verbal and multimodal representations play in (re)establishing dominant ideologies. To expose this role, Van Leeuwen (2008a) argues, CDA needs to consider not only what is or is not represented non-verbally or multimodally (e.g., whether ethnic minorities are represented in the media) but also how such representations are constructed. Van Leeuwen (2008a) presents many examples from his earlier research, including the use of oblique horizontal angle to depict a group of people as 'other', and create detachment between depicted social actors and image viewers, and ways that the visual and kinetic construction of toys can conform to racial and gender stereotypes. To illustrate, Van Leeuwen (2005) has revealed how advertising discourses employ combinations of signifiers such as dress, colour, smell, and so on to construct and sell lifestyle identities that mask mass consumerism, while Machin and Van Leeuwen's (2007) analyses of women's magazines and electronic war games have demonstrated that multimodal genres impose Western values and homogenise the formats used to present local content. This work has highlighted popular culture and discourses (Djonov & Zhao, 2014) as a fertile ground for developing tools for productively uniting the agendas of critical and multimodal discourse analysis. As Van Leeuwen (2013) explains, "the discourses that need the scrutiny of a critical eye are now overwhelmingly multimodal and mediated by digital systems that take multimodality entirely for granted" (p. 5) as "racist [and other] stereotypes persist in visual rather than verbal texts, and in comic strips, advertisements and other forms of popular culture rather than in more factual and 'highbrow' texts" (p. 2).

4. Social Semiotics in the Age of Semiotic Software Technologies

A major focus throughout Van Leeuwen's research has been exploring the ways technologies shape social and semiotic practices. While this focus is evident as early as 1982, in Van Leeuwen's MA dissertation on the intonation of radio announcers, it has intensified significantly over the last two decades, as Van Leeuwen has responded to the ubiquity of software technologies by developing a holistic approach for the critical multimodal study of what he calls 'semiotic technology'—technologies for meaning-making. This approach—charted in Van Leeuwen and Djonov (2013), further developed using PowerPoint as a case study in Zhao, Djonov, and Van Leeuwen (2014), and most recently synthesized in Djonov and Van Leeuwen (in press)—involves examining three dimensions: software's design, its use, and their relationship to broader semiotic, socio-cultural and historical practices. It thus innovates research in applied linguistics, discourse analysis and multimodality, where software is treated primarily as a tool for creating or analysing texts, and these texts, rather than software, constitute the main object of study. By offering a framework for systematically examining ubiquitous software and its use in everyday communication practices, Van Leeuwen's work also builds on composition, cultural, media, and design studies which have raised critical awareness of the need to move beyond views of software as a neutral tool and led to the establishment of the field of software studies, where the focus is almost exclusively on software in the creative industries.

Studies of semiotic software, according to Van Leeuwen's approach, must reflect an understanding of the ways such software resembles and differs from semiotic resources such as language. While semiotic software makes available resources (e.g., typography, layout, colour, texture, etc.) for making meaning, it evolves in response not to the functions it serves in different social practices but to the needs and interests of global software design corporations. A software product such as Adobe AfterEffects is thus best defined as a 'semiotic artefact' (Kress & Van Leeuwen, 2001; Van Leeuwen, 2005), a material resource that makes available certain modes (layout, font and colour) and media (visual, print, aural, electronic), and embodies rules about the ways and semiotic practices in which they should be (co)deployed. To reveal the semiotic regime built into the technology, following Djonov and Van Leeuwen's (2012) model for exploring normativity in software design and use, the analysis of a semiotic software product must therefore examine both the software as a system that makes available certain semiotic resources and choices, and the ways the software interface, as a spatio-temporal arrangement (a syntagm), presents these options and makes some automatic or easier to access and activate than others. These choices and their presentation must also be examined in relation to broader socio-historical and cultural contexts, especially the semiotic sources, technologies and practices that a given software product recontextualises (in the case of Photoshop, for instance, this would include visual arts, photography, and graphic design practices and technologies).

In line with Van Leeuwen's social semiotics, critical multimodal studies of software must also consider software use and the discourses that surround it. This entails examining how the products (i.e., the texts and interactions enabled through software) and practices of software use are shaped by both software design and its use in specific historical, cultural, and institutional contexts. To illustrate, Van Leeuwen's research on PowerPoint has analysed changes in the design of the software itself over time (e.g., all versions of PowerPoint for Windows from 1992 to 2007), slideshows designed with the software and their embodied deployment in university lectures in different disciplines and corporate presentations, and the ways people justify why and how they use PowerPoint (Djonov & Van Leeuwen, 2011, 2013, in press; Zhao et al., 2014; Zhao & Van Leeuwen, 2014). A study within that project (Van Leeuwen, Djonov, & O'Halloran, 2013) has also investigated David Byrne's (2003) use of PowerPoint to create the art exhibition and album *Envisioning Emotional Epistemological Information*. The study argues that Byrne's work can be seen as research on semiotic technology that contributes to all three goals of social semiotics outlined in Van Leeuwen (2005), as it systematically examines different types of semiotic resources available within the software (e.g., the AutoShape menu), reflects an awareness of the ways PowerPoint's design influences its use and imposes and shapes contemporary corporate culture values, and makes creative use of the software "to express new meanings in new ways" (Van Leeuwen et al., 2013, p. 12).

Van Leeuwen has also drawn attention to the role semiotic technologies play in reshaping broader semiotic practices such as writing. One such practice is what Van Leeuwen (2008b) calls 'new writing' (see also Chapter 10, this volume), writing that follows the logic of space, rather than time, and thus resembles visual design and blurs the boundary between written language and visual design. New writing presents ideas through words and/or images, but achieves cohesion and coherence in their presentation increasingly through resources such as layout and colour schemes. New writing is not controlled by and learned from style manuals and explicit teaching, but through rules built into semiotic technologies such as office software, where spelling can be automatically corrected, bullet lists automatically aligned, and so on (see further Djonov & Van Leeuwen, 2013, 2014).

A recent study inspired by Van Leeuwen's approach to examining how software design and its use interact with broader semiotic, socio-cultural, and historical practices is Kvåle (2016), which exposes the inability of Microsoft Word's SmartArt tool to support linguistic students to adopt the minimalist and abstract style expected of morphological tree diagrams. The study demonstrates the power of ubiquitous software products such as Microsoft Office to colonise the representation of knowledge in various academic disciplines by promoting—through easy-to-use templates (e.g., the organisational chart)—the practices and values of office management, where a more decorative visual style, which does not convey specific, technical meanings, is favoured.

5. An Overview of the Book

In this volume, we bring together 12 contributions by Theo van Leeuwen's close collaborators, colleagues, and mentees. The book is both retrospective and prospective in its outlook. It looks back at Theo van Leeuwen's research career through a mixture of personal recounts and in-depth discussions of key concepts in social semiotic theory and multimodal and critical discourse studies. At the same time, it endeavours to open up dialogues and debates about the theory through cutting-edge research on a diverse range of semiotic phenomena and social practices.

The book is loosely organised into three sections. The first four chapters are envisaged as a series of theoretical 'dialogues' between Theo van Leeuwen and leading theorists in multimodality (Kress, Chapter 2), critical discourse analysis (Wodak, Chapter 3), media studies (Bell, Chapter 4), and education (Selander, Chapter 5). Kress's contribution (Chapter 2) recounts a long period of collaborative work with Van Leeuwen, focusing on the making of two classics: *Reading Images* and *Multimodal Discourse*. The recount is both personal, as it provides rare insights into an enduring intellectual partnership, and academic, as it presents a candid and astute analysis of the strengths and limitations of their research and encourages a rethinking of the paradigm in this technologically shaped new world of ours. In her contribution (Chapter 3), Wodak revisits her collaborative work with Van Leeuwen on legitimising immigration control (Van Leeuwen & Wodak, 1999) and demonstrates its relevance for examining the role of discourse in the most recent (2015/2016) refugee crisis in Europe. By integrating legitimation analysis (Van Leeuwen, 2007; Van Leeuwen & Wodak, 1999; Wodak & Van Leeuwen, 2002) with the discourse-historical approach (Wodak, 2015), the chapter points to the shift of mainstream rhetoric, where exclusionary and discriminatory slogans have become normalised and the distinctions between refugees and migrants have been largely neglected.

In Chapter 4, Bell engages with and challenges visual analytical categories developed by Kress and Van Leeuwen (2006 [1996]) by examining visual representation of race in modern newspapers and historic 'science' books. He argues that a critical reading of racial imagery always requires epistemological analysis, not just a semiological theory of how conceptual/analytical representation 'works'. His analysis shows that 'the myth of race' continues to be recycled in Australian media through the illusory epistemological reassurance of digital photographs. Selander's work (Chapter 5) explores what it means to take a social semiotic, multimodal understanding of communication into an understanding of learning. He puts forward two central theses: 1) there is a difference between a multimodal social semiotic perspective on communication, on the one hand, and a knowledge-oriented, epistemic perspective on learning on the other, and 2) the concept of social context is not adequate for understanding communication—an analysis of epistemic contexts, not least in relation to learning, is often required.

The second section of the book includes four papers that examine the meaning-making potentials of a range of (emerging) semiotic resources and artefacts—touch (Jewitt, Chapter 6), community currency (Mooney, Chapter 7), and sound (Gabriel, Chapter 8) and moving images (Tseng, Chapter 9) in complex filmic narratives. Jewitt (Chapter 6) takes inspiration from Van Leeuwen's interdisciplinary and exploratory work on the semiotics of materiality and applies a social semiotic lens on touch, an emerging area of study. Her chapter provides an extensive review of literature on touch and proposes three initial routes into the multimodal analysis of touch, i.e. through concepts of materiality, modal affordance, and semiotic resource. Drawing on Van Leeuwen's work on the semiotics of colour, texture, images, and typography, Mooney (Chapter 7) looks at the semiotics of five community currencies circulated in UK. She argues that the design of community currency draws on the existing semiotic repertoires of national currency but nevertheless creates a modern, local imaginary. The community notes index the hyperreality of money, which provides an invitation to think about what money really is and, in their local instantiations, return money to its sender in its inverted (and true) form.

The following two chapters focus one of Van Leeuwen's favourite media—film (1991, 2005). In Chapter 8, Gabriel examines the notion of artificial intelligence in contemporary cinema. In particular, he offers a detailed analysis of how various subjective experiences of the characters in Alex Garland's *Ex Machina* (2014) are signalled by different configurations of sound, such as pitch, dynamics, volume, and reverberation, and considers how the cultural import of pre-existing music and songs helps 'humanise' a film centred around computers and artificial intelligence. Chapter 9 by Tseng zooms in on van Dormael's *Mr. Nobody* (2010), a film known for its complexity due to its multiple endings. Through a fine-grained analysis of this puzzle film, the chapter demonstrates how social semiotic theories can be employed to effectively deal with significant empirical issues, such as narrative complexity, genre, and intermedial comparisons, which are debated perennially in studies of narrative and the moving image.

The three papers in the final section of the book showcase the ways in which some key concepts from Van Leeuwen's social semiotics, such as new writing (Ledin and Machin, Chapter 10) and recontextualisation (Archer and Björkvall, Chapter 11; and O'Halloran, et al., Chapter 12) can be deployed and expanded in providing understandings of new and emerging social practices. Ledin and Machin (Chapter 10) unpack the neoliberal ideas, values, and identities behind the fitness regime CrossFit. They argue that new writing provides coherence in the CrossFit discourse and has transformed social practices in the interests of neoliberalism. Archer and Björkvall (Chapter 11) question the rise of global consumer movements that critique overconsumption by looking at value adding in artefacts. Specifically, they analyse how resources such as texture, colour, and typography are recontextualised and, to various degrees, recognised in upcycled artefacts that move between South Africa and Europe. In doing so, they demonstrate how the processes of value adding can be described in terms of spatio-linguistic recontextualisation, sensory recontextualisation, and intertextual anchorage as markers of provenance. In Chapter 12, O'Halloran, Tan and Wignell explore the relevance of social semiotic theory in the age of big data and global terrorism. Their study analyses violent extremist propaganda materials produced by the Islamic State and the multimodal recontextualisation of images from these sources across different media platforms. The team aims to develop a mixed-methods approach for integrating qualitative methods of multimodal discourse analysis with quantitative methods of data mining and information visualisation to study discourse patterns in large datasets. Their research establishes the need for digital techniques to develop evidence-based approaches to the study of multimodal recontextualising practices.

The volume ends on a crescendo with a visual essay by Boeriis. Through 11 stunning visual plates, Boeriis engages with visual semiotic theory by displaying the consequences of various available choices and thereby attempting to isolate the parameters, their interplay, and their semiotic consequences in visual meaning-making. Intended as an implicit meta-discussion about what (and how) can be discussed visually, the essay makes a fitting tribute to the theoretic imagination of Van Leeuwen.

A key theme in the more recent development of Van Leeuwen's work—semiotic software technologies—has been deliberately left out from the contributions this volume, as we want this volume to mark not the end of a journey in social semiotics but an invitation to engage with Van Leeuwen's social semiotics. During the editing of this volume, a research symposium on semiotic technologies and social media, organised by Søren Vigild Poulsen (University of Southern Denmark) and Gunhild Kvåle (University of Agder), was being held in Odense, where a diverse group of scholars was passionately debating a range of semiotic phenomena that define the ethos of our age: selfies and social photography, digital aesthetics and curation, Snapchat performances, research content aggregation platforms, data visualisation, online shopping and learning, and many more, and a special journal issue on semiotic technologies is underway.

References

Bernstein, B. (1990). *The structuring of pedagogic discourse: Class, code and control* (Vol.4). London/New York: Routledge.

Byrne, D. (2003). *Envisioning emotional epistemological information*. Print album and DVD: Todomundo.

Caldas-Coulthard, C. R., & Van Leeuwen, T. (2001). Baby's first toys and the discursive construction of childhood. *Critical Discourse Analysis in Post Modern Societies, Special Edition of Folia Linguistica*, XXXV(1–2), 157–182.

Caldas-Coulthard, C. R., & Van Leeuwen, T. (2002). Stunning, shimmering, iridescent: Toys as the representation of gendered social actors. In L. Litosseleti & J. Sunderland (Eds.), *Gender identity and discourse analysis* (pp. 91–110). Amsterdam: John Benjamins.

Caldas-Coulthard, C. R., & Van Leeuwen, T. (2003). Teddy bear stories. *Social Semiotics*, *13*(1), 5–27.
Djonov, E., & Van Leeuwen, T. (2011). The semiotics of texture: From tactile to visual. *Visual Communication*, *10*(4), 541–564. doi:10.1177/1470357211415786
Djonov, E., & Van Leeuwen, T. (2012). Normativity and software: A multimodal social semiotic approach. In S. Norris (Ed.), *Multimodality and practice: Investigating theory-in-practice-through-method* (pp. 119–137). New York: Routledge.
Djonov, E., & Van Leeuwen, T. (2013). Between the grid and composition: Layout in PowerPoint's design and use. *Semiotica*, *2013*(197), 1–34. doi:10.1515/sem-2013-0078
Djonov, E., & Van Leeuwen, T. (2014). Bullet points, new writing, and the marketization of public discourse: A critical multimodal perspective. In E. Djonov & S. Zhao (Eds.), *Critical multimodal studies of popular discourse* (pp. 232–250). London/New York: Routledge.
Djonov, E., & Van Leeuwen, T. (in press). The power of semiotic software: A critical multimodal perspective. In J. Flowerdew & J. Richardson (Eds.), *The Routledge handbook of critical discourse analysis*. London/New York: Routledge.
Djonov, E., & Zhao, S. (Eds.). (2014). *Critical multimodal studies of popular discourse*. London/New York: Routledge.
Gibson, J. J. (1979). *The ecological approach to visual perception*. Boston, MA: Houghton Mifflin.
Halliday, M. A. K. (1978). *Language as social semiotic*. London: Arnold.
Halliday, M. A. K. (1985). Systemic background. In J. Benson & W. Greaves (Eds.), *Systemic perspectives on discourse volume 1: Selected theoretical papers from the 9th international systemic workshop* (Vol. 1, pp. 1–15). Norwood, NJ: Ablex.
Halliday, M. A. K., & Matthiessen, C. M. I. M. (2004). *An introduction to functional grammar* (3rd ed.). London: Arnold.
Hodge, R., & Kress, G. (1988). *Social semiotics*. Cambridge: Polity Press.
Jakobson, R., & Halle, M. (1956). *Fundamentals of language*. The Hague: Mouton.
Kress, G., & Van Leeuwen, T. (2001). *Multimodal discourse: The modes and media of contemporary communication*. London: Arnold.
Kress, G., & Van Leeuwen, T. (2006 [1996]). *Reading images: The grammar of visual design* (2nd ed.). London: Routledge.
Kvåle, G. (2016). Software as ideology: A multimodal critical discourse analysis of Microsoft Word and SmartArt. *Journal of Language and Politics (Special Issue: Multimodality, Politics and Ideology)*, *15*(3), 259–273. doi:10.1075/jlp.15.3.02kva
Lakoff, G., & Johnson, M. (1980). *Metaphors we live by*. Chicago/London: University of Chicago Press.
Machin, D., & Mayr, A. (2012). *How to do critical discourse analysis: A multimodal introduction*. London/Thousand Oaks, CA/New Delhi/ Singapore: Sage.
Machin, D., & Van Leeuwen, T. (2003). Global schemas and local discourses in *Cosmopolitan*. *Journal of Sociolinguistics*, 7(4), 493–512.
Machin, D., & Van Leeuwen, T. (2007). *Global media discourse*. London: Routledge.
Machin, D., & Van Leeuwen, T. (2016). Multimodality, politics and ideology. *Journal of Language & Politics*, *15*(3), 243–258. doi:10.1075/jlp.15.3.01mac
Malinowski, B. (1923). The problem of meaning in primitive languages. In C. K. Ogden & I. A. Richards (Eds.), *The meaning of meaning* (pp. 296–336). New York: Harcourt Brace.
Martinec, R., & Van Leeuwen, T. (2009). *The language of new media design*. London/New York: Routledge.

Van Leeuwen, T. (1982). *Professional speech: Accentual and junctural style in radio announcing.* MA hons. M.A. Honours Thesis, Macquarie University, Sydney, Australia.
Van Leeuwen, T. (1985). Rhythmic structure of the film text. In T. A. van Dijk (Ed.), *Discourse and communication: New approaches to the analyses of mass media discourse and communication* (pp. 216–232). Germany: Walter de Gruyter.
Van Leeuwen, T. (1991a). Conjunctive structure in documentary film and television. *Continuum*, *5*(1), 76–114.
Van Leeuwen, T. (1991b). The sociosemiotics of easy listening music. *Social Semiotics*, *1*(1), 67–80.
Van Leeuwen, T. (1992). The schoolbook as a multimodal text. *Internationale Schulbuchforschung*, *14*(1), 35–58.
Van Leeuwen, T. (1998). Taste in the framework of a semiotics of materiality. In A. Piroëlle (Ed.), *La représentation sociale du goût.* Dijon: University de Bourgogne: PRISM.
Van Leeuwen, T. (1999). *Speech, music, sound.* London: Macmillan Press Ltd.
Van Leeuwen, T. (2000). Visual racism. In M. Reisigl & R. Wodak (Eds.), *The semiotics of racism: Approaches in critical discourse analysis* (pp. 333–350). Vienna: Passagen Verlag.
Van Leeuwen, T. (2003). A multimodal perspective on composition. In T. Ensink & C. Sauer (Eds.), *Framing and perspectivising in discourse* (pp. 23–61). Amsterdam/Philadelphia, PA: John Benjamins.
Van Leeuwen, T. (2005). *Introducing social semiotics.* London/New York: Routledge.
Van Leeuwen, T. (2006a). Towards a semiotics of typography. *Information Design Journal*, *14*(2), 139–155.
Van Leeuwen, T. (2006b). Translation, adaptation, globalisation: The Vietnam News. *Journalism: Theory, Practice and Criticism*, *7*(2), 219–239.
Van Leeuwen, T. (2007). Legitimation in discourse and communication. *Discourse & Communication*, *1*(1), 91–112. doi:10.1177/1750481307071986
Van Leeuwen, T. (2008a). *Discourse and practice: New tools for critical analysis.* London: Oxford University Press.
Van Leeuwen, T. (2008b). New forms of writing, new visual competencies. *Visual Studies*, *23*(2), 130–135.
Van Leeuwen, T. (2009a). Parametric systems: The case of voice quality. In C. Jewitt (Ed.), *The Routledge handbook of multimodal analysis* (pp. 68–77). Oxon/New York: Routledge.
Van Leeuwen, T. (2009b). The world according to Playmobil. *Semiotica*, *2009*(173), 299–315. doi:10.1515/SEMI.2009.013
Van Leeuwen, T. (2010). Discourse and technology. *Journal of Applied Linguistics*, 6(3), 379–392.
Van Leeuwen, T. (2011a). *The language of colour.* Oxon/ New York: Routledge.
Van Leeuwen, T. (2011b). Rhythm and multimodal semiosis. In S. Dreyfus, S. Hood, & M. Stenglin (Eds.), *Semiotic margins* (pp. 168–176). London/New York: Continuum.
Van Leeuwen, T. (2011c). The semiotics of decoration. In L. O'Halloran Kay & B. A. Smith (Eds.), *Multimodal studies: Issues and domains* (pp. 115–127). New York/Oxon: Routledge.
Van Leeuwen, T. (2013). Critical analysis of multimodal discourse. In C. Chapelle (Ed.), *Encyclopedia of applied linguistics.* Oxford: Wiley-Blackwell (Area Editor: Sigrid Norris).

Van Leeuwen, T. (2014). Colour: Code, mode, modality—the case of film and video. In C. Jewitt (Ed.), *The Routledge handbook of multimodal analysis* (2nd ed., pp. 397–410). London: Routledge.

Van Leeuwen, T. (2015a). Creativity in the fourth dimension: The grammar of movement according to Jean Tinguely. In R. H. Jones (Ed.), *The Routledge handbook of language and creativity* (pp. 336–352). New York: Routledge.

Van Leeuwen, T. (2015b). Looking good: Aesthetics, multimodality and literacy studies. In J. Rowsell & K. Pahl (Eds.), *The Routledge handbook of literacy studies* (pp. 426–439). New York: Routledge.

Van Leeuwen, T. (2017). A social semiotic theory of synesthesia?—a discussion paper. *HERMES: Journal of Language and Communication in Business*, *55*, 105–119.

Van Leeuwen, T., & Boeriis, M. (2017). Towards a semiotics of film lighting. In J. Wildfeuer & J. A. Bateman (Eds.), *Film text analysis: New perspectives in the analysis of filmic meaning* (pp. 24–46). New York/Oxon: Routledge.

Van Leeuwen, T., & Caldas-Coulthard, C. R. (2004). The semiotics of kinetic design. In D. Banks (Ed.), *Text and texture: Systemic functional viewpoints on the nature and structure of text* (pp. 355–382). Paris: L'Harmattan.

Van Leeuwen, T., & Djonov, E. (2013). Multimodality and software. In C. Chapelle (Ed.), *Encyclopedia of applied linguistics*. Oxford: Wiley-Blackwell (Area Editor: Sigrid Norris).

Van Leeuwen, T., & Djonov, E. (2015). Notes towards a semiotics of kinetic typography. *Social Semiotics*, *25*(2), 244–253. doi:10.1080/10350330.2015.1010324

Van Leeuwen, T., Djonov, E., & O'Halloran, K. L. (2013). "David Byrne really does love PowerPoint": Art as research on semiotics and semiotic technology. *Social Semiotics*, *23*(3), 409–423. doi:10.1080/10350330.2012.738998

Van Leeuwen, T., & Humphrey, S. (1996). On learning to look through a geographer's eyes. In R. Hasan & G. Williams (Eds.), *Literacy in society* (pp. 29–49). London/New York: Longman.

Van Leeuwen, T., & Jaworski, A. (2002). The discourses of war photography: Photojournalistic representations of the Palestinian-Israeli war. *Journal of Language and Politics*, *1*(2), 255–275.

Van Leeuwen, T., & Kress, G. (1995). Critical layout analysis. *Internationale Schulbuchforschung*, *17*, 25–43.

Van Leeuwen, T., & Wodak, R. (1999). Legitimising immigration control: A discourse-historical analysis. *Discourse Studies*, *1*(1), 83–118. doi:10.1177/1461445699001001005

Wodak, R. (2015). *Politics of fear: What right-wing populist discourses mean*. London: Sage.

Wodak, R., & Van Leeuwen, T. (2002). Discourses of un/employment in Europe: The Austrian case. *Text*, *22*(3), 345–367.

Zhao, S., Djonov, E., & Van Leeuwen, T. (2014). Semiotic technology and practice: A multimodal social semiotic approach to PowerPoint. *Text & Talk*, *34*(3), 349–375. doi:10.1515/text-2014-0005

Zhao, S., & Van Leeuwen, T. (2014). Understanding semiotic technology in university classrooms: A social semiotic approach to PowerPoint-assisted cultural studies lectures. *Classroom Discourse*, *5*(1), 71–90. doi:10.1080/19463014.2013.859848

2 Changing Academic Common Sense

A Personal Recollection of Collaborative Work

Gunther Kress

This is an informal account of a long period of working collaboratively with Theo Van Leeuwen. It is neither strictly 'academic' nor overly 'personal', mirroring a relation which was seriously academic and marked by friendship. Where I might implicate Theo in views which he might not hold or wish to be associated with, I use the personal "I". That is the case, for instance, with my reflections on disciplines as "agencies of socialisation" and my sense of what these make possible and what they make difficult.

1. Encounter

In 1978, *Language as Ideology* was published. Bob Hodge and I had worked on the book when we were colleagues at the University of East Anglia. Our aim had been to make mainstream linguistics socially useful and useable by showing how its categories could reveal the workings of power in shaping language in its constant use. As we were finishing the book, it was clear to us that the theory we had sketched could and should be expanded to all means of making meaning. We promised ourselves to do just that if and when that might become possible. In 1978, it became possible to make a start on that—whenever the small matter of distance between Perth and Adelaide might permit. For the now much-enlarged frame—compared with that of *Language as Ideology*—that we were envisaging, we would need to borrow categories from outside linguistics. Art history for instance, might, amongst others, prove a useful source.

In that context, I encountered a significant piece of research, analysing the speech of disc-jockeys working on different commercial radio stations in Sydney (Van Leeuwen, 1982). The research focused on *phonetic* and *phonological* features of speech, such as *pace* and *intonation* for instance, as well as on aspects of (a 'mid-Pacific') *dialect*. In the descriptions, the clear, ideological positions of the speakers themselves and of the radio stations for which they were working were evident. The research presented was a fine-grained, subtle, detailed, phonetic/phonological account. It was totally persuasive.

These were analyses and accounts of the kind that Bob Hodge and I had outlined in our work, though by making use of the full range of linguistic features—grammatical, syntactic, lexical, and textual. Here, by entire contrast, the accounts were based solely on features of the *sound* of speech. No grammatical, syntactic, lexical, or textual elements appeared. The analyses were virtuoso pieces: precise and plausible accounts both of the speakers' ideological positioning and those of the institution where they were working.

Some years on, in 1984 or so, I came across two occasional papers, published in the Department of Anthropology at Sydney University. The author, again, was Theo van Leeuwen. Here too, the material dealt with was sound; now, though, *sound-as-music* rather than *sound-as-speech*. In their 'take' on meaning, the papers were as astonishing as the earlier research had been. A major, underpinning point of reference was the monumental ethnographic work of Alan Lomax, in the vast world of ethno-musicology (Lomax, 1968). From this Theo had drawn out, extrapolated, and brought into focus semiotic aspects of the music being made, based on the social arrangements evident in the different kinds of music-making.

I had heard a lecture or two by the author of the papers; and had heard his accomplished performances as a (jazz) pianist, both as soloist and playing with a small group. Given my own developing interests at the time and theoretical direction, given the earlier encounter with Theo's work on the speech of disc-jockeys, and now having read his writing on music, it was clear that he and I would find it enjoyable and maybe productive to talk around our interest in *meaning*—beyond what was then the mainstream notion, available in and through 'language'.

Our shared interest in the social-functional approach of Hallidayan linguistics (Kress, 1976) was one point of departure. Theo had come to linguistics as a film-maker and theorist, as well as a practising musician and composer. Bob and I had just been offered a contract for a book to be called *Social Semiotics* (Hodge & Kress, 1989). We had chosen its title to acknowledge the influence of Halliday's work on our thinking. With our new book, we aimed to extend the theory of *Language as Ideology* to encompass all means of making meaning.

The 'social' in Halliday's approach was not a fully elaborated social theory: more a sketched outline of interlocking/overlapping social domains: of *field*, *tenor* and *mode*. As a kind of 'scenic backdrop', it served to characterise the social domain sufficiently for his linguistic theory. Three mediating functions—the *ideational*, the *interpersonal*, and the *textual*—linked the social with the semiotic domain. From the perspective of our beginning work, then, in this sketchy frame, *language* could be readily replaced by any other resource for making meaning. All it would need was to change the material articulations of the three domains and the realisation of the three matching *functions* by the chosen material resource. For Theo and myself, that resource was going to be *image*.

It is worth reflecting on the extent to which a professional socialisation constantly shapes—or twists out of shape—attempts to get to somewhere new. Theo and I had set out to remake an established academic/intellectual—and commonsense—position in fundamental ways; yet all the time, we used the conceptual/theoretical tools that had shaped the world we were trying to get beyond.

2. Joint Work 1: *Reading Images*

By a happy and extremely useful coincidence, at that time Theo and I were living within a five-minute walk in the inner Sydney suburb of Newtown. Talking was going to be relatively easy. In 1986, we decided to turn shared interest and occasional conversations into real work. We knew that we would need to start, pretty well, from scratch. Of course, we had the theoretical frame of Hallidayan grammar, were aware of the writings of art historians, of film theorists and of those who were engaged in visual design. Our aim was to provide an account which would make evident the 'regularities' of image-material due to their social shaping; an account which, while systematic and organised, would not be either 'linguistic' nor 'art historical' (Kress & Van Leeuwen, 1996).

We imagined something akin to a 'grammar', which would describe *elements* and *relations* in the *designs* evident in images; it would provide a basic frame of meaning relations. We had begun to feel uneasy about certain theoretical formulations in linguistics; yet our aim was to provide tools that would serve in the design of semiotic entities of 'the visual', much as a grammar of 'language' gave and even now still does give us indications, for instance, on how to construct a sentence. So—paradoxically, nearly—and with some explanation of our use of the term, we decided to retain, in a renovated fashion, the term *grammar*.

In the conversations we had had before, our assumption had been the Hallidayan one, that if language was the product of social (inter-)action, then the same assumption would apply to images. Hence our mode of working was to get some relevant 'material' as the 'data' that was to be accounted for. We spent much time jointly looking at such bits of data. We asked questions which arose out of a Hallidayan conception of a meaning resource, for instance: "How does the interpersonal function 'work' in respect to this (bit of) image?"

The first larger piece of such material that we looked at in detail—and stayed with over the next few weeks—was a copy of *Australian Women's Weekly*. Serendipitously, it was the first likely 'bit' we had come across as we had gone looking, going from the garden where we had decided to 'work', into the house.

Our 'looking' was founded on a shared theoretical interest and position, which, nevertheless did allow for differences of disposition, experience, and approach. Neither shared interest nor differences made 'things' appear at all readily in the materials on our initial looking. Questions here and there, around things that seemed odd about our materials, were means of slowly prising open what might 'actually' be going on. In conversations with page designers, we had been told, for instance, that advertisements as well as larger images ought to be placed in certain spaces on a page. We were puzzled to note that these 'rules' seemed not to be used by the designers in their own work. Such discrepancies provided a prompt for looking, digging deeper, and thinking further about more plausible accounts.

This was pretty early—and scary—work: going against what seemed the settled professional sense of experienced designers, for instance. Nor did we have any idea how our thinking might be received by our colleagues. We did not know whether our descriptions would provide what we wanted them to provide. In that context, the support and confirming effect of working closely with someone whose judgement one could trust can not be overestimated.

In our joint working over the next ten years and more, we kept to this mode of proceeding. We would start with some material that attracted our interest in some way; we would ask questions: slowly finding ways to get 'closer'. The Hallidayan categories provided both a stable reference 'grid' and a constant prompt. Having decided on the theoretical frame, the 'grid' of categories prompted specific directions and places to look, as much as it provided ways of looking. At times, we stayed with specific issues over quite long periods. Our different backgrounds provided usefully different productive points of view. Differences within a shared theoretical position remained as one constant in our work, the differences proving at least as productively significant as the shared basis and perceptions.

While the categories of Halliday's theoretical frame were a rough and ready even if not solid set of guidelines, nevertheless, from the very beginning, we made use of both frame and categories in a significantly different way to the ways in which others (O'Toole, 1994; O'Halloran, 1998) had used these 'same' categories, much more closely aligned to the linguistic framework. Early on, we realised that the *materiality* of the resources for representation imposed specific constraints on how the *semiotic* categories of the theory might or could be realised.

To exemplify this briefly, a *social* category such as *power* might appear as a matter of *social distance* or *proximity*; as its analogue, it has *semiotic distance*. The *semiotic* category *power* is *realised*—made materially evident—differently due to the constraints of the materiality of each mode. In *speech* or *writing* there is lexis: adjectives for instance, such as *inferior* or *superior*; in grammar as (*temporal*) *distance*, as (*past* or *present*) *tense*; or as (*ontological*) *distance* via the category of *modality*. In speech—in English—there is a large range of intonational contours to realise *power*. While *image* does not have the resource of *lexis*, *power* can be realised in *image* through its specific *semiotic* means, for instance through 'spatial distance' as its metaphoric realisation of 'social distance', or through the signifier of 'angle' in visual representation—as in '*high*' or '*low*' angle—as well as through other (spatial) means.

Our awareness of the effect of *materiality* on the means by which *semiotic* categories are realised never made it plausible for us to use *linguistic* categories as means to account for visual meanings. Halliday (1970, 1983) had shown that *speech* (in English) worked according to different principles than did *writing*. For *speech*, the capacity of human lungs imposes a physiological/physical/material limit: namely, the volume of air available in 'breathing out'. It is this volume of air which is available to shape and utter a *speech-unit*.

In thinking about theoretical relations across modes, our focus was on the *semiotic* categories underlying the *linguistic* descriptions and realisation. We could ask, plausibly, "How is *involvement* realised/materialised in *image*?" or "How does one 'do' *intensity* in the modes of *image*, or *gesture* or *colour*?" In our account of the mode of *image*, categories such as *text, coherence, genre, composition, relations, modality, modification, frame, distance*, and so on all had a place.

With a difference in modal material the categories are realised differently. Consequently, our questions were not: "What is an *adjective* in the mode of image?" or "What *clause types* are there in the mode of image?" We asked, rather, "How does *modification* work in *image*?", "What are the means available in the mode of *image* (or *gesture*, or *gaze*) for realising *states, relations, processes*?" or "How do *cohesion* and *coherence* work in *image*?"

For Theo as a maker and a theorist of film as much as a practicing musician and theorist of music (Van Leeuwen, 1991, 1999), it was clear that it should be possible to account, at a certain level of abstraction, for the semiotic resources of both film and music with the same semiotic categories as for other representational resources. Predictably, given the different materiality, these were not 'captured' in any way by the categories and terms provided by *linguistic* theories. Using Halliday's work in my own thinking about the move children make from speech to writing (Kress, 1982), it had become clear to me that it was increasingly difficult to think of speech and writing as comfortably accommodated under the single label 'language'.

Our work with images had made it clear that the material and semiotic resources of *language* are constantly (re-)shaped in relation with and as a response to the requirements of (inter-)action in social environments. The same was bound to be the case with all resources for making meaning. In our case, it would apply to *image*.

From the outset, we were clear that our model would be the categories, the thinking, and the examples of *Halliday the semiotician* rather than those of *Halliday the linguist*. Clearly, one central question in this was 'the social'. We assumed that his schema would account in the same manner for the relation of the social to the semiotic with all the resources of meaning: for the resource of *image* as well as for those of *speech* and *writing*. With each mode, there would be distinct differences in realisation given the different materiality.

Theo's publications about *speech* and *music* had been written in that vein (Van Leeuwen, 1982, 1999). In earlier publications I had focused on the distinctive differences of speech and writing, and had begun to include visual materials (Kress, 1982). And now Bob Hodge and I were looking at a range of materials in our work for *Social Semiotics*—photos, sculpture, paintings, linguistic materials, of course, architecture, and so on. In the work that led to *Reading Images*, Theo and I occasionally glanced at other modes and their constitution and organisation. Our emphasis however stayed firmly on *image*. We made suggestions about semiotic categories which we felt were applicable to all modes—for instance, the notion of different kinds of 'realism', of kinds of 'modality' in the sense of "proximity to 'truth'". We were conscious that the semiotic landscape encompassed quite different modes; we assumed that most if not all the *semiotic* categories we were identifying and describing in the mode of image would be present in all modes.

What became ever clearer in the course of doing this work on images was that in terms of communicational 'use', compositions involving many modes—*multimodal orchestrations* and *complexes*—were governed by one and the same set of 'social forces' and therefore would be organised by and subject to the same set of semiotic categories as those we regarded as 'monomodal' were.

The move from (the assumed use of) one mode—'language'—to an awareness that all compositions/texts consist of more than one mode, introduced the issue of 'choice'. There was now a decision to be made which was quite different to the question of mere competence: namely, the question of which mode to use in a specific situation, and why. With that question, the category of *design* has become central in every act of meaning-making. The (rhetorical) question now was, "What am I trying to communicate here, for whom, and how are the resources available to me put to best use for this purpose here?" When the presence, availability, and use of more than one mode has become generally recognised as commonplace, the question of *design* has become central. With hindsight it is evident that *design* is a factor in all semiosis.

3. Joint Work 2: *Multimodal Discourse*

Of course, we had talked about 'what next?' Both of us had analysed spoken and written texts over a considerable time, with the tools, for instance, of critical linguistics and critical discourse analysis; these included texts with images. Now we felt that we could complement an analysis of language with a nearly equally clear account of images: We could describe and analyse compositions of *image* and *writing*. We felt confident that we had the means to produce a book in which both approaches could be clearly 'modelled': one approach (more) language oriented, the other (more) image oriented. The book would be a kind of 'how to' manual, which might be useful to students of communication and media studies, and of any similarly 'text-oriented' subjects, education being one.

We spent considerable time debating what a title of such a book might be: we decided to try the term 'multimodality', and so the title we suggested to the publisher was *Multimodal Text*. We fully expected a negative response to the word 'multimodality'. Far from it, the publisher liked the term; she did insist however that the word 'discourse' should appear in the title. Lesley Riddle, our editor/publisher at Edward Arnold's, had plausible and persuasive arguments for that change, mainly to do with various nitty-gritty practices of competition for limited shelf-space in bookshops. Further, at that time the term 'discourse' was likely to 'sell', overcoming the novelty of 'multimodality'.

Now we had a contract for another joint book: joint, again, in authorship; and joint in bringing language and image together (Kress & Van Leeuwen, 2001). Once we started thinking about the potential offered by the title for the kind of book we might produce, we realised from our work on *Reading Images* that multimodal texts were based on and demonstrated 'integration' of various kinds. In our thinking, the scope of the book expanded. It should, we felt, provide a relatively formal and explicit account of 'the multimodal world of meaning', encompassing accounts of objects of all kinds; of buildings—domestic or public; of 'rooms' and their furnishings; an ambitious account of the semiotic world. To give it all coherence and frame, we used the term 'overarching grammar', in that all modes and complexes of modes could be accommodated and accounted for.

For that grammar, we did not expect to find instances of strict rules; rather we expected 'regularities' of certain kinds. A larger range of materials might enable us to deduce this 'over-arching grammar'; it would provide 'indications', 'suggestions' more than rules, on how modes could be used together.

This seemed plausible as an aim. Yet, we did not manage to make it work; it proved impossible to achieve in that book. One question was at what 'level' and with what kinds and 'size' of unit the connections between modal elements could and would be possible. If the minimal meaningful unit of semiotics is the sign, then, with speech or writing some answers to the question, "what is a sign in writing?" or even "what are the signs used in writing?" are not too difficult. But with image, the same questions become difficult. What are the *signs* in an (naturalistic) image of a tree? The leaves of the tree? Its branches? Is each leaf a sign?

There were the accounts provided by art history, or, in different versions of design studies, and so on. But these came from distinctly different paradigms, posing different kinds of questions to those of a social semiotic approach. Without a reasonably firm sense of *entities*—of kinds of signs or of sign complexes, in our case—it is difficult to think about combinations of modes: what would or could be combined with what? These were new questions.

In the face of these difficulties we moved away from attempts to describe phenomena at a 'surface' level, to hypothesising about larger level, general requirements at issue in the making of multimodal complexes. This account would work for all instances of multimodal complexes, though at a quite abstract level. We felt we could make plausible suggestions about principles of composition which were at work in the making of any multimodal complex.

Implied in our work both in *Reading Images* and in *Multimodal Discourse* was a decisive shift of academic paradigm: largely from a *linguistic* to a *semiotic* paradigm, with all the far-reaching implications that such a shift entails. As our first attempt at a set of social semiotic categories that might underpin such an account, we suggested that all multimodal complexes would have to attend to four principles: of *discourse* (in the Foucauldian sense), *design*, *production*, and *distribution*.

4. Looking Back and Looking Ahead

My account of this 'joint history' of working with Theo is skewed in a number of ways. It is skewed being written with the hindsight provided by—in some cases—more than 25 years' distance. Inevitably, my more recent 'insights' have seeped into this account. The more than 25 years since the start of our work have seen profound social—and technological—changes. These can be discerned, with hindsight, in the social and semiotic landscape of 'then'. 'The social' of 2017 is, however, a far remove from what was, in 1986, seen, unremarkably, as a stable social. The clearest indication of the change is the shift from the then still relatively intact nation-state with its aims and givens, to the dominance of the neoliberal market with its entirely different aims.

Reading Images comes, discernibly, from the early part of that twenty-five-year period. It has—and shows—its disciplinary origins in the three centuries' long hegemony of the verbal-written 'Western' culture. *Multimodal Discourse* is (in my view) a product of a much more recent social. To give one example: The subtitle of *Reading Images* is "**The** *grammar of visual design*": not '*a* grammar. . .'. In working on *Multimodal Discourse*, we wanted to provide something resembling—note 'resembling'—a definition of *mode*. What we did provide was a 'condition': namely, that *mode* is that which a community regards as a mode *if* it fulfills the community's semiotic/communicational needs. The move from the certainty, the *definiteness* of the definite article 'the' in the subtitle of *Reading Images*, to the provisionality of "*something resembling a definition*" in *Multimodal discourse*, is one of many instances of an unease the book betrays in parts. It is a response to its much more recent genesis and the profound social instabilities of the contemporary period.

If the semiotic categories of the social semiotic theory are the product of social arrangements, then the fraying of these social arrangements is bound to produce instability of the semiotic categories. Take *genre* as a case in point. If we take genre (as I do) as the *entexting* of social relations of participants in some event, then the semiotic category of *genre* becomes entirely unstable if the social relations have ceased to be stable. Or, as a further example, take *cohesion* and *coherence*. These two categories assume and project known, understood, social relations, and organisation. There is no possibility of a translation of the social relations into epistemological semiotic relations if the former does not exist.

Writing this account has shown me the extent to which—all throughout—our joint work has been shaped by frameworks that we were struggling to leave behind. The tools we had for the task were the tools that had produced what had now become the problem. A theory and its categories (and the disciplines in which they are 'accommodated') are a response to the problems and questions of a specific social time. There comes a time when the problems and questions are quite other, and the tools are no longer apt. This is not to detract in any way from a sense that the two works offer useful ways of thinking and tools, relevant for the analysis or the design of semiotic entities: complex or simple, traditional or contemporary.

I do think that social semiotics has a potential to deal with many of the contemporaneously most pressing problems around *meaning* and *meaning-making*. The accounts we provided in *Reading Images* of the categories of the mode of *image* and the regularities of their use offer insight both for the analysis of images and for their use in the design of texts as multimodal complexes. I do think that the notion of *mode* is relevant and timely; it is in a very early stage of being explored and of being more securely established along a number of different parameters. It also poses questions about what text is, what its elements are. *Multimodal Discourse* takes some steps along that path. The environments and conditions of the use of the mode of *image*, as indeed of all modes, have changed profoundly. These emerging environments and conditions will inevitably change the compositional principles not only of the mode of *image* but of all multimodal composition and meaning-making.

To get a sense of trends around multimodal meaning-making requires a hard, close-up look at the make-up of the contemporary social and its likely development. We know that the pace of social change is not the same as that of technological change, even though educational policies and fashions tend to suggest that they are. Nor does the pace of semiotic change exactly match either of these. Yet the three are entirely linked, though each with its different dynamic and pace.

There is, for me, now, an entirely new question: it is about the relation of 'the social' and 'the technological'. It concerns the speed—near instantaneous—of contemporary *transmission* (even if not necessarily *communication*) of "micro-messages", via the most recent forms of the social media (i.e. post-Facebook) and the likely potential effects of that. The messages are bite-size (though they can be expanded by *links*). This immediately raises two questions: that of representational resources—for instance, what *modes* and what *genres*—are used and in what ways; and entirely related, that of size. The *speed* of exchange/interchange is such that there is no possibility of 'calibration', of checking within and against a known or reliable 'social' to establish what used to be regarded as 'fact' or 'truth'. It is difficult to think what cohesive devices there might be and how *coherence* might be produced in such socially featureless environments.

Older forms of (relatively) instantaneous communication—local gossip, for instance—could be checked, 'weighed', compared against relatively settled understandings by the members of a 'gossip community', which, in its idealised and maybe mythic form, might have been a local neighbourhood, or close variants of this. Current forms of instantaneous communication have a geographic and social reach that is beyond any geographical and social domain—beyond and across all and any such communities. The 'content' of such messages cannot be verified. They stand by themselves and for themselves. It is this feature and the resultant conditions that lend plausibility to notions of a post-fact and post-truth society.

If there is some plausibility to this account, these forms of interaction do look like the constitutive components of a 'new social'. That social would be formed by temporary and transient aggregations and disaggregation of socially un-located individuals. It is a particularly virulent form of MacLuhan's dictum (McLuhan & Fiore, 1967) that the media are the message/massage—that is, a situation where the media constitute the social, displacing former arrangements.

The semiotic consequences of this are difficult to assess, to sketch, to imagine. The kinds of issues which have hovered more recently on the horizon of current developments of social semiotics and multimodality were questions such as the boundaries of 'the semiotic' and the 'physiological/biological'; the description of elements and relations of as yet 'undocumented' modes; making evident 'tacit' and 'embodied' ways of knowing, and making evident means of engagement with the world of the 'tacit' (Van Leeuwen, 2011). All these may fade in the face of this (still seemingly technological) development.

Any attempts to consider ethical, social, and political futures, questions about the kind of social we wish to engender, to foster, and to support become both more urgent and certainly more difficult. No doubt, solutions there will come from traditional forms of social action. Social semiotics can have a significant role in helping make some sense of that world.

In needing to account for a radically changing social, social semiotics will now have to re-orient to deal with a new set of issues. As mentioned earlier, in *Multimodal Discourse* we proposed that meanings are made in four domains (we had called them 'strata'): *Discourse*, as "socially constructed knowledge(s) of (some aspects of) reality"; *Design*, as the arrangement, the composition, of *discursive materials*; *Production*, as the material realisation of a semiotic event or object; and *Distribution*, "the technical 're-coding' of semiotic products and events, for purposes of recording and/or distribution".

Thinking about that now, in 2017, it seems to me that the energy, the emphasis broadly, in thinking and research had largely focused on the first two of these. That too can be seen as a continuation of the 'traditional approach': whether in CDA or in Multimodal Discourse Analysis, the emphasis had been on the "content of the message", to evoke McLuhan (2001) once more. The direction in which the social and semiotic world is moving suggests that the last two categories are bound to come much more into focus (Van Leeuwen & Djonov, 2013).

References

Halliday, M. A. K. (1970). Language structure and language functions. In J. Lyons (Ed.), *New horizons in inguistics*. Harmondsworth, Middlesex: Penguin Books.

Halliday, M. A. K. (1983). *Spoken and written English*. Oxford: Oxford University Press.

Hodge, R. I. V., & Kress, G. R. (1979). *Language as ideology*. London: Routledge.

Hodge, R. I. V., & Kress, G. R. (1989). *Social semiotics*. Oxford: Polity Press.

Kress, G. R. (Ed.). (1976). *Halliday: System and function in language: Selected papers*. Oxford: Oxford University Press.

Kress, G. R. (1982). *Learning to write*. London: Routledge.

Kress, G. R., & Van Leeuwen, T. (1996). *Reading images: The grammar of visual design*. London: Routledge.

Kress, G. R., & Van Leeuwen, T. (2001). *Multimodal discourse: The modes and media of contemporary communication*. London: Edward Arnold.

Lomax, A. (1968). *Folk song style and culture*. St Louis: Transaction Publishers.

McLuhan, M. (2001). *Understanding media: The extension of man*. New York: Routledge Classics.

McLuhan, M., & Fiore, Q. (1967). *The medium is the massage: An inventory of effects*. New York: Bantam Books.

O'Halloran, K. (1998). Classroom discourse in mathematics: A multisemiotic analysis. *Linguistics and Education*, *10*(3), 359–388.

O'Toole, M. (1994). *The language of displayed art*. Leicester: Leicester University Press.

Van Leeuwen, T. (1982). *Professional speech: Accentual and junctural style in radio announcing*. M.A. Honours Dissertation, Macquarie University, Sydney, Australia.

Van Leeuwen, T. (1991). Conjunctive structure in documentary film and television. *Continuum*, *5*(1), 76–114.

Van Leeuwen, T. (1999). *Speech, music, sound*. London: Palgrave.

Van Leeuwen, T. (2011). *The language of colour: An introduction*. London: Routledge Falmer.

Van Leeuwen, T., & Djonov, E. (2013). Multimodality and software. In C. Chapelle (Ed.), *Encyclopedia of applied linguistics*. Oxford: Wiley-Blackwell.

3 "Strangers in Europe"

A Discourse-Historical Approach to the Legitimation of Immigration Control 2015/16

Ruth Wodak

1. Introduction

In 1999, Theo van Leeuwen and I co-authored a paper on 'Legitimising immigration control' in the first issue of the then new journal *Discourse Studies*. Not only has this paper been very well received and widely cited, the topic has remained just as relevant or become even more relevant. Indeed, since the summer of 2015, when thousands of refugees tried to enter the European Union countries because of the terrible wars in Iraq, Syria, Libya, and so forth, the topics of immigration and flight have gained more salience: governments, the EU institutions, NGOs, and the media are debating how to cope with the so-called 'refugee problem', 'refugee crisis', or 'immigration problem'. Ever-new ways of legitimising measures to keep 'strangers' out of Europe (and elsewhere) dominate these debates. Slogans such as 'Fortress Europe' and "we have to protect our borders" have become hegemonic. Although first launched by right-wing populist parties and politicians (Carr, 2015, 5ff.), this rhetoric has influenced both centre-right and centre-left wing parties, and a much more general border-and-body politics has emerged in current political debates (Wodak, 2015, 2016).

In the 1999 paper, we explored the systematic rejection of family reunion applications of immigrant workers in Austria by combining the discourse-historical approach (DHA) with systemic-functional discourse analysis to study a corpus of official letters which notified immigrant workers of the rejection of their family reunion applications. We were able to detect four types of legitimation strategies, which were employed in the rejection of family reunion (Van Leeuwen & Wodak, 1999, 104ff.; Wodak & Van Leeuwen, 2002). Briefly, *authorisation legitimation* is legitimation by reference to authority, i.e., the answer to the implicit or explicit question, "Why is it so?" or "Why must it be so?" is essentially "Because *I* say so", or "Because so-and-so says so", where the 'so-and-so' is someone in whom institutionalised authority is vested. *Rationalisation legitimation* is legitimation by reference either to the utility of the social practice or some part of it ('instrumental rationalisation'), or to 'the facts of life' ('theoretical rationalisation').

It may be established in some form of common sense or by the specialists who elaborate the domains of knowledge used for the purpose of legitimation, i.e. in the way in which economic theory can be used to legitimate contemporary employment policies. Furthermore, we distinguished two kinds of *moral legitimation*: the first based on abstract moral values (religious, human rights, justice, culture, and so forth), and the second established by means of straightforwardly evaluative claims. The fourth major type of legitimation is *mythopoesis*, legitimation achieved through the telling of stories. The telling of stories is one of the most important strategies in racist and anti semitic discourse in non-official contexts (see Table 3.3, Taxonomy of Legitimation Strategies, below).

For example, in the following two quotes (Examples 1 and 2), from former Austrian Chancellor Werner Faymann (from the Social-Democratic Party, SPÖ) and then U.S. Republican presidential candidate Donald Trump, the building of a wall to protect their respective countries is legitimised, albeit in different ways.

Example 1

> There is a difference, whether one builds a border or whether one builds a small door with side-parts. There is no fence around Austria. This is a technical security measure that does not box in Austria.
>
> (Werner Faymann, 28/10/15)[1]

Example 2

> "It's gonna be a great wall", Trump said on the Sunday program. "This will be a wall with a big, very beautiful door because we want the legals to come back into the country".
>
> (Donald Trump, 9/2/2016)[2]

Faymann, who had vehemently opposed the building of a wall for several months (for a chronology of events in 2015–2016, see Table 3.2 below), uses a euphemistic expression which focuses on a door, reframing the wall as 'the side-parts' of the door, thus backgrounding the literal fence. This is legitimation by theoretical rationalisation—furthermore, Faymann euphemistically states that the wall only implies technical security measures (instrumental legitimation). Trump, on the other hand, justifies building of a wall in order to keep 'illegal immigrants', who are presupposed to be dangerous, out, the 'big, very beautiful door' within it only opening for 'legal' immigrants. In this way, Trump presupposes that it should be easy to distinguish between legal and illegal migrants. In both cases, the politics of exclusion has been re-semiotised—from policies to concrete material practices, created by barbed wires, bricks, and mortar.

Legitimation strategies thus justify and legitimise the inclusion or exclusion of migrants in a specific nation state (such as Austria, the UK, or the U.S.) (e.g., Rojo-Martin & Van Dijk, 1997). Legitimation strategies make use of specific argumentation schemes, namely a range of formal- and content-related topoi, which can serve as warrants in such legitimation procedures (Wodak, 2015; Reisigl, 2014; see also Table 3.1 below). Or, one could also claim that argumentation in political debates employs legitimation strategies, as part of strategic maneuvering (Van Eemeren, 2010; Ietcu-Fairclough, 2008; Zarefsky, 2008). I will discuss this dialectic relationship in more detail below insofar as it impacts on the selection of specific immigration-related topoi and fallacies, in particular in the context of the 2015/16 refugee crisis in Austria and Europe more generally.

Table 3.1 Selected list of content-related topoi in discriminatory discourses about immigration (adopted from Reisigl & Wodak, 2001, p. 74–80)

Topos	*Warrant*
Topos of advantage or usefulness	*If an action from a specific relevant point of view will be useful, then one should perform it.*
Topos of uselessness or disadvantage	*If one can anticipate that the predicted consequences of a decision will not occur, then the decision has to be rejected.*
Topos of threat or danger	*If there are specific dangers or threats, one should do something to counter them.*
Topos of humanitarianism	*If a political action or decision does or does not conform to human rights or humanitarian convictions and values, then one should or should not make it.*
Topos of burden or weighing down	*If a person, an institution or a country is burdened by specific problems, one should act in order to diminish those burdens.*
Topos of finance	*If a specific situation or action costs too much money or causes a loss of revenue, one should perform actions that diminish those costs or help to avoid/mitigate the loss.*
Topos of reality	*Because reality is as it is, a specific action/ decision should be taken/ made.*
Topos of numbers	*If the numbers prove a specific claim, a specific action should be taken/ not carried out.*

Below, I first elaborate some aspects of recent border-and-body politics and focus on the concept of the moralisation of borders (Vollmer, 2016) (Section 2.1). There, I also discuss multiple argumentation schemes, exemplified in detail in section 2.2., related to the legitimation strategies identified in Van Leeuwen and Wodak (1999). Section 3 summarises some of the socio-political developments in Austria (the 2015/16 'refugee situation') and analyses examples from media debates about refugees and immigrants in order to distil the (new and old) legitimation strategies and topoi involved. The conclusion (Section 4) discusses continuities and discontinuities as made visible in the media reporting about "protecting our borders from strangers" throughout Europe and beyond.

2. Legitimising Border and Body Politics

2.1 The 'Moralisation' of Borders

The manifold discursive forms of inclusion and exclusion define who are 'Europeans' and create an 'imagined community' (Anderson, 1994) that necessarily excludes 'Others', who are usually represented as 'strangers' (Simmel, 1950; Bauman, 1995) or even 'enemies'. Which 'Europe' is implied? And who are the 'strangers'?

The Schengen Convention, ratified in 1990, was incorporated into the Treaty of Amsterdam in 1997. It allows for the abolition of passport control in the so-called Schengen area, which today, in 2017, consists of 25 member states, a population of 450 million people who are able to move freely across a political space of 4.312099 square kilometres, within a common external frontier of 42,672 kilometres of land borders and 8,826 of coastlines (e.g., Carr, 2015, p. 28). The countries at the periphery of the Schengen zone are responsible for sealing their borders against the aforementioned strangers; it comes as no surprise, therefore, that to accompany the freedom 'inside Europe', ever stricter immigration laws are being established for people coming from 'outside Europe'. Border and identity politics converge to keep specific kinds of strangers out while letting others in. Ever since 9/11, immigration restrictions have multiplied, legitimised by a plethora of security reasons (Wodak & Boukala, 2015).

Accordingly, renationalising tendencies can be observed across many EU member states, a nativist body politics seems to be 'celebrating' a revival, embracing the metaphor of 'The Nation as Body' (Musolff, 2010; Wodak, 2015). Paasi (2010) and Vollmer (2017) maintain that a renegotiation of the concept of the border has been occurring for more than a decade. Increasing measures of securitisation and militarisation are implemented not only at political levels but also at normative levels in what Vollmer (2016, p. 4) labels the "moralisation of bordering":

> Moralisation of bordering takes place when considering the balancing act of excluding a selection of people but at the same time standing on

> the high moral ground that the EU and its Member States stand for. This exclusionary practice has been morally legitimised over the years by an array of policy frames [. . .] but also by a narrative of deservingness, that is, by following the principle that "some people do not deserve to be treated equally or in the way we (the 'host' society) treat human beings".

Moralisation of borders thus necessarily implies a range of justification and legitimation strategies. Territorial borders have become more than a means to provide security and control by also symbolising social meanings that cut to the core of human life. For example, legitimation by authority takes place by reference to 'the regulations' or 'the law', legitimation by rationalisation (Van Leeuwen & Wodak, 1999, p. 105) by reference to some form of common sense ("there are too many refugees", "the boat is full"). Moral legitimation occurs when boundaries and borders are justified in terms of health, leadership, public interest, and so forth. The appeal to 'order' and 'the rule of law' as universal and fundamental values thus also sometimes produces a dehumanising rhetoric, ultimately legitimising the construction of a 'fortress' in a strange, and indeed paradoxical, defense of liberal values.

2.2 *Justifying and Legitimising Exclusion*

Legitimation and Argumentation

Rojo-Martin and Van Dijk (1997, p. 528ff) define legitimation as involving "a powerful group or institution (often the State, the government, the rulers, the elite) which seeks normative approval for its policies or actions [and] does so through strategies that aim to show that such actions are consistent with the moral order of society". They maintain that "the socio-political act of legitimation is usually accomplished by persuasive (and sometimes manipulative) discourse" (ibid.), and distinguish between pragmatic, semantic, stylistic, interactional, and social dimensions of the linguistic realisation of legitimatory acts (ibid, p. 531–532). Importantly for the case in point, they also emphasise that "the propositions of legitimation discourse are usually organised by a complex argumentative schema, with premises that pertain to the nature of the action, and conclusions that pertain to its social, moral or political acceptability" (ibid, p. 532). In their careful microanalysis, they illustrate an argumentative scheme by deconstructing a complex argument and point to the importance of presupposed knowledge, without taking this relevant issue any further (ibid, p. 548–549). It suffices to state that most scholars agree that argumentation and legitimation are inherently related and that the specificities of legitimatory acts depend on various dimensions of context.

Ietcu-Fairclough (2008, p. 133ff) takes the argumentative dimension as the starting point and defines legitimation as "a social, political and argumentative practice, a form of strategic maneuvering which aims to reconcile successfully various conflicting demands and pressures acting on political actors". The concept of *strategic maneuvering* (Van Eemeren, 2010) introduces context into the analysis of argumentation, depending on various domains (fields) of society. "The nature of the political field", Ietcu-Fairclough (ibid, p. 133) concludes, "will create field-specific dialectical constraints on strategic maneuvering, as well as rhetorical opportunities for strategic maneuvering with arguments of legitimation". Zarefsky (2008) lists relevant contextual (historical) constraints in the U.S. political field and elaborates some relevant argumentation strategies, some of which have been extensively discussed elsewhere, such as Lakoff's concept of 'framing' (2004) or Hansson's work on strategies of blame avoidance (2015). Moreover, he points to the importance of latent knowledge of broad and narrow socio-political and historical contexts when attempting to deconstruct the argumentation schemes in specific political debates (Zarefsky, 2008, p. 118): "Not only is the argument messy, but it is very hard to know what sorts of norms and requirements ought to govern the dispute".

Topoi and Common Sense

Legitimatory practices in politics which appeal to an accepted set of normative values, moreover, rely on *endoxon*, the presupposed common-sense knowledge of a specific epistemic community. Questions, however, could be posed here: Accepted by whom? Whose common sense is being appealed to?

The notion of common-sense (or everyday) argumentation is salient for the understanding of more or less explicit preferences of specific electoral groups or political parties. Aristotle uses the concept of *endoxon* in order to describe an opinion that can be accepted by the majority of people, as it represents traditional knowledge but not necessarily true knowledge.

Subsequently, van Eemeren (2010, p. 111) defines endoxa as commonly held beliefs or generally accepted commitments. Van Eemeren's approach supports Habermas's thesis (1992) that legal systems must ultimately always be grounded in moral systems, and that formal procedural law, having cut its connections with sacred law and its larger religious context, was forced to let morality in again through the back door, to infiltrate whatever room for interpretation was left—the more so, the more law became an instrument of governmental control (e.g., Van Leeuwen & Wodak, 1999, p. 111).

Categorising Topoi

Topoi are "search formulas, which tell you how and where to look for arguments" (Kienpointner, 2011, p. 265). At the same time, they are "warrants which guarantee the transition from argument to conclusion" (see Wodak, 2015, pp. 51–54 for an extensive discussion).

Topoi have been categorised in different ways, elaborating and also changing Aristotle's seminal approach. Following the Aristotelian tradition,

Amossy (2002, p. 475) divides topoi into "those that rely on logico-discursive patterns believed to be universal and those built on social and cultural beliefs pertaining to a given ideology", albeit conceding that "in most cases it is difficult, if not impossible to draw a clear-cut difference between the two" (p. 476). Wengeler (2015), on the other hand, differentiates special topoi, or context-specific patterns, which are applicable only within a specific content-related area, such as discourses about migration, from general topoi or context-abstract patterns of conclusion. For Rubinelli (2009, pp. 73–75), too, argument schemes vary in their level of applicability and include: (1) Topoi that are of universal applicability and also appear in topics; (2) topoi that are still of universal applicability, although they are not found in topics; (3) less abstract versions of the *topos of the more and the less*; and (4) topoi that focus mainly on emotional aspects of human relationships or on considerations valid in rhetorical contexts only (for more details see, e.g., Boukala, 2016, p. 255).

In discourse, topoi can be made explicit as conditional or causal paraphrases such as 'if x, then y' or 'y, because x' (Reisigl & Wodak, 2001, pp. 69–80). Focusing on such conclusion rules, Kienpointer (1997) distinguishes between various 'content-abstract', or formal, argumentation schemes (as in Aristotle's taxonomy), such as *topos of definition, topos of the species and the genus, topos of comparison, topos of the part and the whole, topos of authority*, and so forth. For example, the *topos of authority* can be deconstructed as follows (see also Reisigl, 2014, p.76):

Conclusion Rule: If authority X says that A is true, A is true.
A: X says that A is true.
C: Thus, A is true.

It is important to emphasise that topoi are not necessarily fallacious.[3] Some examples discussed in the following section manifest flawed logic, but in particular contexts, arguments using a specific topos could be right, based on formal logic: Topoi are—neutrally speaking—a useful shortcut appealing to existing knowledge in a specific epistemic community. Thus, the use of topoi in specific contexts (which are often very complex), and what they ignore or sidestep, can be fallacious and manipulative.

3. Legitimising Fences and Walls—Examples from Austrian Debates 2015/16

In this section, I present some examples from the Austrian hegemonic political debates about building a fence/wall "to keep illegal migrants and refugees out" in the period from April 2015 until February 2016.[4] I focus on the range of legitimation strategies employed as well as on the related topoi providing common-sense arguments supporting the respective legitimation strategy. The examples are selected from a corpus of 6,701 texts, published between April 2015 and February 2016, all dealing with the so-called 'refugee crisis' compiled from the 11 national newspapers in Austria, (i.e. *Der Standard, Die Presse, Heute, Kleine Zeitung, Kronen Zeitung, Kurier, Oberösterreichische Nachrichten, Österreich, Salzburger Nachrichten, Tiroler Tageszeitung, Wiener Zeitung*), as well as three Austrian and one German weeklies (*Profil, News, Biber, Die Zeit*). The sub-corpus on 'building a fence/wall' was then compiled on a thematic and lexical basis, comprising 1,697 texts. The examples (Section 3.2.) discussed here were chosen due to their salience based on three distinctive criteria. Firstly, a chronology of the important regional, national and more global events which had a huge impact on the discourse about fences and walls in the period from July 2015 to February 2016 was established (see Table 3.2). Secondly, each event was characterised by a specific political statement (by government or opposition politicians), which immediately dominated the headlines in the national newspapers with the widest outreach. Thirdly, these utterances (and the headlines) were recontextualised and repeated most frequently in our entire corpus over several days.[5] The DHA applied here enables the tracing and understanding of the political debate about 'fences and walls' and the emerging qualitative shift in policy-making in Austria in a diachronic and context-dependent way: from a 'welcoming culture' to a 'culture of walls and exclusion'.

3.1 Brief Summary of Regional, National, and Transnational Contexts

As evidenced in Table 3.2, one can identify several national and transnational/global tipping points in the debates linked to specific events, such as the death of 71 refugees, the picture of the drowned child Alan Kurdi

Table 3.2 Periodisation in the debate about borders: July 2015—February 2016

- In July 2015, neighbouring Hungary begins to build its border fence, a move which is at first heavily criticised by the SPÖ (Austrian Social-Democratic Party) and the ÖVP (the Austrian Christian-Social, Conservative Party).
- On 26/8/15, 71 refugees are found dead, locked in an airtight truck near Parndorf, a small town in Burgenland on the route from the Hungarian border to Vienna.
- German Chancellor Merkel famously states on 31/8/2015 that "we will achieve this" [*wir schaffen das*] and that the right to asylum cannot have a maximum quota. Austrian Chancellor Faymann (SPÖ) publicly aligns with Merkel's policy.[1]
- On 2/9/15, the picture of the dead child Alan Kurdi, who drowned near Bodrum (Turkey), dominated the news world-wide and triggered massive shock and empathy amongst governments and the European Union officials. Many governments promised to take in refugees, some of which were never fulfilled.
- Throughout September and October, during regional election campaigns in Vienna and Upper Austria, Vienna's Mayor Häupl (SPÖ) speaks out for 'taking a stand' for refugees,[2] while Austria's right-wing populist Freedom Party (FPÖ) campaigns for a limit to asylum seekers and for cutting their social security.[3]

- On 23/10/15, then Interior Minister Mikl-Leitner (ÖVP) declares, "We have to build the Fortress Europe" to safeguard our security.[4]
- On 26/10/15, Minister of Exterior Affairs and Integration Kurz (ÖVP) proposes building a border fence to trigger a 'domino effect' in other countries along the Balkans route.[5]
- On 28/10/15, Mikl-Leitner (ÖVP) announces that 'technical barriers', including a fence, will be built at the Austrian border.[6]
- On 11/11/15, the government officially decides to build a "border management system" that will include a fence, although Faymann (SPÖ) maintains that it is just "a small door with side-parts" (see Example 1 above).[7]
- On 13/11/16, a horrific terror attack takes place in Paris, simultaneously at several locations, including the Bataclan.
- After numerous reports of sexual assaults by "Arab- or African-looking men" during New Year's celebrations in Cologne,[8] the debate intensifies.
- On 12/1/16, the ÖVP's National Secretary Lopatka argues that distinguishing between 'economic' and 'real refugees' is not possible when there are hundreds queuing at the border; the maximum limit therefore "must apply to both groups".[9]
- On 14/1/16, Vice-Chancellor Mitterlehner (ÖVP) calls for "a drastic reduction of refugees down to zero".[10] The FPÖ's (Austrian Freedom Party's) Vice-Chair Darmann demands an immediate halt to all immigration and closing the borders.[11]
- On 20/1/16, the two governing parties unexpectedly agree to set a maximum limit of 37.500 per year. On 24/1/16, Faymann (SPÖ), having completely reversed his position, says, "Refugee number 37,501 will be turned back at the border".[12] On 24/2/16, Mikl-Leitner (ÖVP) praises the closed borders along the Balkans route as a "chain reaction of reason".[13]

on 2/9/15 near Bodrum and the closing of the Hungarian borders; on a different level, there are regional influences tied to election campaigns in the Austrian regions of Styria, Burgenland, Upper Austria, and Vienna. In these campaigns, the perceived pressure from the Austrian right-wing populist Freedom Party (FPÖ) led all the mainstream parties with the exception of the Vienna chapter of the SPÖ to accommodate more and more to the FPÖ's

Notes:

1 www.ots.at/presseaussendung/OTS_20150912_OTS0032/
2 www.news.at/a/michael-h%C3%A4upl-boot-lange-nicht-voll. This clear stance polarises the Vienna elections, which were won by the SPÖ.
3 http://diepresse.com/home/politik/innenpolitik/4822750/
4 http://derstandard.at/2000024358096/
5 http://kurier.at/politik/inland/kurz-man-ist-nicht-rechts-wenn-man-realist-ist/160.273.015
6 http://orf.at/stories/2306423/2306424/
7 http://steiermark.orf.at/news/stories/2741734/
8 See the report submitted by Interior Minister Rolf Jäger to the regional government after the "Cologne events": www.land.nrw/sites/default/files/asset/document/bericht_innenausschuss_12012016.pdf
9 http://derstandard.at/2000028877483/
10 http://ooe.orf.at/news/stories/2752375/
11 http://diepresse.com/home/politik/innenpolitik/4903499/
12 http://derstandard.at/2000029660627/
13 http://diepresse.com/home/politik/innenpolitik/4932380/

position. The next major tipping point was 'Cologne', 31/12/15, which shifted the debate from 'welcoming refugees' to "protecting our (Austrian/German) women from illegal migrants". Under ever more pressure—none of the policies decided on the EU level being implemented—Austria's foreign minister Kurz (ÖVP) proposed to close the Balkan route. Polarisation in the upcoming Austrian presidential election in 4/16 was the next tipping point for Austria in at least two respects: the disastrous result for the SPÖ candidate would later lead to the resignation of Chancellor Faymann on 15/5/16; and, in the run-off (22/5/2016), the two remaining candidates (from the FPÖ and the Green Party) would manifest diametrically opposed positions dividing the electorate almost exactly in half.

3.2 Constructing 'Fortress Europe'

Semantic and Lexical Analysis of 'border' (Grenze)

Lexical analysis indicates a plethora of border-related terminology, some of which could arguably be considered neologisms. These terms emerge in ever more frequency in the course of the debate's development over time, as though there were a need to lexically highlight the border region and demarcate or reinforce the border itself. In particular, compounding with *Grenze*, i.e. 'border', is shown to be extremely productive in this context (166 unique compound lemmas) (e.g., Rheindorf & Wodak, 2017).

Based on a corpus-linguistic analysis, the lexical items were sorted into six groups: the border region (e.g., people and towns on the Austrian side of the border); the border itself; the border's demarcation (e.g., fence); measures to protect and safeguard the border (e.g., controls, police, soldiers); orderly openings of the border (e.g., regular commuter traffic, gates); and threats to the border (e.g., illegal crossings, riots) (Rheindorf & Wodak, 2017). It is important to note that the word 'border' actually occurs more frequently in spite of having used the search term 'border fence' to compile our corpus; while notions that commonly delineate the "line of the border" are rare, there exist a range of euphemistic terms compounded with 'border', and thus related to the border space. The latter re-semiotise the physical object of the 'fence' as actions such as 'securing' and 'protecting' or such abstractions as 'control' and 'management'.[6] There is also a notable absence of compounds that build further on 'border fence', whereas there exist numerous three-part compounds that build on 'border space' or 'border control'.

The border fence being a highly symbolic referent, due to the Iron Curtain, which once separated Austria from its Eastern Communist neighbours before 1989, there was intense negotiation of terminology between the political actors involved. Since 'border fence' is negatively connoted, those in favor of building a wall or fence—initially only the ÖVP, later on also the SPÖ—employed many euphemisms deeply embedded in moralising and rationalising legitimation. This was undermined, however, by the

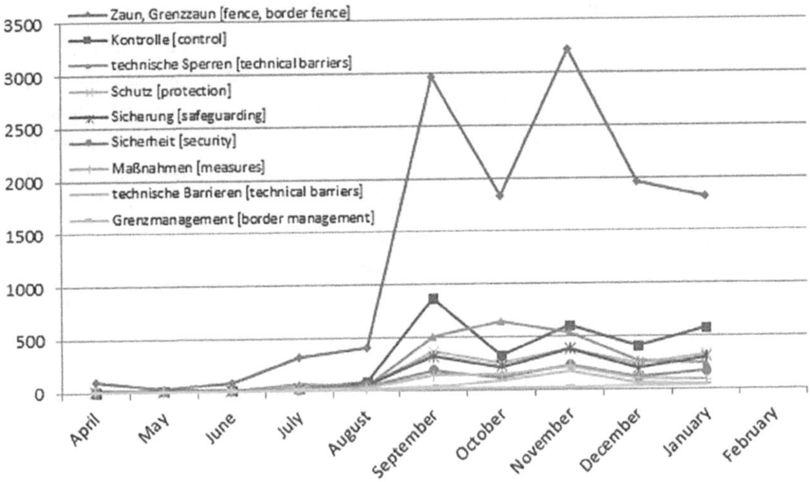

Figure 3.1 The 'border fence' and related euphemisms (frequency by month 2015/16)

Vice-Chancellor and the Minister of Interior Affairs, both ÖVP, who began to appeal explicitly for a '*Festung Europa*', i.e. Fortress Europe (see Examples 3 and 4; Fig. 3.1).

Figure 3.1 shows frequencies per month for 'border fence' and all its major metaphors. It furthermore indicates the correlation between the focus on building a fence and the threat of terrorism, at least for the two initial peaks in September and November. As will be illustrated below, *the topos of danger* is interdiscursively related to the discourses about terrorism and security. This link see ms to disappear after the fence is built (and appears to be ineffective) and as the mediatised threat scenario shifts, in the wake of the incidents of sexual harassment during New Year's Eve in Cologne, from an external to an internal one. A fence is obviously not well suited to protecting the national body constructed as the gendered body of Austrian women. New moral and rational legitimation strategies substantiate the danger posed by refugees and migrants, frequently related to religion (Islam) and to a 'clash of cultures', thus emphasising *the topos of culture.*

Legitimising and Delegitimising Walls

In the following, I illustrate the dynamic of the polarised debate about "protecting Austria from refugees/protecting refugees in Austria" by analysing some of the statements made by prominent Austrian politicians at the successive tipping points of the socio-political developments presented above (in Table 3.2). More specifically, I focus on the range of legitimation strategies and their related topoi, which serve to substantiate legitimation/de-legitimation attempts. Table 3.3 presents a tentative taxonomy of legitimation strategies (e.g., Van Leeuwen, 2008), some of which are salient in this debate. It quickly becomes apparent that overlaps exist between some legitimation strategies and relevant topoi (see Table 3.1), for example 'authorisation' frequently makes use of the *topos of authority*; or the 'authority of tradition' is linked to the *topos of history*. The *topos of comparison* employs moralisation by analogy. Mythopoesis as a legitimation strategy is related to the *argumentum ad exemplum*, and so forth. Of course, the various strategies can be realised by other means as well, for example by specific predication (attributes) and/or nomination (labelling) strategies, or a range of fallacies. In this way, the interdependence of legitimation strategies and argumentation schemes becomes explicit.

Table 3.3 Taxonomy: Legitimation Strategies (extrapolated from Van Leeuwen, 2008)

Authorisation

Authority

- *Personal Authority*: Authority based on institutional status of individuals/groups
- *Impersonal Authority*: Authority originating from laws, policies, regulations, etc.
- *Expert Authority*: Academic, scientific expertise or other type of credible knowledge
- *Role Model Authority*: Popularity and acceptability of positions of "role models or opinion leaders" (p. 107)

Custom

- *Authority of Tradition*: Acceptability of what is claimed to have always been done
- *Authority of Conformity*: Acceptability of what everyone or most people do

Moralisation

- *Evaluation*: Legitimation of positions and practices via evaluative adjectives
- *Abstraction*: "Referring to practices. . . in abstract ways that "moralise" them by distilling from them a quality that links them to discourses of moral values" (p. 111)
- *Analogy*: Relying on legitimating or delegitimising force of comparisons and contrasts

Rationalisation

Instrumental Rationalisation

- *Goal Orientation*: Focusing on goals, intentions, purposes as envisaged by people
- *Means Orientation*: Focusing on aims embedded in actions "as a means to an end"
- *Outcome Orientation*: Stressing "the outcome of actions . . . as something that turned out to exist in hindsight" (p. 115)

Theoretical Rationalisation

- *Definition*: Characterising activities in terms of other already moralised practices
- *Explanation*: Characterising people as actors "because doing things this way is appropriate to the nature of these actors" (p. 116)
- *Prediction*: Foreseeing outcomes based on some kind of expertise

Mythopoesis

- *Moral Tales*: Narrating rewarding decisions and practices of social actors
- *Cautionary Tales*: Associating nonconformist and deviant decisions and practices with undesirable consequences

In example 3, Mitterlehner (ÖVP) employs an instrumental rationalisation legitimation strategy: A list of control measures to be applied immediately, as otherwise, he argues, the EU would fail.

> *Example 3*
>
> Europe will not fail only if we succeed in solving the asylum problem in a solidary and orderly manner. That means: The outer borders [of the EU] must be controlled; hotspots must be established at the outer borders as emergency intake centres, and every asylum applicant who illegally travels onward will be transferred back there. And then there has to be an orderly verification procedure that corresponds to the EU's system of law. That means: Europe, in principle, is becoming the "Fortress Europe".
>
> (Vice-Chancellor Mitterlehner, 19/9/15)[7]

The legitimation is substantiated by the *topoi of danger* (the EU might fail), *responsibility* (governments should act in an orderly fashion), and *control*: only by carefully controlling borders, immigrants, and asylum seekers will the EU succeed. The argument then continues—if all these measures were implemented, the EU would be transformed into a 'Fortress Europe', legitimised by the danger of apparent failure.

While most members of the government were at pains to avoid the term 'border fence' in the discussion of plans to at least partially close the border and strengthen control, the oppositional FPÖ was using the term to signal its hard stance regarding refugees. Everyone involved, however, seemed to be acknowledging that even though they could not call it a fence, what they were really talking about was, after all, a fence. On 23 October 2015, pushed for answers after a cabinet meeting, Mikl-Leitner (ÖVP) lost her composure, implicitly appealing to a moralised conception of bordering (see Example 4).

Example 4

Without better protection of the EU's exterior borders that situation will be impossible to get under control in the medium-run, said the Minister—"We must build Fortress Europe", said the Minister during a visit on-site.

And on 28 October, she stated:

Example 5

Of course this is also about a fence. There is nothing bad about a fence. (Mikl-Leitner, 28/10/15)[8]

In Examples 4 and 5, Mikl-Leitner justifies the building of a fence by theoretical rationalisation, i.e. a fence is the only possible way of maintaining control. Losing control would be dangerous for the EU—in this way, the *topos of danger* is appealed to. Moreover, the moralisation of borders occurs in Example 5: If borders protect the EU, then they are—by definition—good; deontic modality emphasises her point—'Fortress Europe' 'must' be built.

Example 6

In an interview with ÖSTERREICH Werner Faymann heavily criticised the refugee policy in Hungary. Faymann: "The way the Hungarians are treating asylum seekers, that's not the way . . . But above all, it is unacceptable that refugees are coming from Hungary in fear, panic, starving and partly traumatised. When trains meant to lead to freedom are suddenly diverted into camps, I am reminded of dark times in our history. We acted differently during the Hungarian Crisis and put little red-white-and-red flags on the border to take away the fear of the people who were fleeing".[9]

In Example 6, Faymann, former Chancellor of Austria, justifies the nation's open border polices in autumn 2015 by moral legitimation, combined with the *topoi of history* and *comparison*. First, he mentions that the refugees arrive in Austria from Hungary in a state of 'fear and panic', triggering pity. He then compares the fact that the refugees were not told where the trains were taking them to the Holocaust, insinuated by the phrase "dark times in our history". Finally, he reminds the Hungarians of 1956, when Austria took in almost 200,000 Hungarian refugees who were fleeing the Soviet occupation. Thus, Faymann makes a strong case for humanitarian border policies, in contrast to the Hungarian and both the ÖVP and FPÖ politicians. Two ideological positions in respect to the refugee crisis become explicit. Different values are appealed to, legitimised by a range of strategies, evoking fear on the one hand, solidarity on the other.

Compared to Faymann' s later statement of 28/10/2015 (see Example 1, section 1), one is confronted with a significant change of opinion in the SPÖ, except for the Mayor of Vienna, who at the same time repeatedly recontextualises a famous metaphor from the late 1930s, namely that "the boat is not full", an instrumental legitimation strategy substantiated by a *topos of numbers* (if the boat, i.e., our country, is not full, then there is room for more refugees).[10] However, under ever more pressure from the ÖVP and the FPÖ, the humanitarian position is silenced and theoretical and instrumental rationalisation legitimation strategies override any opposition to building a fence/wall/Fortress Europe (e.g., Examples 7and 8).

Example 7

Mitterlehner described the present situation in extremely drastic terms: Until last August, one had thought it possible to handle the refugee movement with the "traditional Austrian attitude". By now, however, there was "an actual mass migration" on the way to Austria, Germany and Sweden. That would constitute an "extreme situation", therefore one would have to act and "set limits".

Here, Mitterlehner evokes a scenario of imminent danger, which forces Austria to abandon its "traditional attitude" and act immediately by setting clear limits. The *topos of numbers* (which can be identified by the vague quantifier of "mass migration") is used to substantiate this instrumental rationalisation legitimation. Similarly, the two ÖVP ministers (Interior and Foreign Affairs) reinforce their responsibility in setting immediate measures in order to protect Austria and the EU.

Example 8

After the summit, it was said they wanted to set joint measures to severely limit the continuing refugee movement along the so-called Balkans route in the direction of central Europe. "We want a chain reaction of reason", explained Mikl-Leitner. Mikl-Leitner said that the streams of migrants had to be stopped and described it as a life-or-death issue for the EU. Europe, she said, was facing "its biggest challenge since the Second World War". Minister Kurz again emphasised that all participating countries would prefer a joint European solution, but in the absence of such a solution were forced to take national measures: "Austria is overwhelmed, plain and simple."

Both Ministers emphasise the imminent danger awaiting Austria and the EU, if "streams of migration" could not be stopped ("a life or death issue for the EU", an exaggeration using a *topos of danger*). Following a comparison with the end of WWII (*topos of history*), Kurz regrets that there is no European solution. This fact then legitimises national measures, via a *topos of burden* ("If Austria is overwhelmed, measures have to be taken"). Moreover, Mikl-Leitner appeals to reason by creating the metaphor of "a chain reaction of reason" which serves as theoretical rationalisation legitimation, that is, other countries will agree with Austria that closing the Balkan route (i.e. building fences and establishing border management) are reasonable actions and thus to be copied. In this way, the ÖVP constructs itself as the part of the coalition government that recognises future dangers in time and is prepared to act responsibly, even if this would imply different values, a 'new Austrian way'.

Finally, the events in Cologne on 31/12/15 serve as further evidence for the imminent danger to the EU and its people, especially women. Apart from the *topoi of burden* and *numbers*, we encounter an interdiscursive overlap of discourses about security and terrorism with discourses about a 'clash of cultures'. Thus, a range of moral legitimation and mythopoesis strategies starts dominating the media, specifically the tabloids, enhanced by the rhetoric of the FPÖ, whereas the government enforces legitimation most frequently by authority and rationalisation.

4. Legitimising Immigration Control—2015/16

Approaching legitimation from a sociological point of view, Abulof (2016, p. 11) claims that populist movements (both on the left and right) manifest a new kind of political and moral legitimacy—*popular legitimacy*. Having studied the Arab Spring and oppositional populist movements in the Middle East, Abulof concludes that "legitimacy has become the 'absolute horizon' of modern politics: increasingly alluring, forever elusive, and dangerously frustrating" (p. 11). Popular legitimacy spans, as Abulof maintains, "identity, polity, authority, and policy" (ibid, p. 4).

Indeed, when analysing the moralisation of borders, the strong appeals to "protect our people and countries against strangers", identity politics "ascended, as people sought to become not only the source of legitimacy but also its object: their 'peoplehood' itself required validation before they could legitimate their politics" (ibid). A discourse-historical analysis of politicians' statements about the necessity/non-necessity of building walls and fences to protect Europe and the EU from refugees and migrants, and their recontextualisation in the media from April 2015 to February 2016, provides much evidence for both a new moralisation of borders and new forms of legitimation, as exposed by Vollmer (2016) and Abulof (2016).

Walls and fences have become the symbols for responsible governance and government. Appeals to common sense and reason reinforce slogans such as "the boat is full" and warn of the imminent danger that the entire post-war project of the EU might fail. In spite of the strong humanitarian oppositional voices from the mainstream left and many NGOs, theoretical and instrumental rationalisation, the authority of experts, and moral arguments cleared the ground for legitimising 'Fortress Europe'. In this endeavour, a 'politics of fear' (Wodak, 2015, 2016), mainly evoked by the extreme and populist right-wing, overrides other voices. The Austrian government gave in to this pressure, thus normalising discriminatory policies, frequently transcending the limits set by the Geneva Convention and the Charter of Human Rights.

The legitimation strategies employed are substantiated and realised by many linguistic, rhetorical and pragmatic devices and argumentation schemes such as topoi. Indeed, it is obvious that legitimation and argumentation are interdependent in many complex ways, on many levels of language and discourse. In order to deconstruct, understand, and explain significant policy shifts, as illustrated in this paper, a context-dependent interdisciplinary in-depth analysis is required, which allows the tracing of discourse strands and their embedded legitimation strategies both quantitatively and qualitatively.

Notes

1 http://orf.at/stories/2306741/2306742/
2 http://talkingpointsmemo.com/livewire/donald-trump-mexico-wall-good-people.
3 I am very grateful to Andrew Sayer to pointing out to me that this differentiation should be made explicit in order to avoid confusion and misunderstandings.
4 These data were collected in a three-year research project funded by the Austrian Science Foundation FWF, P 27153. In Rheindorf and Wodak (2017), we analysed two discourse strands (April 2015–February 2016), while focusing on controversies about the ideology-laden terminology used by the two mainstream parties with respect to labelling borders, fences, and walls, as well as about setting a maximum limit for asylum applications for 2016. There, we also delve into the chronology of events accompanying the struggles over meaning in much more detail which I cannot present in this paper for reasons of space.
5 For reasons of space, I refer readers looking for the entire quantitative analysis and full details of the corpus to Rheindorf and Wodak (2017).
6 See Iedema (2003) for definitions of 'resemiotisation'—basically meaning a recontextualisation of an argument, text, or other form of discursive practice into another (visual, multimodal, material) practice.
7 www.salzburg.com/nachrichten/dossier/fluechtlinge/sn/artikel/mitterlehner-im-sn-interview-bauen-an-der-festung-europa-166324/
8 ZIB2 ORF news, 28/10/15
9 12/9/2015, www.ots.at/presseaussendung/OTS_20150912_OTS0032/oesterreich-interview-faymann-attackiert-orban-und-fordert-eu-sondersitzung
10 Mayor Michael Häupl emphasised in an interview with the magazine *News* before the Vienna election of 11/10/2015 that "the boat won't be full for a long time. During the war in Bosnia we took in 80,000". He employs *topoi of history* and *comparison* (comparing 2015 with the war in Yugoslavia in the 1990s) and referring to the Swiss closing of borders to Jewish refugees fleeing Nazi Germany 1938/39.

References

Abulof, U. (2016). *Absolute horizon*. Princeton, NJ: Princeton University Press.

Amossy, R. (2002). How to do things with doxa: Toward an analysis of argumentation in discourse. *Poetics Today*, *23*(3), 465–487.

Anderson, B. (1994 [1985]). *Imagined communities: Reflections on the origin and spread of nationalism*. London: Verso.

Bauman, Z. (1995). Making and unmaking of strangers. *Thesis Eleven*, *43*(1), 1–16.

Boukala, S. (2016). Rethinking topos in the discourse historical approach: Endoxon seeking and argumentation in Greek media discourses on 'Islamist terrorism'. *Discourse Studies*, *18*(3), 249–268.

Carr, M. (2015). *Fortress Europe: Inside the war against immigration*. London: Hurst Publ.

Habermas, J. (1992). *Faktizität und Geltung*. Frankfurt: Suhrkamp.

Hansson, S. (2015). Discursive strategies of blame avoidance in government: A framework for analysis. *Discourse & Society*, *26*(3), 297–323.

Iedema, R. (2003). Multimodality, resemiotisation: Extending the analysis of discourse as multi-semiotic practice. *Visual Communication*, *2*(1), 29–57.

Ietcu-Fairclough, I. (2008). Legitimation and strategic maneuvering in the political field. In F. Van Eemeren (Ed.), *Examining argumentation in context: Fifteen studies on strategic maneuvering* (pp. 131–152). Amsterdam: Benjamins.

Kienpointner, M. (1997). On the art of finding arguments: What ancient and modern masters of invention have to tell us about the 'Ars Inveniendi'. *Argumentation*, *11*, 225–236.

Kienpointner, M. (2011). Rhetoric. In J. Ostman & J. Verschueren (Eds.), *Pragmatics in practice* (pp. 264–277). Amsterdam: Benjamins.

Lakoff, G. (2004). *Don't think of an Elephant*. Chelsea Green, VT: White River Junction.

Musolff, A. (2010). *Metaphor, nation and the Holocaust*. London: Routledge.

Paasi, A. (2010). Boundaries as social practice and discourse: The Finnish-Russian border. *Regional Studies*, *33*(7), 669–680.

Reisigl, M. (2014). Argumentation analysis and the discourse-historical approach: A methodological framework. In C. Hart & P. Cap (Eds.), *Contemporary critical discourse studies* (pp. 67–95). London: Bloomsbury.

Reisigl, M., & Wodak, R. (2001). *Discourse and discrimination: Rhetorics of racism and antisemitism*. London: Routledge.

Rheindorf, M., & Wodak, R. (2017). Borders, fences and limits—protecting Austria from refugees: Metadiscursive negotiation of meaning in the current refugee crisis. *International Journal of Immigration & Refugee Studies*. http://dx.doi.org/10.1080/15562948.2017.1302032

Rojo-Martin, L., & Van Dijk, T. A. (1997). "There was a problem, and it was solved!" Legitimating the expulsion of 'Illegal' migrants in Spanish parliamentary discourse. *Discourse & Society*, *8*(4), 523–556.

Rubinelli, S. (2009). *Ars topica: The classical technique of constructing arguments from Aristotle to Cicero*. Berlin: Springer.

Simmel, G. (1950). *The sociology of Georg Simmel*. New York: Free Press.

Van Eemeren, F. (2010). *Strategic maneuvering in argumentation discourse: Extending the pragma-dialectical theory of argumentation*. Amsterdam: Benjamins.

Van Leeuwen, T. (2008). *Discourse and practice: New tools for critical discourse analysis*. Oxford: Oxford University Press.

Van Leeuwen, T., & Wodak, R. (1999). Legitimising immigration control: A discourse-historical analysis. *Discourse Studies*, *1*(1), 83–118.

Vollmer, B. A. (2016). A hermeneutical approach to European bordering. *Journal of Contemporary European Studies*, *25*(1), 1–15. doi:10.1080/14782804.2016.1148591

Wengeler, M. (2015). Patterns of argumentation and the heterogeneity of social knowledge. *Journal of Language & Politics*, *14*(5), 689–711.

Wodak, R. (2015). *Politics of fear: What right-wing populist discourses mean*. London: Sage.

Wodak, R. (2016). *Politik mit der Angst. Zur Wirkung rechtspopulistischer Diskurse*. Hamburg: Konturen.

Wodak, R., & Boukala, S. (2015). European identities and the revival of nationalism in the European Union: A discourse historical approach. *Journal of Language & Politics*, *14*(1), 87–109.

Wodak, R., & Van Leeuwen, T. (2002). Discourses of un/employment in Europe: The Austrian case. *Text*, *22*(3), 345–367.

Zarefsky, D. (2008). Strategic maneuvering in political argumentation. In F. Van Eemeren (Ed.), *Examining argumentation in context: Fifteen studies on strategic maneuvering* (pp. 115–130). Amsterdam: Benjamins.

4 The Limits of Semiotics—Epistemology and the Concept of 'Race'

Philip Bell

1. Introduction

Theo van Leeuwen was teaching film production in 1980 when I became his colleague at Macquarie University, in Sydney. His academic interests led him to develop the innovative ideas of Michael Halliday and Raqiaya Hasan (the latter a Macquarie colleague) to the study of broadcast radio speech, then to media interviews understood in functional social semiotic terms (Bell & Van Leeuwen, 1994). With Gunther Kress, Theo published *Reading Images: The Grammar of Visual Design*, in 1996 (RI, hereafter).

My contribution to this celebration of Theo's distinguished career develops several arguments about the representation of 'race' from the insights of that ground-breaking book—a richly detailed and adventurous discussion that helped to move Systemic Functional Semiotics (SFS hereafter) out from the linguistic field in which it was born and into the general analysis of diverse contexts of communicative practice, that is, practices by which people could be said to create and transact meaning. Its revolutionary insight was that meaning-making did not have to be seen as analogous to, certainly not as reducible to, language. This was despite the use of 'grammar' in Kress and Van Leeuwen's title.

My tribute to RI's ground-breaking approach to visual semiotics argues that questions of the truth of a visual/verbal text are always semiotically relevant. My examples are taken from newspaper reports about 'scientific' studies of race and from photographic 'evidence' in policy discourse about Australian Aboriginal people 'dying out'. Epistemology is the study of truth claims and their justification, raising questions seldom explicitly canvassed in semiotic analysis.

2. Photographic Truth, Context

Umberto Eco famously called semiotics the study of anything "that could be used to lie" (Eco, 1975). It follows that semiotics studies utterances or representations that purport to be 'true', regardless of the physical modality of the medium in which they are realised. Photographs implicitly make truth claims in most of the contexts in which they circulate. Indeed, their usually unquestioned use as evidence in forensic and scientific contexts attests to just this assumed epistemological innocence.

I want to question this common-sense assumption, not by discussing examples of putative photographic evidence that has been 'doctored' or manipulated (although this is important in an age of digital media), but by investigating the general claim that semiotic analysis can facilitate judgements of truth/falsity without also considering epistemological issues that are independent of semiotics as such. To anticipate why I make this claim, let me assert that how an image-text is read may presuppose the very knowledge that it seems to claim (even allowing for 'context' in the expanded sense proposed by SFS). I discuss several examples of images that ask to be read as representing the concept of 'race'. I argue that when a photographic text ('a unit of meaning', to oversimplify) makes theoretical claims to which the empirical indicators of race membership are thought to be relevant, it invariably *begs the question of the truth or otherwise* of the text's claims.

Susan Sontag (1967) famously argued that a photograph of the Krupp factory taken in the 1930s could only be communicative if it is given a narrative, historical context (and that means, usually, a verbal context). Otherwise, its connotations are open and indeterminate when it is viewed in the usual semiotic circumstances in which it is likely to be found (history books, photographic compendia, etc.). Sontag's example is an image of *a particular* factory, albeit one that metonymically links to the Nazi German industrial complex when understood historically. It is not an *abstract* or *conceptual* image in the sense that Kress and Van Leeuwen (2006) use these terms, and which I discuss below. Nevertheless, while it is not textually 'abstract', the Krupp factory image reminds us that all images are read in terms of abstract categories, or at least in terms of general concepts (not just history as in Sontag's example, but in other unstated terms such as 'beauty', 'nostalgia', 'power', etc.). However, such presupposed concepts are only made explicit when people discuss an image, and hence sometimes propose contrasting contexts for understanding it. Such contexts might be called 'theoretical' because they draw implications from the particular photograph for abstract, general interpretation.

Having made this observation, and despite Sontag's forceful point, I want to emphasise that 'formal' semiotic analysis is an invaluable first step in defining the genre and the communicative intention of a diagrammatic/photographic 'text' (SFS isolates 'units of meaning' as 'texts' for the purposes of analysis, and these are not necessarily verbal). Functional semiotic analysis highlights what Kress and Van Leeuwen (2006) call the 'coding orientation' that a text invites its readers to adopt in reading it. For example, to see a text as 'scientific' rather than as 'artistic' is to ask very different questions about the way it claims to be true, veridical or unarguable. So I am concerned with the limitations (or boundaries) of semiotic analysis insofar as photographic texts appear to 'represent', 'mean', 'imply' (presuppose), or 'refer to' abstract concepts. My example is the biological/social concept of 'race'.

3. Visualising Abstractions—Kress and Van Leeuwen's Semiotic Analysis

Consider the newspaper article below, presented as my Figures 4.1 and 4.2, that explicitly claims to present by word and illustration ideas of 'scientific' significance. It was published on the *front page* of a contemporary Australian 'quality' or 'broadsheet' newspaper, *The Sydney Morning Herald* (25 June, 2005).

I present below an abbreviated semiotic analysis that might be advanced for the contentious image in Figure 4.1. I do this as a way of exemplifying the subtle methods developed by of Kress and Van Leeuwen (2006). I will then consider what might be called the epistemological limitations of semiotic theory. Figure 4.1, above, and Figure 4.2, below, make up the one news article.

The series of nine images that make up Figure 4.1 exemplifies what Kress and Van Leeuwen (2006) term a 'temporal analytical process'. Here "a set of participants ('possessive attributes') is ordered linearly on a horizontal [. . .] time line of successive stages of a temporally unfolding process" (p. 107). (The SMH timeline actually begins at each end and meets in the middle, so to speak, an important subtlety discussed below.) Its modality Van Leeuwen defines as 'abstract'. It exemplifies "[a] type of modality in which the truth criterion is cognitive, based on whether the representation represents as general pattern underlying superficially different instances, or deeper 'essence' of what is represented" (Van Leeuwen, 2005, glossary). 'Modality' in SFS "refers to semiotic resources for expressing as how true or as how real a given representation should be taken (sic)" (Van Leeuwen, 2005, glossary). So the above example is best described as representing *a temporal analytic process of abstract modality, within a context that invites a 'scientific coding orientation'*, albeit in the paradoxical situation of a quality newspaper rather than the more usual textbook or academic journal.

The photographic exemplar of beauty, ('the look') and additional verbal text make up the remainder of the newspaper article: The text line below

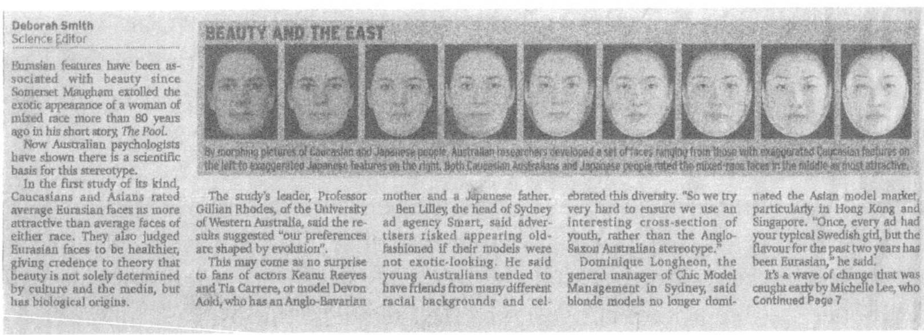

Deborah Smith
Science Editor

BEAUTY AND THE EAST

By morphing pictures of Caucasian and Japanese people, Australian researchers developed a set of faces ranging from those with exaggerated Caucasian features on the left to exaggerated Japanese features on the right. Both Caucasian Australians and Japanese people rated the mixed-race faces in the middle as most attractive.

Eurasian features have been associated with beauty since Somerset Maugham extolled the exotic appearance of a woman of mixed race more than 80 years ago in his short story, *The Pool*.

Now Australian psychologists have shown there is a scientific basis for this stereotype.

In the first study of its kind, Caucasians and Asians rated average Eurasian faces as more attractive than average faces of either race. They also judged Eurasian faces to be healthier, giving credence to theory that beauty is not solely determined by culture and the media, but has biological origins.

The study's leader, Professor Gillian Rhodes, of the University of Western Australia, said the results suggested "our preferences are shaped by evolution".

This may come as no surprise to fans of actors Keanu Reeves and Tia Carrere, or model Devon Aoki, who has an Anglo-Bavarian mother and a Japanese father.

Ben Lilley, the head of Sydney ad agency Smart, said advertisers risked appearing old-fashioned if their models were not exotic-looking. He said young Australians tended to have friends from many different racial backgrounds and celebrated this diversity. "So we try very hard to ensure we use an interesting cross-section of youth, rather than the Anglo-Saxon Australian stereotype."

Dominique Longheon, the general manager of Chic Model Management in Sydney, said blonde models no longer dominated the Asian model market, particularly in Hong Kong and Singapore. "Once, every ad had your typical Swedish girl, but the flavour for the past two years has been Eurasian," he said.

It's a wave of change that was caught early by Michelle Lee, who
Continued Page 7

Figure 4.1 Beauty and the East—'race'

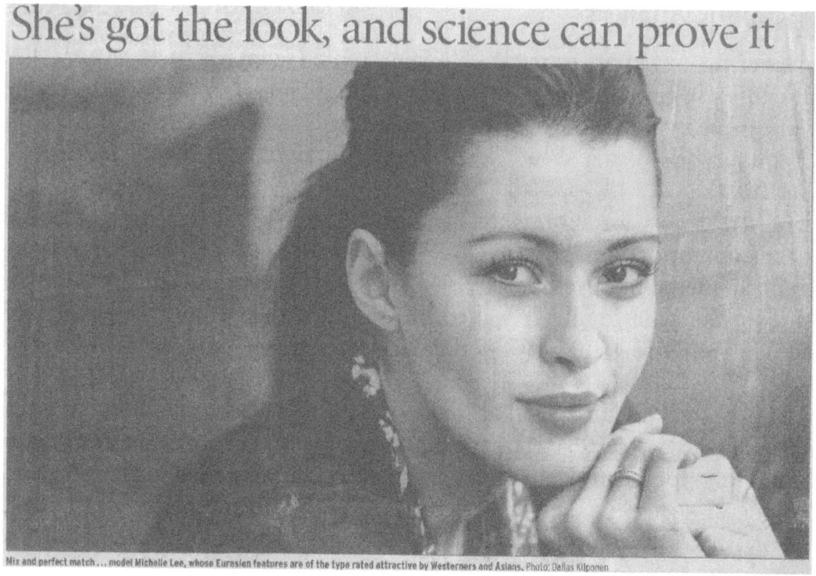

Figure 4.2 'Eurasian' Michelle Lee—she's got the look and science can prove it

Michelle Lee's image reads: "Mix and perfect match [. . .] model Michelle Lee, whose Eurasian features are of the type rated attractive by Westerners and Asians".

It is important to stress that in Figure 4.1, the superficially different instances in the image series are 'anchored' to a highly tendentious verbal text, without which it would at best be ambiguous.[1] Significantly, this verbal anchorage explicitly invokes 'science' to heighten its modality: 'Truth', in this newspaper feature, is *scientific, abstract, expert-guaranteed* truth. The 'essences' which are to be inferred as uniting the exemplars semiotically are 'race' and 'beauty', both popularly understood as qualities of individual people that can be observed, represented and described. Hence the head-canting photograph of the model, "whose Eurasian features are of the type rated attractive by Westerners and Asians" (sic).

So, extending my analysis, I would claim that to make sense of Figure 4.1—an 'analytic diagrammatical representation'—the reader must bring to it a 'scientific' coding orientation (although the verbal text invites an aesthetic judgement as well). The nine portraits must be seen as a *series* so that the *sine qua non* of science—*quantification*—can be accepted as part of the discourse. The series must represent exemplars of the same logical kind, asking to be judged as 'same but different', so to speak. To this end, the verbal text assumes that the inferable essence—'race'—is quantifiable (hence its exemplars can be *averaged* to yield the melded instances of heterogeneous ancestry at the centre of the analytic series of photographs). Perhaps the same is true of 'beauty'. After all, beauty pageants award numerical scores to contestants as though they can be ranked on a single quantitative dimension (as do equally problematic 'intelligence' tests, for example). The young women's faces are representations of what might be called 'degrees of their ancestry' (which ancestry, it is implied, must have been a 'purer', more 'concentrated' or more 'extreme', version of a selection of the attributes that define the young models). That is, the attributes carried by the depicted models are 'moderate' or 'less extreme' versions of these assumed (visible, photographable) ancestral attributes. We need to accept this conceptual schema, and also to accept the meaning of ancestry (and arguably 'race') that it implies, if we are to understand and to accept that what the newspaper article presents is true. We must believe that photographable features such as skin colour, eye shape, nose shape, face shape, hair colour, etc. are *racially relevant attributes for classifying* the individual models as members of different ancestral populations. When we do this, the beautiful exemplar will emerge from the genetic soup and be recognised as 'Eurasian'. So, by implication, Michelle Lee also illustrates the putative mid-point of 'European' and 'Asian' ancestry. Clearly, these categories are neither geographically nor biologically precise, even allowing for the vague 'common-sense' lexicon of race classification in English on which the journalist relies.

Interestingly, the SMH showcases a named, *individual*, woman to illustrate genetically determined 'beauty'. This seems to deflect the possible criticism that the newspaper regards populations of people as 'beautiful-in-general', and therefore, the uncomfortable logical corollary that populations could be judged to be '*ugly*-in-general'. To allow the latter implication might be criticised by SMH's readers as 'racist'. So the journalist is careful to write that the model is 'judged' beautiful. This much at least is subjective, although the *causes* of the model's physical attributes are presented as *objective* biological aspects of her hypothetical origins.

Kress and Van Leeuwen's approach draws our attention to what they call the 'gaze' of the models. Each woman 'addresses' the viewer in an 'affiliative' way as she looks at the camera and invites inclusion in her world, so to speak. The larger image of Michelle Lee poses her in a slightly submissive way, canting her head and looking 'back at' the viewer's gaze, thus confirming the connotations of her feminine 'beauty' label while consolidating an affiliative relationship with the viewer. Following Kress and van Leewuen (cf. 2006, p. 119–130), we could argue that the models 'demand' an 'affective' response from readers. The images do not merely 'offer information' as evidence, as might be expected in a 'scientific' illustration. They also demand an emotional response, one that trades on a stereotypically 'feminine' pose (Goffman, 1976).

In his foundational semiotic writings, Roland Barthes (1973) pointed out that the photographic image conveys meaning 'at one stroke'—it hides the semiotic choices made in its production and so appears to be 'natural' and ideologically 'innocent'. But Barthes also emphasised that interpretations of photographic images could be guided by the written texts that accompany them, and in Figures 4.1 and 4.2, biological and aesthetic discursive contexts are patent in limiting the 'preferred' readings of the article. Michelle Lee's beauty is presented as 'natural' in the literal sense of that term, but it is also 'scientifically' validated. Her beauty is, in Barthes's sense, immediate (un-*mediated*) by the means used to select and print the photo.

Semioticians such as Umberto Eco have shown the value of a simple 'commutation', or 'substitution' test in exposing the arbitrariness of our readings of images and words alike. So one way of seeing how the Figure 4.1 diagram 'works' semiotically is to substitute for the faces of the young women, faces of, say, old men from European and Asian geographical backgrounds, and to 'average' these very different faces (e.g., wizened, lined, discoloured, balding) to yield an alternative scientific specimen as the ideal product of the genealogical confluence. Amusingly, this commutation test will only appear to be 'scientific' if *an odd, and not even, number* of such venerable physiognomies is chosen for the purpose of 'averaging', as has been done in the SMH for youthful models. An *even* number of images could not result in an idealised 'average', or mid-point 'blend', for purely mathematical reasons. The point of my satirical comment, of course, is to highlight as pseudo-scientific the quantitative interpretations offered in the newspaper. Photographs of 'ugly', 'old' men might also give the journalist pause about implying that there exist (or once existed) 'pure (or pur*er*) races' from which we are all mixed, so to speak. I would ask: if beauty is quantifiable and can be averaged, why not ugliness? Whether beauty is at stake or not, readers' interpretations still need to be guided by verbal sign-posts so that feminine features, and not, say, age itself, are read as the variable being visually 'quantified'. In all these actual and hypothetical cases, it seems fair to say that readers could only 'see' photographic 'evidence' for concepts that *they already had been prompted by the verbal texts to believe were depicted* (that is, concepts that they believed referred unproblematically to attributes of, or to valid classifications of, *real phenomena*). Readers would have to believe that such phenomena must *exist independently of the words and images used to depict or describe them*. I take up this ontological/epistemological issue in later sections.

4. Race Concepts—Abstraction, Classification, and Observability

The individual models in the SMH series are exemplars of an implied class, indicated by the attributes they 'carry'. That is, they are presented as *depicting* racially 'mixed' types, and as *illustrating* varying degrees of the putatively more 'extreme' versions of themselves that their ancestors (if only we could in turn depict *them*) would exemplify. Of course, the SMH cannot depict these ancestral exemplars. This is a logical, not a technological point: To show actual ancestors would highlight the logical problem that *an infinite regress* of the photographic evidence could be generated. How many instances/generations would we need to see photographs of before we agreed that we were seeing the 'average' (presumably the *mean*, not the *median* or the *mode*) of an implicitly unobservable/un-photographable concept? 'Unobservable' in the sense of being itself abstract—indeed, a concept that *can not logically be applied to individuals* in biological scientific discourse (*pace* my discussion of Ashley Montagu below).

It follows that when we read the SMH's diagrammatic series of portraits, we can only see what we already believe—that 'race' is an empirical concept that applies to individuals; that, in the past, races were more homogenous, maybe even 'pure'; and that racial background/origins are exhibited to varying degrees in each person's facial features. The only way 'purer' versions of the chosen models can be depicted is by *making the very assumption that the photographs purport to show*—that is, the series is part of a *circular argument* when seen in its context. I would go further and say it is an ideologically naïve instance of racism, because it trades on ignorance about the nature of (indeed the existence of) differences amongst, within, and between isolable, interbreeding groups of humans. But this critical point requires further discussion of the concept of 'race' itself, for it is this that is the 'essence', degrees of which the models in Figures 4.1 and 4.2 are claimed to exhibit. This discussion will lead me to consider further epistemological matters, because I believe that considerations of what it means to know an abstract concept are *logically prior* to semiotic analysis.

Semiotic analysis alone cannot ward off the ubiquitous tendency to what philosophers call the 'reification' of abstract terms like 'race'. 'Reification' is a shorthand linguistic practice of referring to abstractions as 'things'. In the social sciences, examples of such verbal 'thingification' of qualities are usually labelled 'essentialist' because they *hypostatise* (or posit as materially 'real') features of people, personalities or experiences. Reification usually implies that the quality that is 'thingified' is a physical entity 'in' a person, or is a material consequence of membership of a nominated group—so (to propose a ludicrous but illuminating example) 'red-heads' are short-tempered *because* there is something in them that is part of, or is correlated with their membership of this (rather 'race'-like) group; or, an African-American athlete runs fast *because* she is African-American. *Membership of the group implies a universal characteristic that is located, so to speak,* ***in*** *all members of the group.* Most egregiously, such essentialist attributions underpin everyday racism, so academic discussion of 'race' issues has sought to displace the biological (material) connotations of 'race' by adopting a less reifying term, 'ethnic group' or 'ethno-linguistic group'. Most recently, the more euphemistic terms 'people of difference' or 'difference' have become fashionable. These locutions seem to avoid biological essentialism which is seen as scientistic, reductive, and deterministic. Of course, this theoretical or linguistic move is important, because racism had usually been coded in claims of unchanging and unchangeable biological/psychological differences between groups of different-looking people, differences such as those supposedly measured by 'intelligence' tests, observable morphological features of individuals (Figures 4.1 and 4.2), or, at times, differences in psychological dispositions of whole populations (to aggression, etc.).

Politically, the belief in fixed biological differences based on uncritical reification, has had pernicious consequences, as the history of even 20th Century racism attests. Racist discourse is replete with assumed racial (i.e. biologically-determined) 'inferiority' or other intrinsic, essential, 'difference'. But 'different' is an adjective, and it is implicitly *relational*. Something can only be different ***from*** something else. 'Difference' *is not a quality* of anything any more than is 'taller' or 'better'. So, to attribute 'difference' as a quality to someone is also a form of reification, albeit one hidden in the shadows of euphemism and 'political correctness'. This is clear if one asks to whom a person of 'difference' is being compared. Any answer to this question shows that someone or something must be assumed to be the norm against whom the putatively different person or entity is defined. 'People of difference' can only *be different* if one uses language ethno*centrically*. When difference is adjudged it is from the assumed position of the judg*er*, so different may just mean 'different from me'! (Speakers do not attribute 'difference' to themselves, only to others).

In the digital age, the SMH series of computer-generated, blended faces can be made to represent the abstract idea that the article constructs. Its nine shades of beauty could have been manufactured from a couple of images 'morphed' to show gradations of the assumed concept. A simpler mode of manipulation could show gradations of skin colour (hue or intensity) consistent with the abstract aims of the proponent. The photographic verisimilitude of the resulting images would be indistinguishable from the series in Figure 4.1. If race 'membership' is naively or tendentiously defined in terms of skin colour, then photographic manipulation for racist ends is a very simple matter, as the example of President Barak Obama's Photoshopped face attests in Figure 4.3, below. Hyphenated euphemisms notwithstanding, recent examples abound of journalists and politicians reifying and spuriously quantifying an individual's qualities in relation to putative race/colour continua, especially one ranging from 'black' to 'white'. Race-connoting labels and the assumptions they encode persist in the most blatant ways.

In the USA, 'dark skin' implies membership of a particular ethnic minority (albeit a very large minority) of 'African-Americans'. The manipulation of the 'darkness' of Obama's skin in advertising aimed at discrediting him therefore trades on the racist notion that skin colour principally or alone reflects what I have called 'degrees of racial heritage'. Colour, however, is never mentioned by *name* in the US advertising; instead it is represented as *visible* evidence of racial membership. Note especially the contrast between Obama's skin tone and his pearly white teeth. It seems that the president and the proletariat alike are members of one of the non-overlapping populations

SMH 2-3/1/16

Tone of ads under scrutiny

United States
Max Ehrenfreund
Washington

A new study shows that negative advertisements targeting US President Barack Obama in 2008 depicted him with very dark skin, and that these images would have appealed to some viewers' racial biases.

The finding reinforces charges that some Republican politicians seek to win votes by implying support for racist views and ethnic hierarchies, without voicing those prejudices explicitly, what is called "dog-whistle politics".

A study published online this month in *Public Opinion Quarterly* analysed 126 advertisements from the presidential campaign in 2008, digitally measuring the darkness of the two nominees' skin in each spot, then sorting the ads into categories based on themes. Mr Obama and his opponent, Senator John McCain, looked very different in various advertisements depending on how the footage was produced.

When Senator McCain's campaign aired spots that connected Mr Obama with alleged criminal activity by liberal groups, the producers almost always used images that made Mr Obama's skin appear very dark.

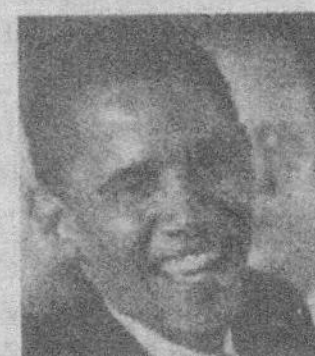

Barack Obama in a 2008 attack ad. Photo: Washington Post

Similarly, as the election approached, images of Mr Obama in spots aired by Senator McCain's campaign became gradually darker. Images of Senator McCain, meanwhile, became somewhat lighter. Whether this was a conscious strategy is impossible to say.

Yet a large body of evidence shows that racial prejudices are stronger against African-Americans with darker skin. For example, jurors are more likely to sentence to death defendants with stereotypically African features.

Washington Post

Figure 4.3 Manipulated photograph—Barack Obama

Note that "*[W]hen Senator McCain's campaign aired spots that connected Mr Obama with alleged criminal activity by liberal groups, the producers almost always used images that made Mr Obama's skin appear very dark*". (SMH, 1st–3rd January, 2016)

of people who share certain characteristics, most egregiously, skin tone. So by manipulating Obama's photograph his opponents implicitly endorsed several commonly held beliefs. In summary:

1. That *discrete races exist*, and that one sufficient criterion for membership is skin 'colour'. Other criteria can also be invoked to suit particular purposes—face shape, eye shape, lip thickness, and so on indefinitely, each selected to suit a particular prejudice (literally, a *pre*-judgement).
2. That *individuals* can unambiguously be assigned membership of such 'races' on the basis of meeting certain physical criteria.
3. That groups, and the individuals who comprise them, have other common attributes that can be inferred from their 'racial' membership based

on these supposed observable features. (Otherwise why make 'colour' salient?)

4. That race is *quantifiable*: people exhibit 'degrees of race'. Hence, the photographic manipulation making Obama '*more* black'. Interestingly, this could not be claimed in words, but, as seen above, images allow *degrees* of some variables to be surreptitiously represented.

To refer back to my earlier discussion, it might be said that the Obama example presents *a corollary of the view of race* exemplified in Figure 4.1: If Republican propagandists exploit degrees of prejudice (negative) that they hope are correlated with values on an assumed 'black-white continuum', then are not the proponents of degrees of 'mixed-race' beauty ('scientists' and their subjects, as well as journalists and editors of the SMH) equally ignorant? Recall that 'beauty' or 'attractiveness' was also judged to be correlated with visible degrees of 'race'.

Epistemology is the study of knowledge claims and their justification—what it means to claim to *know*, rather than merely to *believe*, some proposition about reality. More than 70 years ago the eminent anthropologist Ashley Montagu (1942) led the attempt to shift the understanding of 'race' away from its 'essentialist' presuppositions, arguing that as commonly employed it sustained a dangerously misleading 'myth'. 'Race' was a 'myth' principally because the term *did not refer to any definable groups of humans all of whom shared a finite number of identifiable physical characteristics*. Many anthropologists subsequently refused to use the term 'race' at all.

Montagu argued that 'race' was not an empirically observable feature of people, as it was a *concept* that could *not be applied to individuals*, as discussed above. Its invocation was often, if not always, problematic, and of little or no scientific value. At best, race labels could be useful as *relative* and *comparative* terms that referred provisionally to differing 'gene pools' (i.e. to interbreeding *populations* of humans) but such populations were only meaningful for the sake of comparison with other populations for the purposes of describing the *relative frequencies* of hypothesised traits (e.g., the relative frequency of genetic predispositions to particular diseases in the populations chosen for comparison). So 'race' labels could be chosen to refer to groups of any scale, from 'macro' to 'micro' populations, depending on the point of a particular comparison being made between or amongst them. It follows that, as it is a *relative term*, it makes little sense to assume there exists *a finite number of races*, and therefore there are *no ancestral, and no 'pure races'* between which to make *absolute* empirical comparisons.

Montagu made these arguments in the face of assimilationist and eugenic arguments which had been powerful since the late 19th century and influential in colonialist social policy and its 'scientific' justification. In Australia, for example, as Figures 4.4, and 4.5 (below) attest, photographs seemed to provide unarguable evidence for the ease and desirability of 'breeding out' indigenous populations over a few generations. These pages are taken from A.O.

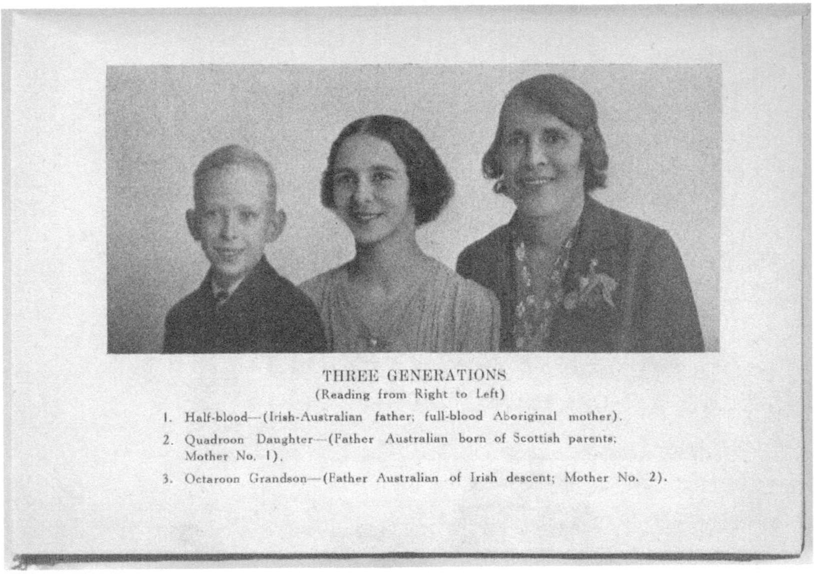
THREE GENERATIONS
(Reading from Right to Left)
1. Half-blood—(Irish-Australian father; full-blood Aboriginal mother).
2. Quadroon Daughter—(Father Australian born of Scottish parents; Mother No. 1).
3. Octaroon Grandson—(Father Australian of Irish descent; Mother No. 2).

Figure 4.4 Assimilation—photographic 'evidence' #1

Neville, *Australia's Coloured Minority—Its place in the Community*, published in 1947. (The Australian Prime Minister, Ben Chifley, owned a copy.)

Australia's Coloured Minority was published in the year that Theo van Leeuwen was born. Today, it appears blatantly colonialist, if not embarrassingly 'racist', in a number of ways. However, I want to argue that these photographic constructions exemplify an interpretation of the concept of race that is remarkably similar to the *assumed reality* of race that underlies the examples I have already discussed, cf. Figures 4.1, 4.2, and 4.3. Most obviously, Neville's tendentious photographs assumed that 'pure' races exist (comprised, if one wants to be as literal as Neville, of '100% aboriginal' people and 100% some other category that he labels in modern national terms—'Scottish', 'Irish', 'Australian'). He proposed that members of (his) designated populations can be 'crossed' (as sheep 'breeds' are in Scotland and Australia) to give progeny that is 50%, then 25% Aboriginal, and presumably over future generations, could be 'bred *out*' (at least 'asymptotically'—12.5%, 6.25%, and so on). But Neville begged the question by depicting his specimens to reflect his pseudo-scientific preconceptions.

5. Words, Images, Concepts—Truth

Adopting the semiotic analyses presented in RI (see pp. 79–108, 164–174), Figures 4.4 and 4.5 can be classed as visual realisations of 'analytical temporal processes' (akin to the Eurasian series in Fig 4.1) and, like it, can

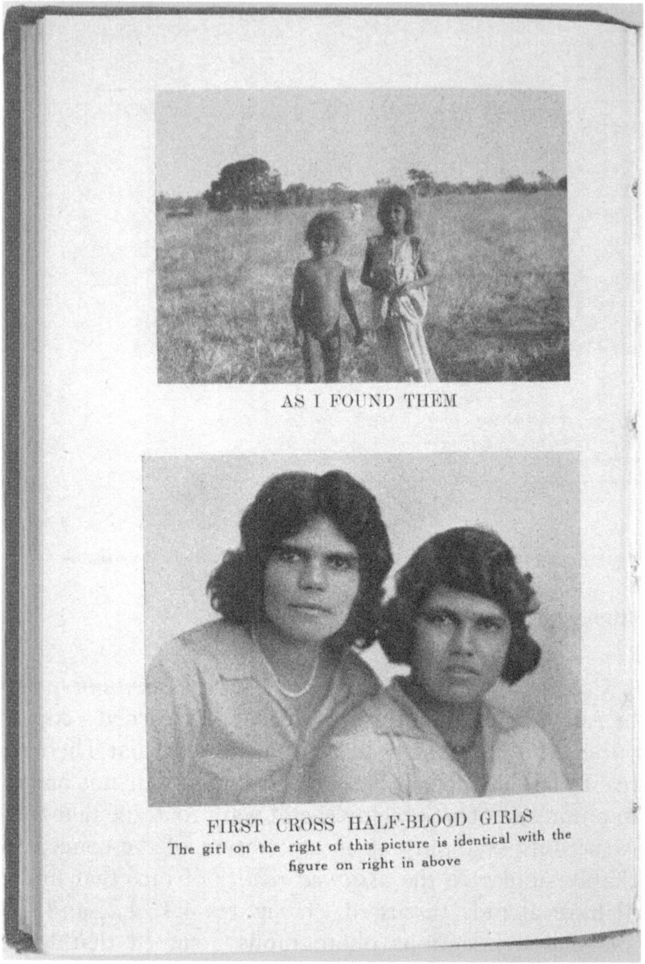
AS I FOUND THEM
FIRST CROSS HALF-BLOOD GIRLS
The girl on the right of this picture is identical with the figure on right in above

Figure 4.5 Assimilation—photographic 'evidence' #2

be read via what Kress and Van Leeuwen (2006) call a 'scientific coding orientation'. Neville's illustrations therefore implied that an abstract and conceptual 'essence' united the exemplars, or more accurately each depicted individual model carried a different degree or 'amount' of the 'essence' that was at stake in the diagrammatically organised photographic series.

My examples of Australian visual representations of 'race' raise, as I believe all semiotic analysis should, the question of whether and how particular texts claim to be true. Without ascending into metaphysical speculation, I want to assert that *to know how and what a text-in-context **means*** *must involve understanding what it claims to be true.* Trivially, had A.O. Neville's analytical photographs not been understood as making claims about real biological phenomena then their meaning cannot be determined. Similarly, although the Eurasian beauty series (Figure 4.1) asks to be understood in cultural/aesthetic terms as well, its meaning depends on it being accepted as depicting a *scientific* truth. Its implicit truth claim is a *sine qua non* of understanding its intended 'meaning'. The same set of photographs, arranged at random, would not make the same, or perhaps any, claim about 'race' and more general biological/genetic reality (contrast Figure 4.6, discussed in the concluding section, below). The contextual assumption (the implied 'coding orientation') that newspapers present visual evidence and verbal propositions as true is what makes this example so problematic and so semiotically interesting. When the added appeal to 'science' is made in the article, the warrant for its veracity is heightened even further.

Verbally, Figures 4.3 and 4.4 exemplify another cultural/political practice so common that it is seldom noticed. This involves assigning people labelled in race terms to the *minority option* available. To be called 'half-caste' in 20th-century Australia was to be assumed 'half-caste *Aborigine*', not 'half-caste *European*'. Tellingly, no-one could be labelled 'half-caste *Australian*', which alone shows the ideology at work in the vernacular register of race categories. Consistent with this practice, Neville's subjects were classified in terms of their assumed *percentage of Aboriginal* ancestry ('blood'), not as exhibiting the reciprocal percentage of 'Anglo-celtic' or 'European' ancestry. 'Quadroon' labels the woman who had one 'quarter' of Aboriginal ancestry (one grandparent who was 'black'). 'Octaroon' was the 'scientific' class into which the small boy was assigned because he had one great-grandparent who was non-European, as judged by Neville's informants. (Of course, Neville had chosen photographs of models and dressed them to illustrate his judgement of their ancestry.)

Labelling the models using a pseudo-scientific lexicon (involving quantification, as science seems to require, see Figure 4.1) and selecting formal, posed photographs that emphasise hair and skin colour, Neville's images mounted an argument in terms of the abstract concept that it named only euphemistically or hid within a scient*istic* register. But without this assumed concept, the photographic evidence makes no sense. Neville's images seem to show the truth of the successive 'dilution' of something like Aboriginal 'essence'. They *show concretely* what they *imagine abstractly* as their cause. However, *the photographs are evidence only of Neville's beliefs*, not the truth of their theoretical presuppositions.

6. The Limits of Semiotic Analysis

Epistemologically, the examples I have analysed suggest that communication through visual imagery is always contentious. Leaving aside the problems of deliberate manipulation and misleading contextualisation of photographs,

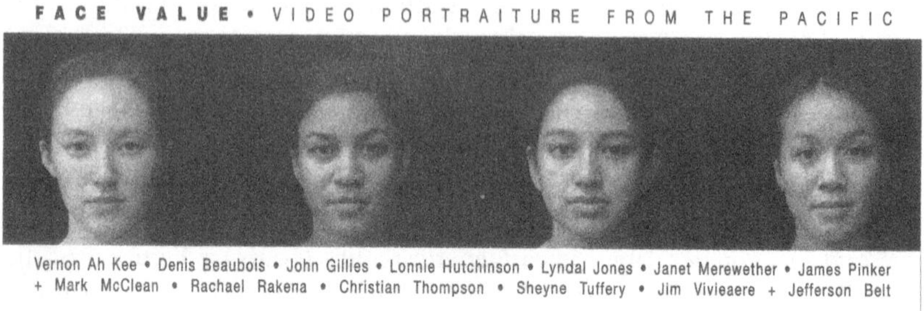

Figure 4.6 'Face value'—art, not science, as coding orientation

the apparently ***un***-mediated ***re-presentation*** of reality by photographic media poses in acute ways the epistemological paradoxes of semiotic analysis: *If photos simply record pre-existing reality, they raise no semiotic issues, being transparently meaningful.* However, *photos seem unambiguously to represent abstract ideas, and to do so through culturally determined codes.*

Alert to this methodological problem I have highlighted the need for semiotics to be grounded in epistemological understanding so that representation can be evaluated in terms of *knowledge claims* and *therefore of the ontological assumptions* that are implicit in particular texts, whether visual or verbal. A text cannot be understood unless its truth claims are also understood, and that means its implicit theoretical/conceptual meanings have to be addressed to augment semiotic analysis. A counter-example to Figure 4.1 reinforces this point: In Figure 4.6 the context within which the series of young women's portraits is presented is 'art' rather than 'science'. Here, the even number of exemplars guards against any sense of 'averaging' the models' facial features. Instead, diversity is celebrated as independent of race classifications—labels are deliberately avoided by the artists in this recent postcard advertising a photography exhibition. The artists' notion of what I would call 'diversity' informs this flyer, which seems to ask the viewer to see the individual models as just that—individuals from various and varying indefinite population(s). Compared to Figure 4.1, Figure 4.6 might be analysed in Kress and Van Leeuwen's (2006) terms as representing an 'analytical process', but not one 'ordered' to invite the essentialist meaning of the SMH article.

The second point of my methodological/theoretical discussion is to highlight the conceptual confusions and incoherencies that persist in current discussions of 'race'. 'Race' continues to be a mystifying concept when it is invoked implicitly in popular media and even in 'scientific' discourse. When Media Studies carved out a 'disciplinary' niche in the academy during the 1970–80s, it embraced semiotics as a way of legitimising its practices of textual analysis. Semiotics offered a precise vocabulary for analysing 'texts', 'discourses', and 'representation' in the soon-to-be multimedia world. But, like their predecessors, new means of representation, insofar as they are intentionally representational, may perpetuate ideologically mystifying (literally, illusory) claims to 'knowledge' just as much as their analogue predecessors. This is especially true in contexts where 'information' is assumed to be 'truth', where 'representation' begs the question of the veracity of verbal claims. Digital media re-imagine notions of 'news' and 'representation', and hybrid modes of image production continue to ground the claims to representational veracity—in scientific, cultural, and in global-political fields of news reporting. Yet, old illusions persist. Across various media photographic depictions of individual people labelled members of discrete 'races', or shown as exemplars of racial 'essence', are still presented as self-evidently true.

7. Conclusion

I have argued that 'race', *qua race*, cannot be *seen* in the literal sense of the word, even in photographic images where differences amongst people on certain physical variables such as skin colour, hair distribution, or the eye shape can be observed. It follows that race cannot be deployed as a positivist, empiricist concept. However, my analyses support the value of a *realist* conceptualisation of 'race'. Epistemology implies ontology. The mystifications of race representation can only be exposed by going beyond explicating how word and image mean, and by asking questions of their theoretical truth. 'Race' is best thought of as a 'relative', comparative and non-essentialist term. But this point can be made only if one avoids *epistemological relativism*. Empirical comparisons between specified *populations* can be made, and these populations might be termed 'races' *for the purposes of the comparison in question*. But that is as far as the epistemological licence extends. So, given the confusions and positivistic uses to which the term has been put, not to mention its use in racist discourse and argument, the term might best be avoided insofar as it is thought to *describe* individuals, groups, or even geographically isolated populations, non-comparatively. The term is mired in 'essentialism' and reification. At best, our culture works with more than one understanding of 'race': We both assume and deny that it is refers to observable features of actual people.

I believe that analysts must consider more than represented texts and implied contexts. To avoid incoherence and/or trivial semiotic display, they must also bring to their analysis *conceptual/theoretical knowledge relevant to the domains in which the particular text is 'uttered'*. To the extent that a text makes claims about reality, it must be understood in terms of realist epistemology. Otherwise, neither the text nor an analyst's commentary can claim to be more than self-referring semiotic games. As a corollary, there could be no reason for preferring one semiotic analysis to another—of race representations or of anything else.

The principal limitation of semiotic analysis, 'functional' or other, may be that abstract knowledge claims remain contestable even after the question has been answered of how a particular text 'works' semiotically. So in relation to my examples, I have emphasised that semiotic analysis demands attention to the epistemological status of presuppositions that both *readers* and *semioticians* bring to a text. Analysts need to ask what knowledge is presupposed in each text and to accept the responsibility of highlighting the truth claims made in it. To do this, they need to be clear about their own epistemological assumptions. Kress and Van Leeuwen (2006), following Halliday, distinguished between the 'context of situation' in which a text is realised (a newspaper and a family photo-album are different situational contexts) and the 'context of culture' that it presupposes (its historical-cultural context). I hope to have shown that to understand what 'race' terms mean in particular texts, especially in photo-realist texts, requires a critical understanding—and that means an *historical* understanding—of its many uses.

Notes

1 Verbal text for 'Beauty and the East' morphed photo series, Fig 1.
2 "By morphing pictures of Caucasian and Japanese people, Australian researchers developed a set of faces ranging from those with exaggerated Caucasian features on the left to exaggerated Japanese features on the right. Both Caucasian Australians and Japanese people rated the mixed-race faces in the middle as most attractive". The linked news item claimed *inter alia* that the research gives "credence to theory that beauty is not solely determined by culture and the media, but has biological origins", because 'Caucasians' and 'Asians' rated average Eurasian faces as 'healthier 'as well as more attractive. The author of the scientific (?) paper on which this was based asserted that such 'findings' suggested "our preferences are shaped by evolution".

References

Barthes, R. (1973). *Mythologies*. London: Paladin.
Bell, P., & Van Leeuwen, T. (1994). *The media interview—Confession, contest, conversation*. Sydney: UNSW Press.
Eco, U. (1975). *A theory of semiotics*. Bloomington, IN: Indiana University Press.
Goffman, I. (1976). *Gender advertisements*. London: Macmillan.
Kress, G., & Van Leeuwen, T. (2006). *Reading images: The grammar of visual design*. London: Routledge.
Montagu, A. (1942). *Man's most dangerous myth—the fallacy of race*. New York: Harper.
Neville, A. O. (1947). *Australia's coloured minority—its place in the community*. Sydney: Currawong publishing Co.
Sontag, S. (1967). *On photography*. Harmondsworth: Penguin.
Van Leeuwen, T. (2005). *Introduction to social semiotics*. London: Routledge.

5 Can a Sign Reveal Its Meaning?

On the Question of Interpretation and Epistemic Contexts

Staffan Selander

1. Prologue: The Beginning of a Question

The first time I met Theo van Leeuwen (and Gunther Kress) was at a conference in London in 1989. After this occasion, I invited both of them to a conference on pedagogic texts in Härnösand (at what is now Mid-Sweden University). Theo came a few days earlier to Stockholm from Sydney, and the two of us started to discuss how one could analyse school textbooks. We talked eagerly about the differences between knowledge representations and semiotic signs in two history textbooks, one Swedish and one Australian, starting at my kitchen table in Stockholm and continuing on the train to Härnösand and then again on the train back to Stockholm.

Two things struck me when I met Theo: first, his curiosity to scrutinise and understand differences in many areas, such as the meanings and functions of the different shapes of doorknobs on a train, or the meanings of colours in paintings from different periods of time. Second, his ability to ask insightful questions, for example, if (as was stated in the Swedish textbook we analysed) humanity came from Africa, why the people represented visually in it are freezing and clothed like Nordic hunters, and why the Swedish textbook starts with people, whilst Australian textbook starts with land that drifted apart from its continent (Van Leeuwen & Selander, 1995)?

Theo's ability to systematise observations, and ask new questions, became essential in our international project *Toys as Communication* (1997–2000, financed by the Swedish Foundation for Humanities and Social Sciences; see Caldas-Coulthard & van Leeuwen, 2003; Van Leeuwen, 2009). Inspired by Theo's approach, I have continued to ask questions concerning different ways to look at things and at concepts that often are taken for granted. This led me further into the question of the sign and its context, and how we can understand a text, or a sign, produced in contexts we do not know, for instance, historical texts or texts from other cultures.

Context is, of course, a tricky term, although precise enough within a specific scientific tradition. It can be used as the co-text in terms of what surrounds a specific paragraph as well as intertextuality—the relation of a specific text to other texts, may it be books, articles, films and so on. Furthermore, context can be understood as the expression of social interests and as a mirror of the power relations construed in a text, and as the ways in which a text can be interpreted and used in a specific social environment. Context can as well be described as the surrounding social mechanisms or the social or political conditions of a situated communicative act.

As I see it, the terms *social context* and *cultural context* are (for a social scientist) ways to make context more a precise term within a given social setting, but perhaps not specific enough for understanding what happens in the communication and interaction between people from different social spheres or cultures. We also need—if we are interested in content—an analysis of *epistemic* context, by which I mean paradigmatic frames or strong traditions of mentally organising and classifying the world. My argument is that the social relations between people (the inter-personal framing) are not only related to a social context, but also to an epistemic context of significant representational models, such as the knowledge emphasis, central concepts, analytical procedures, and metaphors in an institutional domain of knowledge. In the following sections, I will discuss this in relation to Todorov's accounts of the meeting (and the war) between Spanish conquerors (for example, Columbus and Cortés) and South-American Native Americans, here the Aztecs (Montezuma). I will show that this approach is also needed if we want to understand learning and the conditions for learning within different domains of knowledge and performative spaces in different institutional settings.

2. The 'Event' of Multimodal Social Semiotics

Encountering social semiotics in the 1990s, I was struck not only by its richness but also by its roots in sociolinguistics. This perspective was new to me, coming from a psychological-pedagogic and sociological tradition. The book *Reading Images* (Kress & Van Leeuwen, 1990) was not only new to me, it was what the French philosopher Alain Badiou calls an *event* "which compels us to decide a new way of being" (Badiou, 2012, p. 41). In other words, if researchers say that they align to a multimodal, social semiotic approach, they cannot continue conducting analyses of representations (and communication) based on a restricted understanding of text. This approach calls for a new being, a fidelity in a new truth. From this point of view, a text is no longer to be understood 'only' as a something written, but as a 'visual' representation (Björkvall, 2009). The concept of 'text', in its extended meaning, might include drawings, paintings, photographs, moving images, toys, and digital games (although not everyone in the field of multimodality would like to extend the concept of text that far).

To enter a new theoretic and methodological field is like immigrating to a new country—you become the new one, not understanding the language, the eye-on-things, the social environment, the gestures, the jokes, etc. After years of practice, I (almost) became like one in the field (cf. Selander & Kress, 2010; Danielsson & Selander, 2014, 2016; Selander, 2017), only to find myself again asking new question.

3. The Question of Text *and* Context

In the 1970s, a heated discussion about 'text and context', and 'school and society' took place in educational research (cf. Lundgren, 1983). However, this separation of text and context, as well as school and society, should be questioned. At a seminar in Bristol 1990 about teacher education, someone commented: "I understand the word school, and I understand the word society, but what does *and* mean?" Of course, this was not a frivolous remark. The school and society were at the time discussed as two different, objective entities, and consequently we used to discuss the relations between them. Today, we might have a more advanced approach when we discuss how, for example, communication within different institutions and traditions constitutes a society, and, at the same time, how social relations and technical systems constitute the conditions of communication.

This was, of course, no isolated phenomenon. In many sciences, there has been a shift from the analysis of structures of various sorts to situated and communicative events. In sociology and social psychology, for example, the focus shifted from economical and class-related structures (Karl Marx) and structural conditions of reproduction (Bourdieu & Passeron, 1977) to an interest in social distinctions (Bourdieu, 2010), via social representations of groups (Moscovici, 2000; Jodelet, 1995) and then to situated communication and meaning-making (Marková, 2005; see also Gustavsson & Selander, 2011).

From a CDA perspective, Kress (1993) outlined a social semiotic approach to signs and context, arguing that "all signs are metaphors, hence code ideological positions in that they realize the social, cultural and therefore political position of the producer" (ibid, p. 174). He takes his position further, emphasising that "[. . .] a social semiotic approach would attempt to dissolve the category of context itself, preferring to speak of series of interrelating semiotic systems" (ibid. p. 187).

My original assessment of this utterance, coming from the discussions concerning text vs. context, was that it was very inspiring. However, today I do not think that this is enough. We have to spell out our understanding of context and the institutional framing of communication and learning (cf. Björklund Boistrup & Selander, 2009). In sociological terms, we would thus speak of the importance of the meso-level, between the communcative practice on the one hand (the micro-level) and the overarching class and power relations on the other (the macro-level). This also calls for a multiple understanding of context(s) (also see Van Leeuwen, 2008).

4. Context in Texts

It seems obvious that contextual conditions are represented in texts, as to what is taken for granted, what stands out as salient, and in terms of voices as well as power relations, etc. However, as has been discussed in many ways, to interpret a text is not only a question of reading a text and revealing its meaning, as if everything were to be found *in the text*. The French philosopher Paul Ricœur (1979) has discussed this question, with a focus on the interpretation of texts in terms of what develops *between* the reader and the text. The meaning of the text can, from this perspective, neither be found in what the author meant (Schleiermacher, 1959) nor in the text itself as a whole or as a meaningful unit (Gadamer, 1988), but from an understanding of interpretative interest, how the reader positions himself or herself, and how he/she frames the text in the situated act of interpretation.

In many analyses of texts, a specific context is often taken for granted, where the understanding of the text develops from what utterances, objects, symbols, etc. mean in a specific context. An utterance without any context is of course not possible to interpret. Does, for example, the phrase "Close the window, please!" mean that it is too cold in the room, that someone talks to much, or is it a mere grammatical example? Knowledge about the context helps us to understand the utterance. As Bezemer and Kress (2016) write: "[. . .] the sign is always shaped by the environment in which it is made, and its *place* in that environment [. . .]" (Bezemer & Kress, 2016, p. 9).

The question, then, is how we can understand a text, or a sign, produced in contexts we do not know, as is the case of historical texts or texts from other cultures? Is a text to be understood from general features of its time, and if so which ones? It is not difficult, for example, to outline 'typical' power relations from specific historical 'periods' and then 'find' its presence in any text from this time. The problem is that the text in such case will be more like a coherent and illustrative example of what we expect to find, rather than an entity for analysis. Although any text has a certain kind of rhythm, composition, and information linking (Van Leeuwen, 2005), it also has flaws and ruptures, contradictions and different voices (Bakhtin, 1988), or as van Leuuwen expresses it in relation to colour: "Colour codes with a restricted semantic reach have always proliferated, and sometimes contradicted each other. But there are also broader, longer lasted, and more widely distributed trends, such as the reign of 'puritan black' " (Van Leeuwen, 2011, p. 97).

The understanding of texts in contexts thus has both an interpretative and a performative aspect, i.e. meaning occurs both in the reader's (or the viewer's, player's and so on) engagement with, and use of, the text (cf. Kress,

2010). However, as discussed earlier, it would be difficult to avoid such aspects as symbolic values, worldviews, and basic theoretic and organisational principles. Van Leeuwen also touches upon this in his book about colours. For instance, the white clothes of Cistercian monks and the black clothes of the Benedictine order were both used to honour God during the Middle Ages (Van Leeuwen, 2011, p. 16). These colour codings can only be understood in relation to a symbolic universe, transcending each specific communicative act.

5. Epistemic Contexts

My interest in epistemic context relates to an interest in understanding basic organisational principles of knowledge representation, with its significant representational models, knowledge emphasis, central concepts, analytical procedures, and metaphors in an institutional domain of knowledge.

In this case, my interest goes beyond what Fairclough called 'discourse'. On the one hand, Fairclough makes a sophisticated linguistic analysis in relation to (hegemonic) political and ideological discourses (Fairclough, 1992, 1995). On the other, his analysis misses such aspects as the concrete and situated interpretation, as well as the role of genres over time (Ajagán-Lester, Ledin, & Rahm, 2003). I will rather use *discourse* in the way Michel Foucault used the term, both as socially valid categories, including the power of the speaker to exclude certain things, and as the specific procedures that limit and control what is seen as relevant (Foucault, 1965, 1970; Sheridan, 1981; Börjesson, 2003).

I would now like to show some of Tzvetan Todorov's (1985) rich analysis of the conquest of (South) America. The meeting between people from different cultures can be read from different points of view, in terms of technology, ways of making wars, and diseases and so on. What seems most striking in his analysis is the role of signs, which in my interpretation relates to the epistemic dimension of how the world is to be understood.

The Spanish conquistadors had, of course, not one single mission. Although their primary goal was to take gold and bring it back to Spain, there were other interests involved, namely religious missions and political control. Interestingly, the Spaniards related to the Aztecs—'the Other'—equally and unequally at the same time since the Christian worldview puts every man in the same position; everyone was supposed to be treated 'the same way'. Many of the first comments regarding the Native Americans showed some appreciation for their culture, sophistication, behaviour and ability to speak well (in line with the rhetorical tradition at the time in Europe).[1] At the same time, as the Spaniards came into closer contact with the Native Americans, these people were defined as different, as barbaric and not fully human, especially when the Native Americans contradicted the interest of the conquistadors. Once the Spaniards had taken control of the situation, they set up rules, for instance, that Aztecs had to obey the

Spanish crown, or they would be imprisoned and punished, whether they understood this rule or not. In other words, a mere power control of 'the Other' was established.

Todorov asks the following question: "[H]ow are we to account for the fact that Cortés, leading a few hundred men, managed to seize the kingdom of Montezuma, who commanded several hundred thousand?" (Todorov, 1985, p. 53). And his answer is that the 1519 war and the conquistadors' control of the situation has to be understood not only in terms of the superiority of the Spanish war technology, but also the different symbolic universes: "The whole history of the Aztecs, as it is narrated in their own chronicles, consists of the realizations of anterior prophecies, as if the event could not occur unless it has been previously announced" (Todorov, 1985, p. 66). And Durán, one of the best observers of the Aztec society, according to Todorov, writes:

> One day I asked an old man why he was sowing a certain type of small bean so late in the year, considering that they are usually frostbitten at that time. He answered that everything has a count, a reason, and a special day [. . .] This regulation impregnates even the minutest details of life, which we might have supposed were left to the individual's free decision; ritual itself is only the most salient point of a society that is ritualised through and through; yet the religious rites are in themselves so numerous and so complex that they mobilise an army of functionaries.
>
> (Quoted in Todorov, 1985, p. 67)

Hence "the individual himself does not represent a social totality but is merely the constitutive element of that other totality, the collectivity" (p. 67). Central to Todorov's analysis is the interpretation of signs through two different epistemic views of the world:

> The characteristic interrogation of this world is not, as among the Spanish conquistadors (or the Russian revolutionaries), of a praxeological type: "what is to be done?"; but epistemological: "how are we to know?". And the interpretation of the event occurs less in terms of concrete, individual, and unique content than of the preestablished order of universal harmony, which is to be reestablished.
>
> (ibid, p. 69)

As everything has to be interpreted in relation to an already established order, it can only be read by omens and indices, and as the whole society is hierarchical, steady, and cyclic, everything that happens has to be interpreted in its 'right' place. Thus, it was the case, argues Todorov, that when the first Spaniards came, this event had to be interpreted as already foreseen. Montezuma's communication was "made in the context of the world, not at that with men" (ibid, p. 72). Todorov also underlines that "everything suggests that the omens were invented after the fact" and this "is so well adapted to the situation that, hearing the narrative, everyone believes he remembers that the omen had indeed appeared *before* the conquest" (ibid, p. 74).

A single event loses its singularity and is integrated into an order of already existing beliefs. This cyclical world, where everything happens again and again at its right time, is a complex construction of the religious year of 260 days, the astronomic year of 365 days, and then the years themselves in cycles of 20 years, 52 years, etc. To be able to maintain this universe of mind, the Aztecs (as the Incas and the Mayas) had to build up a vast system for the education of interpretation. This is impressive when seen in the light of the fact that the Incas had almost no written language, the Aztecs had pictograms and the Mayas only had certain rudiments of phonetic writing. Todorov (1985) also emphasises that "we see how reluctant Montezuma is to admit that an entirely new event can occur" (p. 86), and he concludes this part as follows:

> Masters in the art of ritual discourse, the Indians are inadequate in a situation requiring improvisation, and this is precisely the situation of the conquest. Their verbal education favours paradigm over syntagm, code over context, conformity-to-order over efficiaty-of-the-moment, the past over the present.
>
> (ibid., p. 87)

I will now take this idea of epistemic context into a final discussion about learning by relating the understanding of learning to the organisation of epistemic principles.

6. Learning in Context

I would like to start by highlighting some differences between a multimodal and a design-oriented approach to communication and learning. When I first started to think about social semiotics in relation to the socio-cultural perspective, it became obvious for me that these approaches operated on different levels of analysis. Whilst the socio-cultural analyses are conducted at a macro level (for example, mediated learning, collective memory, institutional context, etc.), social semiotics (often) operate with a close analysis of a micro-situation, such as a communicative event or the layout of a page, even though this often relates to a social and cultural environment as found in the production and presentation of food, jewellery, and symbols (McGovern, 2010; Salaam, 2014).

Inspired by the French philosopher Paul Ricœur—who studied the concept of narrative in Aristotle and the concept of time in Tomas ab Aquino and then asked what happens if we take the concept of time into the understanding of the narrative (Ricœur, 1983–85)—I started to think about how we could incorporate a multimodal social semiotic understanding of *communication* into the understanding of *learning*. Out of this, I (and my research group in Stockholm) developed the concept of 'designs for learning' (Selander, 2008a, 2008b, 2008c, 2008d; Rostvall & Selander, 2008; Selander, 2017). Instead of simply criticising psychological research in the learning sciences, as was common then, we could offer an alternative understanding by using central concepts from multimodal communication, for instance,' meaning potential', 'prompt', 'transformation', 'sign-making', 'information value', 'information linking', and so on (Kress, 2010; Van Leeuwen, 2005) to analyse learning as sign-making in terms of 'Learning Design Sequences' (Insulander, 2010; Johansson, Verhagen, Åkerfeldt, & Selander, 2014; Kjällander, 2011; Selander, 2008a, 2008b, 2008c; Åkerfeldt & Selander, 2011; Åkerfeldt, 2014). Meanwhile, we continued to elaborate on the differences between a *social semiotic and multimodal* perspective on *communication*, on the one hand, and a *knowledge-oriented, epistemic* perspective on *learning* on the other (Leijon & Lindstrand, 2012; Selander, 2017).

Seen from this point of view, learning something is not only meaning-making, it is also a question of possessing the capability to use different semiotic resources in a refined and elaborated way, developing the capacity to make even more refined distinctions in a field of knowledge, as well as utilising an elaborated capability to take part in the field and employ relevant theories and methods to conduct analyses. Learning always includes a *content* aspect, a *time* aspect, as well as *new situations*, as in the case of becoming a full member of a profession (Lave & Wenger, 2002). This also means that learning will always be related to a *culture of recognition* that frames what is possible to see *as* learning, and thus to develop *as* assessment criteria.

Multimodal analysis of learning tends to focus on the (general) *communicative* aspects, and seems to look upon communication and learning as two sides of the same coin, where learning becomes an aspect of communication. This broader view on learning also entails aspects such as *agency* and *achievements* (Bezemer & Kress, 2016). From a *design-oriented* point of view, learning is not only related to a social context but also to a context of representational models, including knowledge emphasis, central concepts, analytical procedures, and metaphors in relation to an institutional domain of knowledge—in other words an *epistemic* context. Sign-making is here not only seen as a *communicative resource* but also as an *epistemic resource* in relation to a specific field of knowledge. Learning is always learning *something—in* a context (see also Gee, 2014).

But not only epistemic context of importance to learning, so is the engagement and the activities of the learner. This *performative* context can be described in terms of *activity linking*—a category inspired by Van Leeuwen's concept *information linking* (Van Leeuwen, 2006), which relates both to what the reader/user is supposed to do with the information, in terms of either implicit expectations or explicit demands, and what he or she actually does in the transformative work with information to create an own representation.[2]

Even though both approaches are interested in the signs of learning, a design-oriented perspective also asks *what* can be seen as learning and *how* this is measured. A full evaluation of learning can only be made by a person who knows the specific field of knowledge. To understand learning entails both the more general aspect of increased capacities and capabilities, and the more specific aspect related to a specific field of knowledge, which I would call *significant* learning. The term significant does not simply relate to a narrow type of curriculum or to specific course goals, but to a wider understanding of the knowledge domain established outside the narrow context of schools. In the following table (Table 5.1) (inspired by Halliday's communicative metafunctions), I provide a summary of knowledge-oriented context:

Table 5.1 Knowledge-oriented context

	Knowledge-oriented context
Epistemic framing	Specific focus on scientific models, typical examples, knowledge emphasis, central concepts, analytical procedures and metaphors
Interpersonal framing	a) How the individual reader/user is addressed and positioned; b) the voices in the text/ visual representation
Representational framing	The kind of knowledge (of all possible knowledge) in a knowledge domain that is salient in a specific knowledge representation
Institutional framing	The framing of the learning situation and of learning resources, culture of recognition and assessment criteria
Performative framing	Activity linking and (spaces for the learner's) agency

7. Concluding Remarks

Context—this useful albeit vague concept—has been the focus of this chapter. Although many important analyses have been done with a focus on the *social* or *cultural*, as well as on the *ideological* and *political* context, these are not specific enough for understanding what happens in the communication and interaction between people from different social spheres or different cultures. My argument is that we also need an analysis of *epistemic* contexts. Todorov's analyses of the meeting (and war) between Spanish conquerors and the Aztecs has been uses as an illustrative example of the importance of epistemic contexts and understandings. In arguing that the role of epistemic context is central to our understanding of learning, I am, of course, well aware of other aspects of importance as well as the *affective* aspects of learning and meaning-making (see, for example, Lund & Chemi, 2015; Van Leeuwen, 2000). That, nevertheless, is another story.

Notes

1 Todorov mentions letters by the conquistadors to the Spanish king, as well as chronicles from Catholic priests, etc.
2 This also includes the role of *collaborative* learning (Hansen, Shah, & Klas, 2015) and analyses of *epistemic patterns* (Shaffer, 2009).

References

Ajagán-Lester, L., Ledin, P., & Rahm, H. (2003). Intertextualiteter. In B. Englund & P. Ledin (Eds.), *Teoretiska perspektiv på sakprosa*. Lund: Studentlitteratur.

Åkerfeldt, A. (2014). *Didaktisk design med digitala resurser: En studie av kunskapsrepresentationer i en digitaliserad skola*. Diss, Stockholm University, Stockholm.

Åkerfeldt, A., & Selander, S. (2011). Exploring educational video game design—meaning potentials and implications for learning. In P. Felicia (Ed.), *Handbook of research on improving learning and motivation through eduactional games: Multidisciplinary approaches*. Hershey, PA: IGI Global.

Badiou, A. (2012). *Ehics: An essay on the understanding of evil*. London/New York: Verso.

Bakhtin, M. (1988). *Det dialogiska ordet*. Gråbo: Anthropos.

Bezemer, J., & Kress, G. (2016). *Multimodality, learning and communication: A social semiotic frame*. London/New York: Routledge.

Björklund Boistrup, L., & Selander, S. (2009). Coordinating multimodal social semiotics and an institutional perspective in studying assessment actions in mathematics classrooms. In V. Durand-Guerrier, S. Boyd R. & Wertsch, J. (Ed.) *Memory in mind and culture*. Cambridge, MA: Cambridge University Press.

Björkvall, A. (2009). *Den visuella texten: Multimodal analys i praktiken* (Ord och stil). Uppsala: Hallgren och Fallgren.

Börjesson, M. (2003). *Diskurser och konstruktion: En sorts metodbok*. Lund: Studentlitteratur.

Bourdieu, P. (2010/1979). *Distinction: A social critique of the judgement of taste*. London/New York.

Bourdieu, P., & Passeron, J-C. (1977). *Reproduction: In education, society and culture*. London: Sage.

Caldas-Coulthard, C. R., & Van Leeuwen, T. (2003). Teddy bear stories. *Social Semiotics*, *13*(1), 5–27.

Danielsson, K., & Selander, S. (2014). *Se texten! Multimodala texter i ämnesdidaktiskt arbete*. Malmö: Gleerups.

Danielsson, K., & Selander, S. (2016). Reading multimodal texts for learning—a model for cultivating multimodal literacy. *Designs for Learning*, *8*(1), 25–36. doi:http://dx.doi.org/10.16993/dfl.72

Fairclough, N. (1992). *Discourse and social change*. Cambridge: Polity Press.

Fairclough, N. (1995). *Critical discourse analysis*. London: Longman.

Foucault, M. (1965). *Madness and civilisation*. New York: Pantheon.

Foucault, M. (1970). *The order of things*. New York: Pantheon.

Gadamer, H-G. (1988/1960). *Truth and method*. London: Sheed & Ward.

Gee, J. P. (2014). Decontextualised language: A problem, not a solution. *International Multilingual Research Journal*, *8*, 1–15. doi:10.1080/19313152.2014.852424

Gustavsson, A., & Selander, S. (2011). Transformation and changes in social knowledge—towards the dynamics of meaning making. In M. Chaib, B. Danemark, & S. Selander, (Eds.), *Education, professionalisation and social representations*. London: Routledge.

Hansen, P., Shah, C., & Klas, C-P. (2015). *Collaborative informations seeking: Best practices, new domains and new thoughts*. Cham Heidelberg/New York/Dordrecht/London: Springer.

Insulander, E. (2010). *Tinget, rummet, besökaren. Om meningsskapande på museum*. PhD Dissertation, Stockholms universitet: Institutionen för didaktik och pedagogiskt arbete.

Jodelet, D. (1995). *Folies et représentations sociales*. Paris: Presses Universitaires de France.

Johansson, M., Verhagen, H., Åkerfeldt, A., & Selander, S. (2014). How to design for meaningful learning—finding the balance between learning and game components. *ECGBL 2014*, 9–10 October, Berlin, Germany. Retrieved from http://academic-conferences.org/ecgbl/ecgbl2014/ecgbl14-home.htm

Kjällander, S. (2011). *Designs for learning in an extended digital environment*. Diss. Stockholm: Stockholm University.

Kress, G. (1993). Against arbitrariness: the social production of the sign as a foundational issue in critical discourse analysis. *Discourse & Society*, *4*(2), 169–193.

Kress, G. (2010). Multimodality: A social semiotic approach to contemporary communication. London: Routledge.

Kress, G., & Van Leeuwen, T. (1990). *Reading images*. Victoria: Deakin University.

Lave, J. & Wenger, E. (2002/1993). Situated learning. Legitimate peripheral patterns for learning and technology. London: Roudledge.

Leijon, M., & Lindstrand, F. (2012). Socialsemiotik och design: Två multimodala teorier om lärande, representation och teckenskapande. *Pedagogisk forskning i Sverige*, *17*(3–4), 171–192.

Lindstrand, F., Insulander, E., & Selander, S. (2016). Mike the Knight in the neoliberal era: A multimodal approach to children's multimedia entertainment. *Journal of Language and Politics*, *15*(3), 337–351.

Lund, B., & Chemi, T. (Eds.). (2015). *Dealing with emotions: A pedagogical challenge to innovative learning*. Rotterdam/Boston, MA/Taipei: Sense Publishers.

Lundgren, U. P. (1983). Between hope and happening: Text and context in curriculum. Victoria: Deakin University.

Marková, I. (2005). *Dialogicality and social representations: The dynamics of mind*. Cambridge: Cambridge University Press.

McGovern, S. W. (2010). *Semiosis in Japanese culture: Sign-making practices across modes*. PhD Dissertation, Institute of Education, London.

Moscovici, S. (2000). *Social representations: Explorations in social psychology*. Cambridge: Polity.

Ricœur, P. (1979). *Fortolkningsteori*. Köpenhamn: Vinten.

Ricœur, P. (1983–1985). *Temps et récit I-III*. Paris: Éditions du Seuil.

Rostvall, A.-L., & Selander, S. (Eds.). (2008). *Design för lärande* (2nd ed., 2010). Stockholm: Norstedts Akademiska Förlag.

Salaam, S. (2014). Jewellery students as designers of meaning: A multimodal approach to semiotic resources. In A. Archer & D. Newfield (Eds.), *Multimodal approaches to research and pedagogy: Recognition, resources and access* (pp. 192–206). London: Routledge.

Schleiermacher, F. D. E. (1959/1805–1833). *Hermeneutik. Nach den Handschriften neu herausgegeben und eingeleitet von Heinz Kimmerle*. Heidelberg: Carl Winter Universitätsverlag.

Selander, S. (2008a). Designs for learning—a theoretical perspective. *Designs for Learning*, *1*(1), 10–24.

Selander, S. (2008b). Designs for learning and the formation and transformation of knowledge in an era of globalisation. *Studies in Philosophy and Education*, *27*(4), 267–283.

Selander, S. (2008c). Designs for learning and ludic engagement. *Digital Creativity*, *19*(3), 145–152.

Selander, S. (2008d). Tecken för lärande—tecken på lärande. Ett designteoretiskt perspektiv. In A-L. Rostvall & S. Selander, S. (Eds.), *Design för lärande*. Stockholm: Norstedts Akademiska Förlag.

Selander, S. (2017). Didaktiken efter Vygotskij: Design för lärande. Stockholm: Liber.

Selander, S., & Kress, G. (2010). *Design för lärande—ett multimodalt perspektiv*. Stockholm: Norstedts.

Shaffer, D. W. (2009). Epistemic network analysis: A prototype for 21st century assessment of learning. *Massachusetts Institute of Technology: Foundations & Findings*, *1*(2), 1–22.

Sheridan, A. (1981). *Michel Foucault: The will to truth*. London/New York: Tavistock Publications.

Todorov, T. (1985). *The conquest of America: The question of the other*. New York/Cambridge/Philadelphia/San Fransisco, CA/London/Mexico City/São Paulo/Singapore/Sydney: Harper Colophon Books. [*La conquête Amerique*, 1982]

Van Leeuwen, T. (2000). It was just like magic—a multimodal analysis of children's writing. *Lingustics and Education*, *10*(3), 273–305.

Van Leeuwen, T. (2006). *Introducing social semiotics*. London: Routledge.

Van Leeuwen, T. (2008). *Social representations: Explorations in social psychology*. Oxford: Oxford University Press.

Van Leeuwen, T. (2009). The world according to Playmobil. *Semiotica*, *173*(11/4), 299–315. doi:101515/SEMI.2009.013.

Van Leeuwen, T. (2011). *The language of colour: An introduction*. Milton Park, Abingdon: Routledge.

Van Leeuwen, T., & Selander, S. (1995). Picturing "our" heritage in the pedagogic text: Layout and illustrations in an Australian and a Swedish history textbook. *Journal of Curriculum Studies*, *5*, 501–522.

6 Towards a Multimodal Social Semiotic Agenda for Touch

Carey Jewitt

1. Introduction

In this chapter, I set out a multimodal social semiotic agenda for understanding touch communication practices. I outline how multimodal social semiotics can provide a framework that can be used to explore the materiality of touch, how these are shaped into touch based semiotic resources and modes, and how their take up by people to communicate is culturally and socially patterned and regulated. To do this I build on emerging multimodal studies on touch, and draw inspiration from Theo van Leeuwen's early interdisciplinary explorations of emergent modes (i.e. sound and colour) by asking how a multimodal social semiotic approach might be complemented by insights on touch from psychophysics, anthropology of the senses, and sociology. I articulate the relationships across these increasingly blurred disciplinary boundaries towards mapping the landscape of touch as 'semiotic resource' and 'mode(s)'.

2. A General Introduction to Touch Communication

Touch can provide people with significant information and experience of the world. Touch is the first sense through which humans (and other animals) apprehend our environment, and it is central to our development (Field, 2003). Touch is crucial for tool use (Fulkerson, 2014) and to communication: "Just as we 'do things with words' so, too, we act through touches" (Finnegan, 2014, p. 208). Indeed, knowing how to infer meaning from touch is considered to be the very basis of social being (Dunbar, 1996). Touch has many social functions in the everyday life of societies and has been honed to be a specialised form of communication within some social cultural groups. Touch is one means of enacting social relations (interpersonal meaning) and creates a stance to the world. These include greetings—shaking hands and embracing—intimate communication—holding hands, kissing, cuddling, and stroking—and more negatively in correction—punishment or restraining. Touch is commonly used to communicate emotions and has a role in communicating complex social messages of trust, receptivity, and affection as well as nurture, dependence, and affiliation (McLinden and McCall, 2002). Touch has been shown to be an effective means of influencing people's attitudes and creating bonds with people and places (Krishna, 2010). In clinical and professional situations, for example, interpersonal touch has been shown to improve information flow and to result in a more favourable evaluation of communication partners and to increase compliance (Field, 2010). Touch also fulfills social functions related to experiential (or ideational) meaning that serve to construct our experience of the world—providing people with information about objects, for example, interpreting texture, temperature, and perceptual understanding.

Despite the centrality of touch to people's lives there is limited social science engagement with and understanding of touch. The neglect of touch can be tied to the social-historical value and positioning of touch within social science:

- Touch is given considerably less value and attention than sight and speech as a consequence of the (Cartesian) association of the resources of sight and speech with 'the mind' and the resources of touch with 'the body'
- Touch communication is associated with marginalised groups, including the visually and hearing impaired
- Touch does not 'belong' or 'map' to any one specific discipline (cf. language to linguistics).

One result of this relative neglect is that social science understanding of touch-based communication is less developed than that of other communicative forms (modes from a multimodal social semiotic perspective), such as speech, gesture, or gaze. Linguists have largely ignored touch, although there are a few studies on it within socio-linguistics that have extended the role of hand gestures in interaction to consider touch. In his seminal book *Gesturecraft* (2009), Streeck explores the communicative ecologies in which hand gestures appear. He analyses gesture as embodied communicative action grounded in the hands' practical and cognitive engagement with the material world. He argues that the hands are (with the possible exception of the eyes) the most important part of our body in "providing us with knowledge of the world, and no organ (except the brain) has played a greater part in creating the world that humans inhabit" (p. 4). Streeck goes on to state that we need to understand gestures as physical touch, rather than visual phenomena:

> Because gestures are visual phenomena for interlocutors and are often looked at and seen by the people making them, it is often falsely assumed that gesture is a medium which transforms visual experience into visual representations. Rather, as a medium of understanding, gesture incorporates haptic epistemology: it is driven by the body's

> practical acquaintance with a tangible environment that it has forever explored, lived in, and modified. The beholder, the recipient of conversational gesture, also draws upon an undisclosed background of haptic understandings, couplings of motor-schemata and things in the world; otherwise, they would be unable to recognize the action patterns that the gestures instantiate.
>
> (p. 208)

Multimodality has also largely overlooked touch, with a few notable exceptions that I will return to later in this chapter. As a consequence, touch is a relatively unchartered social semiotic terrain.

3. Turning a Multimodal Social Semiotic Lens on Touch

Multimodal social semiotics examines everyday interactions with other social beings and/or with artefacts (this term is used to refer to semiotic materials produced by people, that is anything that bears the traces of semiotic work, e.g., an object, a digital touch device, etc.) to understand processes of meaning-making. Multimodal analysis provides insight on these processes and their outcomes through micro observation and the comparison of the semiotic and modal features of an artefact or the flow of interaction in a given social moment and place. A common analytical starting point is to generate a general description of an artefact or sequence of interaction (e.g., its genre, materiality, and general structure) to locate it in the wider world of representation and communication, to identify and describe the modes and semiotic resources (defined below) that are available in a given situation, how people use them, the choices they make and what motivates these, and how their in situ choices are shaped by (and realise) power. Within a multimodal social semiotic framework both artefacts and interaction are positioned as semiotic material traces—the outcome of a person's or people's actions, imbued with the sign maker's interests mediated through the environment in which the sign was produced and newly encountered. In other words, this approach is concerned with understanding the social world as it is represented in/through interaction and artefacts.

To theorise the contingent and fluid boundaries of 'modes of touch', I suggest that it is necessary to situate the social process of producing and using semiotic resources and modes within the bodily, material, and sensory possibilities of touch and their cultural histories. I will take sound as an illustrative example to provide a starting point for the process of exploring touch. The materiality of sound (sound waves, oscillation in pressure through air and water) in the form of vibrations travels (through air or water) to the ear or is produced via the vocal chords and diaphragm. The perception of these vibrations is linked to the physiological, psychological, and neurological capacity of a person (or an animal). The experience of sound at this level is named as pitch, duration, loudness, timbre, spatial location, and sonic texture (Van Leeuwen, 1999). We can use this approach to explore the materiality of touch, its take up, and the dimensions of how it is experienced. How and what specific meaning functions these elements come to mean (that is, semiotically), is shaped by human sensory capacities in concert with the material potentials of sound or touch, etc., and their use in specific social contexts. In other words, the semiotic meanings of elements of sound such as pitch or loudness come to have situated social cultural meanings—rather than being universal or static meanings. What is classified and dismissed as 'noise' (unwanted sound) or celebrated as 'sound' (what included/excluded?) is culturally situated, not universally the same. A multimodal social semiotic approach can contribute to the exploration of touch, by examining what is counted as touch by a social group in a given context and what semiotic meanings are associated with the dimensions of touch (e.g., location, duration, or pressure). For instance, to place one's hand on the shoulder of another person, to hold it there for a long time, with pressure, can communicate intimacy and reassurance, or power and control. Modes come about by the regularisation and organisation of sets of semiotics resources to realise Halliday's three 'metafunctions' (ideational, interpersonal, intertextual meanings). It is important to note with regard to the relationship between sense and mode: sense does not map directly in a 1:1 way to mode. The aural sense is a basis of sound and its modal shaping into, for example, speech, music, and sound effect. Similarly, touch as sense, and the physical dimensions of touch are shaped to realise different modes: I will return to this later in the chapter in more detail. It is productive to start to map the modal qualities, materiality, and semiotic potential of emergent touch-based modes and to ask under what social conditions and in what social contexts are touch-based resources shaped through their use by people to become semiotic resources or fully articulated modes? What do people use touch to achieve in multimodal complexes? Who uses them? And how are they used and what established conventions inform their use? In the case of touch, this might take us from the contexts of therapy (e.g., massage) to the specialist touch of crafts (e.g., ceramics) to tactile hand signing (e.g., Pro-Tactile ASL) for DeafBlind communities. Finally, multimodal social semiotics is concerned with how technologies re-shape semiotic resources, modes, and practices through their digital production, broadcasting/dissemination, and consumption. At this point in time, touch communication technologies are at an early stage in their development, their digital remediation herald new possibilities and practices for touch.

In the remainder of this chapter, I propose a multimodal social semiotic agenda for touch communication to:

- Describe and document the materiality of touch and how these are experienced
- Map the semiotic resources and affordances of touch
- Identify and examine touch-based modes: their semiotic principles and meaning potentials

- Explore who can touch: agency and power
- Characterise people's use of touch for communication with attention to the cultural and social norms and power relations that shape their use.

In doing so, I argue for the benefits of complementing multimodal analysis with social research on the physical, material, sensory possibilities, and cultural histories of touch.

Social semiotics has been used to develop detailed and systematic descriptive frameworks for the analysis of images (Kress & Van Leeuwen, 2006), colour (Kress & Van Leeuwen, 2002; Van Leeuwen, 2010), and sound (Van Leeuwen, 1999), among other modes. While there is some debate as to whether modes are experienced and (perceived) interpreted as singular, they are usually encountered as components of multimodal complexes and have many shared semiotic features and principles, hence the term 'multimodal'. Nonetheless, there is value in focusing in on a mode, in this chapter, touch, to understand its particular features and functions. To date there has been little multimodal attention on touch—either in relation to specific touch-based mode(s) or to touch as a part of a multimodal ensemble. The research that has been conducted can be characterised as exploratory and theoretical.

Documenting the Materiality of Touch

Within multimodality the body is understood as a semiotic resource for meaning-making. Multimodality pays analytical attention to how people use and interpret specific modes (e.g., gesture, gaze, posture, movement) and how these interact to represent and communicate meaning (e.g., about a person's identity). Stein (2012, p. 26), working within the multimodal semiotic tradition, argues that the body and the senses are integral to multimodal communication:

> The materiality of semiotic modes is related to the sensory possibilities of the body [. . .] The concept of multimodality is inseparable from bodies. Bodies produce multimodality through how they are constituted sensually and how these senses act on the world and are acted on.

Materiality can be physical—marks, textures, shapes and forms—in the sense that it can be felt, heard or touched: in this way we can understand materiality as a direct "interface between the natural and cultural world" (Stein, 2012, p. 26). However, materiality can also have a non-physical appearance, such as spoken words or notes in which sounds have been culturally worked on to produce particular aural modes, speech and music. Stein connects the material—what Kress (2010) refers to as 'stuff'—that is what a society makes available to be shaped into semiotic means for the expression of its meanings, with the sensory capacities of people to 'take up' or 'take in' these meanings. This brings the physical and sensory body clearly into view and complements a multimodal social semiotic perspective by re-focusing attention on how materiality and 'stuff' gets brought into the social domain and socially worked into semiotic resources and principles. In doing so, I seek to connect multimodality with the senses and processes of perception, domains of the biological, psychological, and neurological, that are generally seen as sitting outside of the concerns of multimodality and social semiotics.

It is important to understand how the physical, material, and sensory aspects of touch are a part of when and how touch-based resources are taken up (or excluded) and how they can shape—or are shaped by—people to become semiotic resources. Multimodality can draw insights on the dimensions of touch from a psycho-physical and neuropsychological account of the physical experience and perception of touch and its methodological focus on the skin as an organ, its sensory receptors (nerve endings and corpuscles), and the somatosensory area of the brain (using EGC, Galvanic Skin Tests, MRIs, and neuroimaging technologies) (Spence, 2013). These accounts are limited through their focus on the individual and understanding of the senses as fixed and universal, and not recognising "the role that culture plays in the modulation of perception senses function" (Howes, 2011, p. 161). While sensation is more than a biological process, insights on the physical dimensions of touch and the physiological processes through which 'signals' or tactile sensations (e.g., pain, temperature, pressure) are perceived are the 'stuff' of semiotics.

Mapping the Semiotic Resources and Affordances of Touch

As already noted, a common starting point for a multimodal social semiotic analysis is to identify and describe the semiotic resources that are available in a given situation, and how people choose and use them. 'Semiotic resources' is a term used to refer to the meaning potential of material resources, which developed and accumulated over time through their use in a particular community and in response to certain social requirements of that community. Affordance, when used in social semiotics, is a term that refers to the idea that different modes offer different potentials for making meaning. Modal affordances affect the kinds of semiotic work a mode can be used for, the ease with which it can be done, and the different ways in which modes can be used to achieve broadly similar semiotic work. Modal affordances are connected both to a mode's material and social histories, that is, the social purposes that it has been used for in a specific context.

The example I present here shows how semiotic resources can serve as a multimodal social semiotic entry point for touch and to expand our limited terms to describe touch and tactile experiences. Djonov and Van Leeuwen (2011) conducted an exploratory study of the meaning-making potential of 'tactile surface texture' and 'visual texture', in the presentation of texture (as a fill option for shapes and backgrounds) in PowerPoint from 1992 to 2007. I include this somewhat tangential study in this chapter as it demonstrates the usefulness of examining semiotic resources in the context of 'tactile experience'. The study explored how tactile sensation can translate into meaning through a focus on the materialisation of texture in different media and "developing parameters for describing tactile and visual surface texture" (ibid: 542) and their meaning-making potentials through the exploration of three factors.

First, the *provenance* of texture, that is, the question of where a signifier 'comes from', comes to be associated with values and meaning. They use the example of 'denim' a material with a distinct texture which is associated with blue jeans, the heavy-duty trousers for labourers, and came to be used to signify an 'imagined identification with' and assigned the values of "American cowboys and pioneers, a preference for simplicity and functionality, a choice of equality and against class society" (ibid: 546).

Second, *experiential meaning potential* which is a meaning potential that is based on people's prior physical, bodily experience of, in this instance a texture. For example, the "rough and coarse" texture of denim, qualities which "depending on the context of interpretation [. . .] can receive positive or negative interpretations" (ibid: 547). Mapping the experiential meaning potential of texture involves:

> Extracting the qualities that will allow a given texture to be described and compared with others. Such mapping is a sensory exploration which not only identifies what these qualities are, but also how they are associated with one or more different senses.
>
> (ibid: 548)

They explored the experimental meaning potential of tactile texture—that is, a texture that can be sensed by moving a finger lightly over the surface of an object and which can also involve shape, volume, and weight and proposed that "analyzing tactile sensations into their components can help us understand how tactile sensation translates into meaning" (ibid: 548). The study of semiotic perceptions is both subjective and comparative, because a person

> brings to consciousness the sensations that accompany the human act of feeling textural qualities [. . .] By feeling, with our fingertips, a large number of material surfaces and asking, not "is it soft?" but "is it softer or harder than other similar surfaces?", by recording and describing our observations [. . .] and by benchmarking them against the material qualities described in the literature.
>
> (ibid: 549)

Building on this exploration of texture a *system network* of six primary qualities was designed to describe tactile surface texture as 'clines' or matters of degree rather than as 'binary opposites': liquidity from wet to dry; viscosity from sticky to non-sticky; temperature from hot to cold; relief from flat to relief; density from dense to sparse; rigidity from soft to hard.

The meaning of each of these qualities is "a product of the inherent qualities they represent (e.g. the idea of softness), the other textural, visual and aural qualities with which they co-articulate, and the context in which they occur and are interpreted" (ibid: 549). For example, with reference to the quality of liquidity, they suggest that all textures have a value on "a scale that runs from wet to dry" and draw on their own experiences and associations of liquidity to explore its meaning potentials (e.g., wetness is linked to positive associations with 'water and life' for beauty products and foodstuffs, and negative ones with 'rot and decay', while dryness may connote aging but also cleanliness and comfort) (ibid: 549).

Building on sensory anthropological research (Howes, 2014), I would counter that the social cultural context is central to understanding the qualities themselves. That is that what counts as touch, both as a sense and as it is socially worked into a mode varies and is culturally specific and historically fluid. This example shows how a focus on material and semiotic qualities, resources, and affordances can help to get at touch. In the context of digital touch communication for instance a focus on semiotic resources and affordances could be used to generate a descriptive inventory of the resources and types of touch made available.

Identifying and Exploring Touch-Based Modes

The questions of how touch as a sense is socially shaped to become touch-based modes and when touch is (or can be) considered a mode are a productive starting point for a multimodal social semiotic agenda for touch communication. Within a multimodal social semiotic approach what counts as a mode is: a set of semiotic resources with a regularity of use (i.e. 'a grammar') that fulfils the communication purposes (meaning functions) of that community (Kress, 2010). Returning to the example of sound, for instance, sound is not a mode rather it is the material realisation of modes. In other words, sound has been shaped through people's social usage to produce a variety of modes: sound as speech, sound as music, etc. A key way that Kress and other social semioticians establish whether or not something is a mode is to ask whether it can realise the three 'Hallidayan' semiotic (meta) functions, namely to deal with interpersonal, ideational and textual meanings. Using this modal 'test', Bezemer and Kress's (2014) expectation is that for touch to become the material basis of a mode, to be considered a mode, it needs to be able to realise meanings in the three meta-functions. It is important to note, however, that within this broad expectation, each mode differs in its materiality, semiotic features, and cultural histories and, therefore, how and what meanings are realised in different modes also differs across modes. Applying these criteria touch is clearly already a mode:

(a) Touch is designed for one or more specific others and someone is addressed (e.g., a handshake); this meets Halliday's interpersonal metafunction
(b) Touch communicates something about the world (e.g., touching an object to bring it into the realm of attention, to show its temperature or texture); this meets Halliday's ideational metafunction
(c) Touch is coherent with signs made in the same and other modes in forming a complete semiotic entity, an interaction (e.g., a handshake accompanied by saying 'nice to see you again'); this meets Halliday's (inter)textual function.

At least, it is a mode for certain social groups—e.g. 'tactile signing' also known as hand signing or more recently Pro-Tactile ASL. However, Bezemer and Kress (2014, p. 80) suggest that:

> We can distinguish between communities in which touch is weakly developed, has limited semiotic reach or "communication radius" and communities in which touch has been developed into a mode which is highly articulated, with extensive reach.

The question of whether and when touch can be considered a mode resonates with early multimodal social semiotic explorations of sound as the material realisation of mode (Van Leeuwen, 1999) and colour (Kress & Van Leeuwen, 2002). This question has been taken up to explore touch in a range of contexts (see Walsh & Simpson, 2014), including touch in the context of learning with iPads (Crescenzi, Jewitt, & Price, 2014; Price, Jewitt, & Crescenzi, 2015). In some social contexts, people's usage of colour and sound fitted the definition of a fully articulate mode; in others, they exhibited 'mode-like' qualities and potentials when used in combination with other modes. The same appears to be the case for touch, at least at this moment in time. However, I anticipate that this will change through technological innovation that will extend and reconfigure touch capacities and practices.

Exploring Who Can Touch: Interest and Agency

Who and what can be considered to have the capacity to touch (or respond to touch) are significant to exploring touch. Whilst accepting touch can be a mode, Bezemer and Kress (2014) question what counts as communication with respect to touch, and the interconnected question, who or what can be counted as a communicator and to whom. They distinguish between touch as a resource for 'inward' meaning-making and touch as 'outward' meaning-making—they classify the later as touch-as-mode. Further, they suggest two types of 'inward' touch, that is, 'implicit' or 'tacit touch' and 'explicit touch'. They use the term implicit touch to refer to types of touch that are taken for granted (e.g., kneading dough, typing, tapping links on a touch screen). While this type of touching may be meaningful to the person touching (they can derive meaning or understanding about an object), they suggest it is not intended to represent or communicate meaning (though, of course, it may be interpreted as being meaningful by an observer).

Nonetheless, they suggest it is not addressed to a communicational *other*—that is, they distinguish between meaning-making via touch and communication. Bezemer and Kress use the term 'explicit touch' to describe "touching to 'explore' the world—surfaces, temperature, structures, textures, and so on" (ibid, p. 78). They suggest that this has an effect on the "explorer who feels the tangible characteristics" (ibid) of the world under investigation and that as a result, meaning-making is involved, although they argue communication is not present because there is no addressee for the touch. For Bezemer and Kress, it is only 'outward' touch that has the potential to meet the criteria of becoming a mode because it can be 'designed as a message', 'addressed' to a community, with the capacity to be 'treated as having meaning' to be 'interpreted' (ibid, p. 80–81), suggesting that this is touch that happens between people (or perhaps primates). I find this definition of communication as always between two *people* too restrictive and the demarcation between communication and meaning-making to be too solid.

I argue instead for a definition of communication that considers (at least the potential of) artefacts and digital technologies as potential 'participants' in meaning-making and communication. Multimodal social semiotics understands artefacts and interaction as material traces of the work of those who made them. Both artefacts and interaction are the outcome of a person's (or people's) action, imbued with their sign maker's interests as they are mediated through the environment in which the sign was produced and newly encountered. In other words, the social (world) can be understood as it is represented in/through interaction and artefacts. I am not arguing that objects are agentive (as in Actor-Network Theory); rather, I contend that artefacts 'participate' in interaction, as they are full of meaning potentials that can be activated via interaction.

Norris (2012) offers a framing that I think may be useful for thinking this through that is underpinned by the idea of 'responsive objects'. She distinguishes between acts of 'touch', 'response', and 'feel' and notes that a sequence of touch-response-feel happens between two social actors, where a social actor may be either another human, an animal, or an object. She gives the example of two people shaking hands or a person holding the handles of a wheelbarrow walking downhill:

> The (touching) social actor feels the response of the other social actor whose hand he or she is shaking or the pull of the wheelbarrow.
>
> (ibid, p. 8)

In a multimodal ethnographic study of horse riding, she observes lessons in which a rider communicates with a horse primarily through the mode of touch. A key aspect of learning to ride is to learn how to touch the horse and how to feel the horse's response to the rider's touch. Norris explores touch via a focus on foot, leg, and hand movements within the broader multimodal frame of interaction in the horse-riding lesson. This highlights that touch is a mode that can involve the whole body. She shows a sequence in which the riding instructor demonstrates both the incorrect and the correct 'touch-response-feel' expected. (This formulation shies away from equating human and horse by maintaining a focus on the human who touches, the horse who responds and the human who feels the horse's response—touch remains the purvey of the human—though the horse interprets touch.)

The potential of artefacts to participate in communication is of particular interest to research on touch as it is digitally mediated. The idea of 'responsive objects' is a feature of Cranny-Francis's work on technology and touch who suggests:

> "[meanings are] potentially activated when we touch [objects or others], although the nature of the particular interaction determines which meanings are deployed and to what ends." She goes on to suggest that "by exploring those meanings we are able to map the potentials that are available in every tactile encounter and how they might be mobilised to create the most effective and/or rich interaction".
>
> (Cranny-Francis, 2013, p. 465)

I argue that it is useful to extend touch communication to refer to contact that is human-to-human, human-to-animal, and human-to-object (including the digital). This enables three interconnected aspects of communication to be brought into focus:

1. The production of communicative touch artefacts: The process of producing an artefact itself is understood as a communicative one, the device is seen as designed with an imagination of its communicative context and user, and the traces of the designer's work are embedded in the design of devices as a set of meaning potentials—that are a part of shaping communication.
2. Their interpretation: The ways in which people *interpret* these touch artefacts, what it is possible and not possible to communicate via them are aspects of communication.
3. The use of an artefact to engage with others, that is, how a user's engagement with it is constrained/shaped though not determined by its design, by their user's interests and purpose, and it's the context of use.

Understanding who can touch and how touch is shaped by this condition is one part of a multimodal social semiotic agenda for touch.

People's Use of Touch for Communication: Cultural and Social Norms

Importantly, social semiotics is concerned with issues of power and the ideological functions of modes, that is, modes are understood as a part of the construction of 'reality'. This enables an analysis to explore how aspects of touch are represented as the social norm and what is placed outside of this norm, for instance, how the social use of touch confers particular gendered qualities and roles.

Classifying the social and cultural significances and meanings "generated by the embodied experience of touch" (p. 2) provided the starting point for Cranny-Francis's (2013) exploration of touch. Her focus is on how touch articulates the "values, assumptions, and beliefs of individuals and of their culture and society" (ibid, p. 2). Building on (auto-ethnographic) observations and a review of the literature she posits five 'fundamental properties of touch'.

1. *Connection*: That is, touch creates a connection between people and objects. Touch is regulated (e.g., norms related to touch and gender, touch in a crowd), and particular meaning is given to specific touches by societies and cultures—what Cranny-Francis refers to as the "established tactile regime of a society or culture".
2. *Engagement*: Touch is signified by 'intentional touch' between individuals as compared, for example, to unintentional touch (e.g., the contact on a crowded train that signifies connection only).
3. *Contiguity*: Touch signifies contiguity when we become aware of the boundary that separates us from others, objects, and the world around us.
4. *Differentiation*: Touch signifies the difference between the self and the other.
5. *Positioning*: Physically, touch creates an awareness of our location (via proprioceptive and vestibular senses) in space/time through embodied engagement with the world around us.

These five 'properties' of touch offer a socially orientated way into thinking about touch as a social semiotic practice. I would suggest further work on the functions of touch (e.g., compliance, control and regulation, evoking memory, learning, etc.) may help to generate additional categories. Considering touch as a set of social properties is a useful starting point for the analysis of touch interactions. Cranny-Francis analysed the visual and linguistic metaphors and narratives that people use to understand, interact with and embed touch in their everyday lives (e.g., extension, engagement, connection) to gain access to discourses about touch as well as discourses realised and communicated through touch in order to deconstruct and map their values, beliefs and assumptions about touch. The distinctions and classifications afforded by a social semiotic approach, such as those described above, serve to generate questions about the character of touch communication, ideas of intention, and processes of interpretation, as well as questions concerning the potential for touch communication with digital objects.

Research from anthropology of the senses on the sociality of the senses and ethnographic tools attuned to the sensory (Howes & Classen, 2014; Finnegan, 2014) has the potential to complement multimodal research on the cultural and historical aspects that inform the social semiotics of touch. Howes and others understand the conceptualisation and organisation of the senses as the outcome of an ideological framing related to social-cultural historical contexts. Anthropology of the senses points to the need to understand the sensory material possibilities of touch, the different sensory expressions and practices of cultures and epochs, and how communities demarcate and understand the sensorium in different ways. For example, Classen's (2012) seminal works on touch maps the cultural functions of touch to social change from the Middle Ages through to the current day. She maps the regulation and 'removal' of touch to changing kin relationships, the rise of the individual, the industrial revolution, the management of health and hygiene, and capitalism and points to the parallels drawn between the removal of touch and notions of civilisation. This understanding of the senses as "culturally constructed (and not always stable) categories" (Fors, Bäckstrom, & Pink, 2013, p. 175) provides a useful backdrop to multimodal social semiotic investigation of touch.

While multimodal social semiotics provides a descriptive framework that is sensitive to power relations it can be complemented (and strengthened) by a sociological interpretation of the configurations of power that it makes visible. For instance, a social semiotic analysis of the interaction between two people may make visible (describe) that the position and posture of a man is dominant in relation to a woman and it can theorise that configuration as power, but it does not provide a theory of gender. To adequately interpret the social meaning the analyst would need to draw on additional theoretical frameworks (e.g., feminist theory, theories of power). In other words, while social semiotics (multimodality) is sensitive to power, it can describe how touch is being used, who is using it, what they are doing, patterns in the use of touch in a given context and therefore move towards a notion of norms of touch practices, it cannot answer the question of *why* they are doing it, or the social historical practices that specific touches are related to. However, despite the turn to the body and the sensory, sociology has a rather patchy engagement with touch, and there is a surprisingly small literature on the social aspects of touch (Linden, 2015) beyond a few classic studies linking the senses to urban living, and sociality (Simmel, 1997; Bourdieu, 1986) and exploration of 'feminine' touch (Goffman, 1979). Nonetheless social semiotic concern with power and the ideological function of modes makes it a useful framework for examining how people's situated use of semiotic resources is constrained by and challenges social norms and power.

4. Next Steps

In this chapter, I have set out an emerging multimodal social semiotic agenda for touch. I have discussed the importance of not conflating touch as a sense and touch as the material realisation of mode(s), that is, touch as a social means for communicating. Nonetheless I have argued that there are important relations to be explored between them. Multimodal social semiotics provides a framework through which to explore the cultural and the social shaping of sensory resources into semiotic resources for making meaning. Using the concepts of materiality, modal affordance, and semiotic resource, we can ask how are the sensory, material, and physiological aspects of touch drawn into a social system of signifiers, shaped through people's situated usage, and made to mean? That is, multimodality provides a framework through which to explore the intersection (and boundaries) between the physiological, the semiotic, and the social. Understanding this relationship will become increasingly pertinent in the context of touch in digital environments in which the sensory resources of touch are being newly brought into social practices and the boundaries between touch as sense, touch as mode, and technologies of touch are increasingly blurred and remade.

References

Bezemer, J., & Kress, G. (2014). Touch: A resource for making meaning. *Australian Journal of Language and Literacy*, *37*(2), 77–85.

Bourdieu, P. (1979/1986). *Distinction*. Cambridge, MA: Harvard University Press.

Classen, C. (2012). *The deepest sense: A cultural history of touch*. Urbane, IL: University of Illinois Press.

Cranny-Francis, A. (2013). *Technology and touch*. London: Palgrave Macmillan.

Crescenzi, L., Jewitt, C., & Price, S. (2014). The role of touch in preschool learning. *AJLL*, *37*(2), 86–95.

Djonov, E., & Van Leeuwen, T. (2011). The semiotics of texture: From tactile to visual. *Visual Communication*, *10*(4), 541–564.

Dunbar, R. (1996). *Grooming, gossip and the evolution of language*. London: Faber and Faber.

Field, T. (2003). *Touch*. Cambridge, MA: MIT Press.

Field, T. (2010). Touch for socioemotional and physical well-being: A review. *Developmental Review*, *30*, 367–383.

Finnegan, R. (2014). *Communicating*. London: Routledge.

Fors, V., Bäckström, Å., & Pink, S. (2013). Multisensory emplaced learning: Resituating situated learning in a moving world. *Mind, Culture, and Activity*, *20*(2), 170–183. doi:10.1080/10749039.2012.719991

Fulkerson, M. (2014). *The first sense: A philosophical study of human touch*. Cambridge, MA: MIT Press.

Goffman, E. (1979). *Gender advertisements*. Boston, MA: Harvard University Press.

Howes, D. (2011). Hearing scents, tasting sights: Toward a cross-cultural multimodal theory of aesthetics. In F. Bacci & D. Melcher (Eds.), *Art and the senses* (Ch. 9). Oxford: Oxford University Press.

Howes, D. (2013). *Ways of Sensing: Understanding the Senses In Society*. London: Routledge.

Howes, D., and Classen, C. (2014). *Ways of sensing: Understanding the senses in society*. London: Routledge.

Kress, G. (2010). *Multimodal communication*. London: Routledge.

Kress, G., & Van Leeuwen, T. (2002). Colour as semiotic mode: Notes for a grammar of colour. *Visual Communication*, *1*(3), 343–368.

Kress, G. and Van Leeuwen, T. (2006). Reading Images: The Grammer of Visual Design (2nd Edition). London: Routledge.

Krishna, A. (2010). *Sensory marketing: Research on the sensuality of products*. London: Routledge.

Linden, D. (2015). *Touch: The science of hand, heart and mind*. London: Random House.

McLinden, M., & McCall, S. (2002). *Learning through touch: Supporting children with visual impairments and additional difficulties*. London: David Fulton Publishers.

Norris, S. (2012). Teaching touch/response-feel: A first step to an analysis of touch from an interactive perspective. In S. Norris (Ed.), *Multimodality in practice* (pp. 2–19). London: Routledge.

Price, S., Jewitt, C., & Crescenzi, L. (2015). The role of iPads in pre-school children's mark making development. *Computers & Education*, *87.C*, 131–141.

Simmel, G. (1997). *Simmel on culture: Selected writings* (D. Frisby & M. Featherstone, Eds.). London: Sage.

Spence, C. (2013). The multisensory perception of touch. In F. Bacci & D. Melcher (Eds.), *Art and the senses* (pp. 85–106). Oxford: Oxford University Press.

Stein, P. (2012). *Multimodal pedagogies in diverse classrooms*. London: Routledge.

Streeck, J. (2009). *Gesturecraft: The manu-facture of meaning*. Amsterdam: John Benjamins.

Van Leeuwen, T. (1999). *Speech, music, sound*. London: Routledge.

Van Leeuwen, T. (2010). *The language of colour*. London: Routledge.

Walsh, M., & Simpson, A. (Eds.). (2014). Special Issue on touch. *Australian Journal of Language and Literacy*, *37*(2).

7 Reading That Which Should Not Be Signified

Community Currency in the UK

Annabelle Mooney

Return to sender: the semiotics of community currency[1]

> Australian money is printed on plastic, a shock still to the returning expatriate, as if it is too boldly a signifier of what should not be signified.
>
> (Kress & Van Leeuwen, 2006, p. 225)

1. Introduction

Whether it cannot or should not be signified, one thing is clear: Money is a floating signifier. Money means different things, depending on who holds it, to whom it is given, where it comes from, and what it is used to do. In this chapter, I analyse the semiotic choices made by in the design of community currency paper notes from the UK in order to consider what money is and how it signifies. Van Leeuwen's works on colour (2011), typography (2005, 2006), visual grammar (Kress & Van Leeuwen, 2006), texture (Djonov & Van Leeuwen, 2011), and semiotics generally are crucial in this analysis. Moreover, as Van Leeuwen's (1999, 2009) work has consistently sought to draw connections between language and other semiotics, very often in unusual places for linguists, his research has inspired this chapter not only at the analytical level but also in choosing to look at community currency at all.

Community currency, also known as local or complementary currency, is used around the world and, if one includes systems not backed by legal tender, dates from around the mid-19th century (North, 2010, p. 59). While it does not have legal tender status, it functions in the same way as a complement to national currencies. It can be used to pay for goods and services, usually in a local area. Unlike 'normal' money, however, community currency is designed to stay within the local economy and therefore supports local business, builds the local community, and decreases the environmental impact of consumption. Businesses are not obliged to accept community currency, but as a sign of commitment to the local economy, they may choose to do so. In some areas, the use of community currency is even more extended. For example, Bristol pounds can be used to pay council taxes. In the British examples examined in this chapter, it takes the form of paper notes, though Totnes, Brixton, and Bristol have electronic versions as well.

As community currency is often novel and not legal tender, design is important in two ways. First, the currency *system* needs to be designed so that it is accessible to stakeholders, including businesses and individuals (Longhurst, 2012, p. 174). Second, the notes need to be designed visually and haptically to be legible and trustworthy.[2] In this chapter, I describe the semiotics of community currency. This helps us understand not only what community currency is, but also what money is. Community currency presents an invitation to think about the social contracts and trust that underlie all currency systems.

In the remainder of the chapter, I first define community currency and then introduce North's (2010) concept of 'moneyness' in order to provide a focus for thinking about value and the semiotics of community currency. I then describe how community currency notes draw on and develop existing conventions for money in relation to naming, denominations, security features, and the paper on which the notes are printed. The local imagined community (Anderson, 1983) that is constructed by the notes is then considered in the light of research about what is depicted on legal tender before describing the hyperreal elements of design. I conclude by suggesting that community currency returns money to its sender, in its true inverted form.

2. Community Currency

The New Economics Foundation notes that community currencies:

> are tied to a specific, demarcated and limited community. This community could be, for example, geographical (local currencies); business-based (mutual credit systems); or even online (digital currencies). As such, a community currency is designed to meet the needs of this defined community, typically on a not-for-profit basis.
>
> (2015, p. 32)

Community currency is often designed to have a local circulation, but it is also possible to extend networks across a large area and range of participants (see Longhurst & Seyfang, 2011). They may prioritise different goals and aims, including supporting SMEs (small and medium-sized enterprises), supporting the local economy, reducing reliance on oil, and protecting the environment (Graugaard, 2012, p. 244). The various forms of community currency all seek to break with existing global patterns of finance and trade. Whether geographically local or oriented towards some other kind of community, they resist both national economies and global markets. They can be understood as glocal phenomena, as while they are local currencies, they are nevertheless caught up in global money processes.

While the community currencies examined here are all linked to and backed by the legal currency of the nation state, i.e., pounds sterling, they are not legal tender. They do not pretend to be. Nevertheless, such backing is crucial to uptake, as lowering perceived risks eases stakeholder participation, especially from business (see Longhurst, 2010, p. 154). The close link to 'real' money also means people are more likely to accept community currency as money even though trade with community currency is extremely marginal in the UK economy (Naqvi & Southgate, 2013, p. 322).

The marginal status of community currency makes its design central to its being accepted and used as money. Peter North, in his book on how to set up and run a community currency system, notes that a community currency has to have the 'intangible quality' of 'moneyness'.

> The notes should be of a high-quality design, on appropriate paper, and have security features designed in. They should have images and language on them that encourage potential users to associate them with value.
>
> (North, 2010, p. 106)

The quality of 'moneyness' is closely connected with that of 'value' as forms of money need "to have an elusive characteristic of 'valuableness'" (North, 2010, p. 36). North provides a great deal of information about the questions to consider when setting up a community currency system, for example, who will run it, how large or small the geographic area of operation should be, and how easy it is to convert to legal tender. But the advice on design is less detailed. As indicated in the quote above (with the use of 'appropriate'), North's lack of detail about what constitutes 'moneyness' visually is perhaps attributable both to the variation in money's physical appearance (internationally speaking) as well as what is considered valuable (at a more local level).

3. The Five Currencies

The five currencies examined in this chapter, together with their launch dates, are as follows (see Figure 7.1 for examples of the currencies):

- **Totnes Pound**: May 2007; now in its fourth issue. The current series of notes designed by Rick Lawrence of Samskara Design[3] (Totnes pound, n.d.; see also Granger, Wringe, & Andrews, 2010; North, 2010; Longhurst, 2012).
- **Lewes pound**: 2008 (Lewes Pound, n.d.; see also Graugaard, 2012; Murray, 2015; North, 2010).
- **Stroud pound**: September 2009 (Transition Culture, 2009; see also Scott Cato, 2010). This scheme is currently in abeyance but may be relaunched (Cooke-Black, 2015).

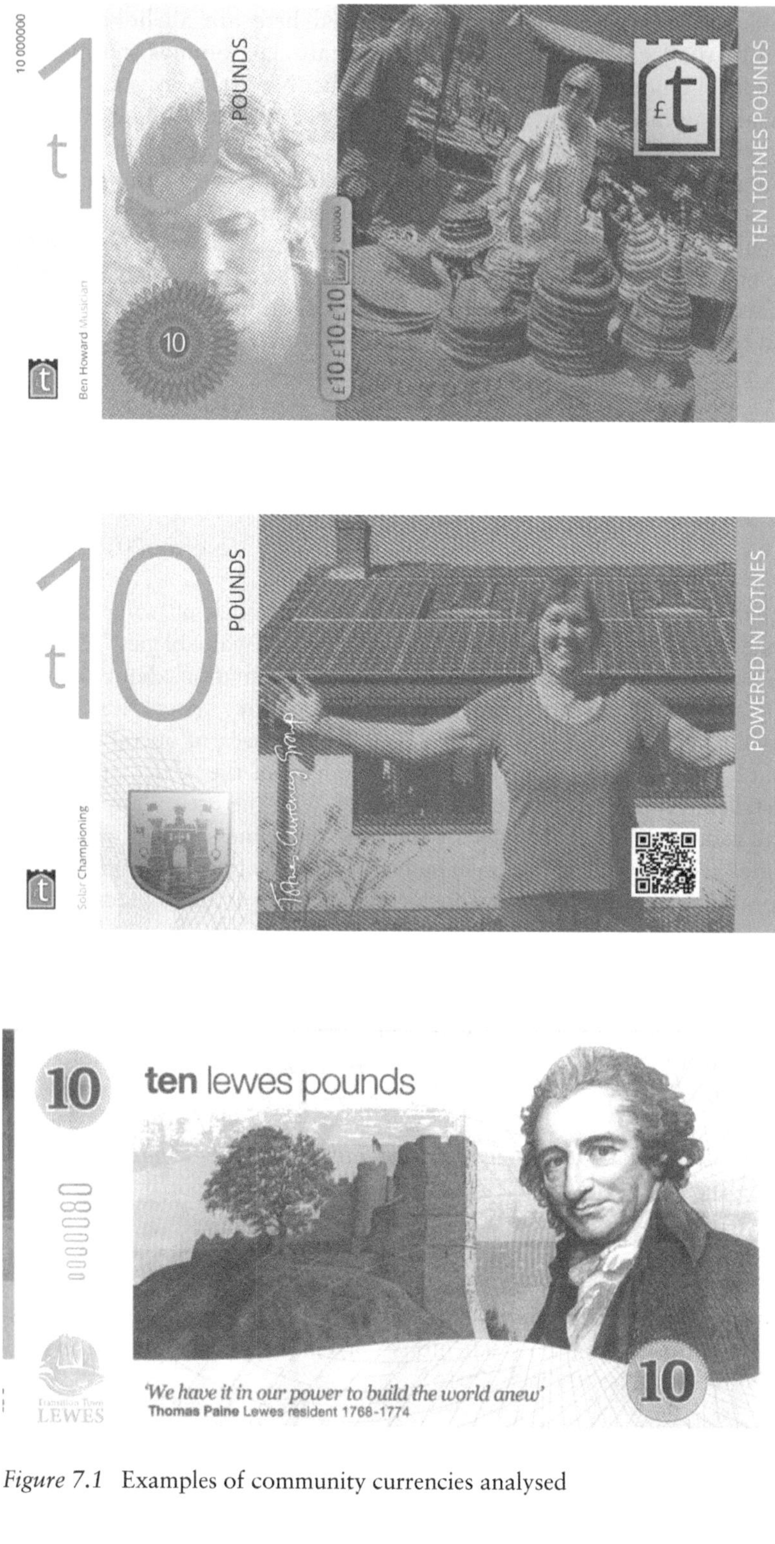

Figure 7.1 Examples of community currencies analysed

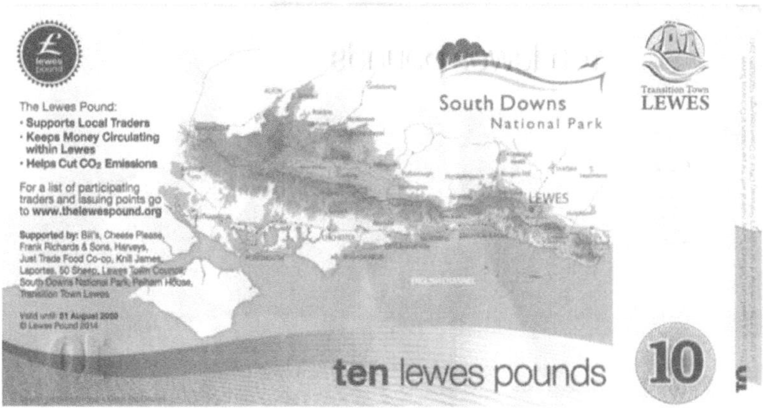

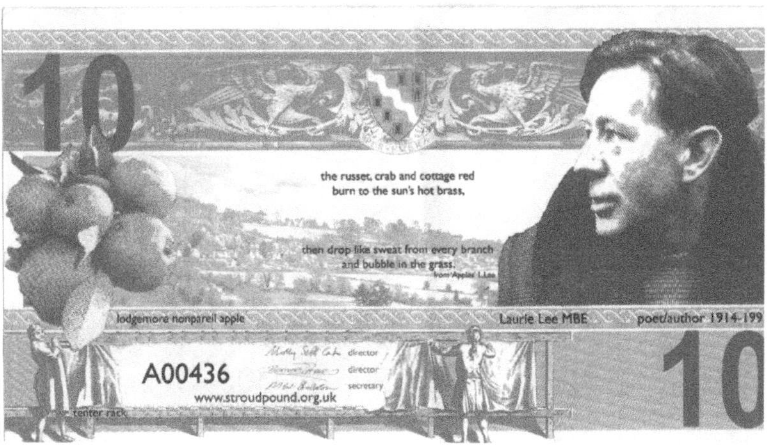

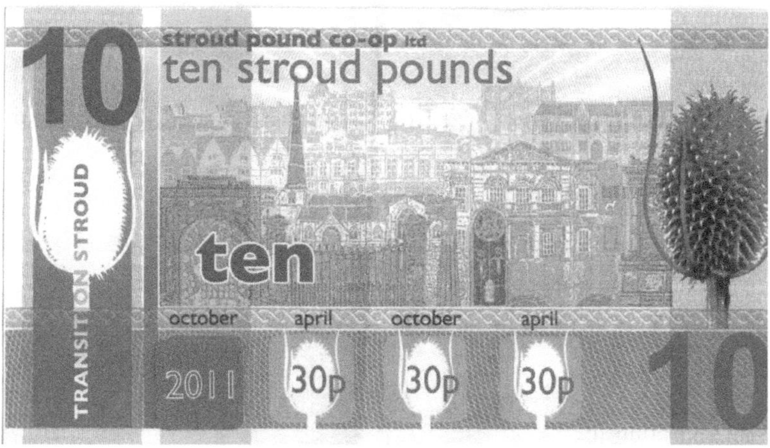

Figure 7.1 (Continued)

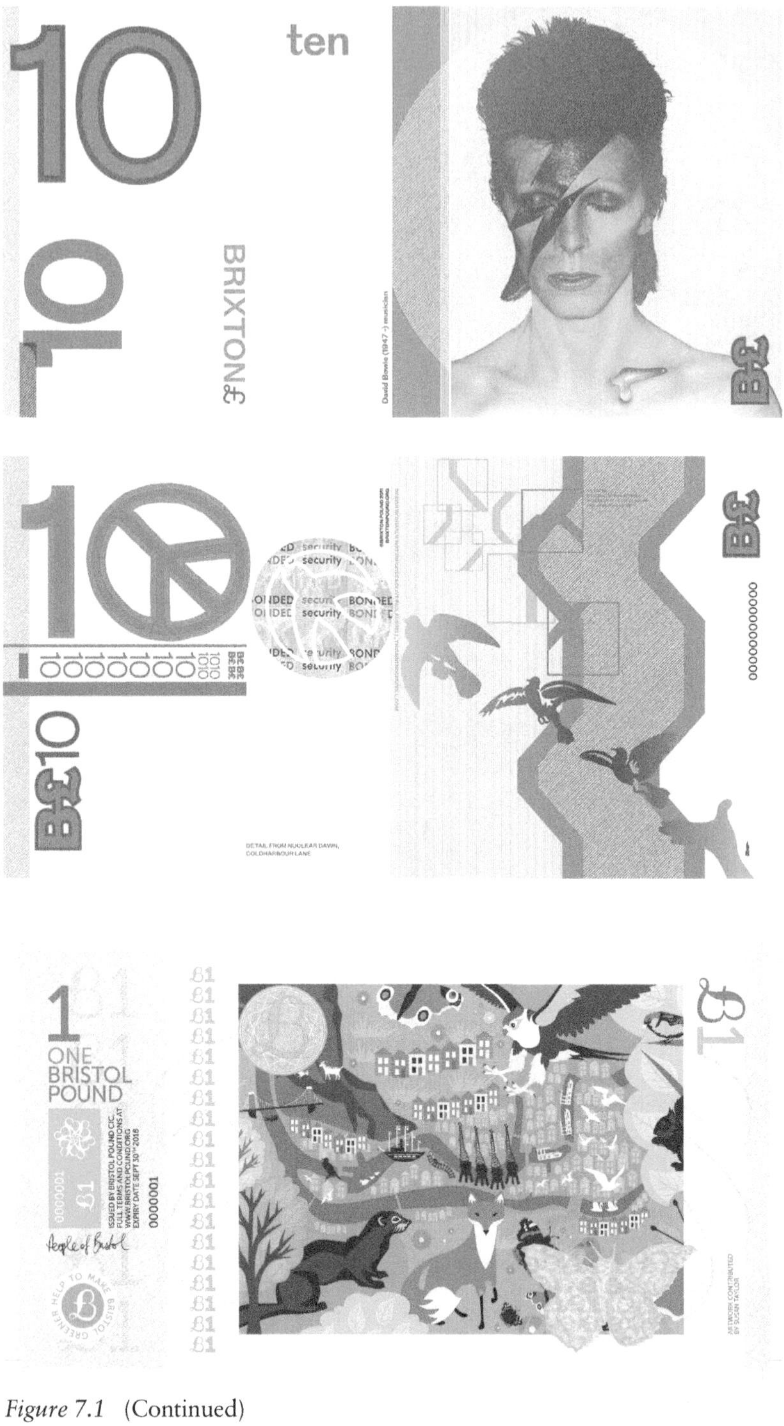

Figure 7.1 (Continued)

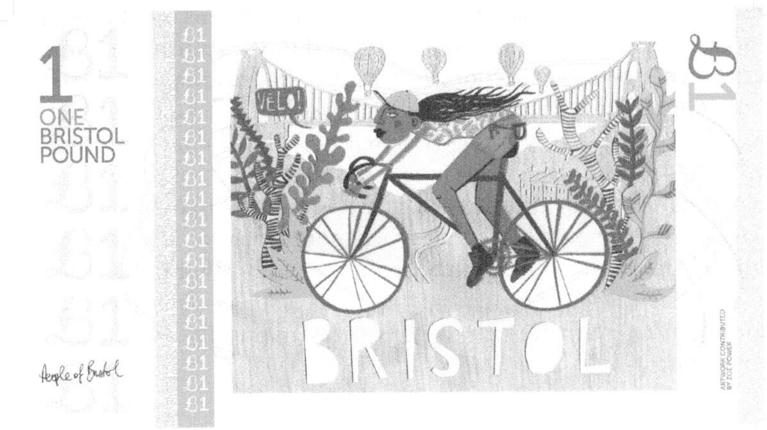

Figure 7.1 (Continued)

- **Brixton pound:** September 2009, now in its second issue designed by Charlie Waterhouse and Clive Paul Russell of This Ain't Rock'n'Roll[4] (see also North, 2010, p. 183–191, Ryan-Collins, 2010). The first community currency cash machine was launched 11th April 2016.[5]
- **Bristol pound:** September 2012 (Sunderland, 2014). It is in its second issue.

As is evident from these names, they all orient to the dominant sterling currency in the UK (pounds). As mentioned above, they are all backed by sterling in that the equivalent value is held in trust in banks or credit unions. Why community currencies developed in these places is a complex question. Brixton cites its "famous local economy", "diverse high street and local market", a "strong community spirit", a diverse community of residents and a history "revolution, activism, change, dynamic people and attracting the avant-garde" (Brixton pound). Bristol, too, cites its diversity, civic pride, and local community commitment as key reasons for founding a community currency.[6] In practical terms, the development and launch of a currency requires the co-ordinated efforts of a range of people, including participation from local business. It would seem that having diversity either in population or traders, a sense of community, and a commitment to quality of life or alternative ways of life are a necessary though not sufficient precondition for a community currency.

The notes examined here were sourced in two ways. First, detailed images from the homepages and other visual sources on-line were examined. Second, in order to be able to analyse the actual colours and the haptic elements of the currency, souvenir issues of the Bristol, Brixton, Totnes, and Lewes pounds were purchased from source. A set of Stroud pounds was sourced from a Canadian currency trader on eBay.

Notes were examined paying attention to the details of the template, text, choice of colour, what was depicted (and how), security features, and typeface. In the following section, I present some detail about these semiotic choices in relation to their broader function. That is, I deal first with the choices that orient to existing national and global conventions around money. Second, I argue that these notes construct and communicate a social imaginary that is local and thus distinct from both national and global financial systems. Finally, like some other money objects, the notes reverse modality. That is, instead of making semiotic choices that index verisimilitude or mimesis, they rather tend to the hyperreal. Through these features community currency invites us to consider semiotically and functionally what money is.

4. Innovating Tradition

All the five series of community currencies examined here rely on, and yet develop, existing conventions for bank notes. This is evidenced by the name and symbol used for the currencies, the denominations chosen, the security features used and the paper on which the notes are printed.

Choosing to call these currencies 'pounds' may seem to be an unmarked and unremarkable choice. But it should be understood in relation to choices LETS (Local Exchange Trading Systems)[7] have made in naming their units of account: "For example, Bristol had Favours, Bath had Olivers, Bradford had Brads, Lewisham has Anchors, and Ilkley had Wharves (named after the local river)" (North, 2010, p. 72). While the name of all notes is the same, three different strategies are used to identify the notes as *local* 'pounds': words, single letters, and new symbols. The Stroud pound simply writes the word 'pound' and uses numbers on their own for denominations (Figure 7.1.a). The Totnes pound uses a single letter, a lower-case 't', as a supplement to the pound sign "t£". On the notes themselves, a lower-case 't' with 'pounds' spelt out is used (Figure 7.1.b). The lower-case 't' used by Totnes is apparent in other aspects of note design and is sometimes more prominent than the pound sign itself. For example, a turret with a £t is found on the bottom of left of all Totnes pounds (obverse and reverse).

The third strategy involves a fusion of a letter and the pound sign, creating a new sign. Lewes (Figure 7.1.c), Bristol (Figure 7.1.d), and Brixton (Figure 7.1.e)[8] all adapt the pound sign in the direction of their town's initial letter. The Brixton pound recently changed their sign, enclosing a pound sign within the outline of a capital letter B. Bristol alters the conventional shape of the pound sign extending its upper arm down to meet the lower arm which is extended up. The right-hand profile thus follows the line of an upper-case B fully enclosing the space. The left-hand profile remains that of the pound sign. The Lewes pound adopts a similar strategy but extends

Table 7.1 Denominations and size

	denominations	*size*
Totnes	1, 5, 10, 21	7 cm × 13.5 cm
Lewes	1, 5, 20, 21	7 cm × 13.5 cm (one and five) 7.5 cm × 14 cm (ten and twenty-one)
Stroud	1, 2, 5, 10	7.7 cm × 13.1 cm (increasing in length up to 14 cm)
Brixton	1, 5, 10, 20	7.2 cm × 14 cm
Bristol	1, 5, 10, 20	7.5 cm × 14.3 cm
Sterling	5, 10, 20, (50, 100)	6.9 cm × 13.4 cm up to 8 cm × 14.9cm

the upper arm down to join the cross bar of the pound. This creates a figure that can be read as a pound sign, an upper-case L with a cursive flourish (creating a counter at the top) or as an upper-case P with an extra lower arm (Figure 7.1.c). Thus Lewes includes within the conventional pound sign both its own local identity (L = Lewes) and the name of its community currency (P = pound).

The same exploitation and development of tradition can be seen in the denominations provided in each series of notes (see Table 7.1). While all currencies provide a one, five, and ten, only Stroud produced a two-pound note. Totnes and Lewes opted for a 21-pound rather than a 20.[9]

As they are part of a series, they have to be recognisably connected and yet individually distinct. Some use small increments in size for this. Note, however, two very obvious things: The notes are all roughly the same size as each other and as sterling, and they are also all rectangular pieces of paper.

Community currency also draws on existing security features used for fiat currency. As community currency can be used to trade and operate in an economy (albeit a local one), it is important for the supply of the currency to be monitored, adjusted, and controlled. It is not possible to provide great technical detail about the security features in the notes (as these details are kept secure exactly for security reasons), but it is possible to catalogue the techniques used (see Table 7.2). All series use serial numbers as unique identifiers as well as a range of other security features. Holograms, foil elements, guilloches, and watermarks are used not only to prevent forgery but also as design elements (see below). The inclusion on some notes of dates of issue and expiry indexes the management of the currency system. Stroud is particularly interesting in this regard, as every six months notes have to be validated with a sticker in order for them to continue to be useful in the scheme.[10] This feature, 'demurrage', is intended to keep notes circulating (rather than have them hoarded) and used (Godschalk, 2011; Scott Cato, 2010).

Table 7.2 Security features

	Serial number	*hologram*	*foil*	*Watermark*	*Issue date/ valid until*	*Other*	*Signature*
Totnes	Twice: black on white and reverse gold matt	Turret silver; raised embossing (obverse) Castle; depressed embossing (reverse)	Engraved serial number reverse iridescent ink (obverse); pointed edging left (reverse)	yes	No	QR code (obverse) links to directory of traders; Guilloche	"Totnes Community Group" obverse
Lewes	Yes	no	Castle and water 'Lewes' (obverse)	Yes	Yes (year) / yes	Embossed number denomination raised (obverse); Guilloche; url	No
Stroud	Yes	no	no	Yes	Yes/yes	Demurrage; Guilloche; url	Three: two directors and one secretary (reverse)
Brixton	Yes	Yes (various on reverse)	Yes (various on reverse) and Engraved serial number and denomination reverse iridescent ink (obverse);	Yes	Yes/no	UV light illustrations; embossed numbers; Guilloche (though square); url	None
Bristol	Yes	Yes—two on reverse. One Bristol pound sign other varies	Engraved serial number and denomination reverse iridescent ink (obverse);	Yes	No/yes	Fluorescent ink on strip; Background image red under UV light; thermochromatic ink; heat sensitive symbol; Guilloche; url	"People of Bristol" (reverse)

Table 7.3 Paper feel

Totnes*	Smooth as though coated; heavier than 80gsm; overall textured pattern; foil; embossed/heat pressed holograms; hard to score
Lewes	Smooth, more papery than coated; embossed hologram; embossed denomination (number and letters); easier to score
Stroud	Smooth with some texture from inking; similar paper stock to Lewes; no embossing or other texture
Bristol*	Smooth as though coated; heavier than 80gsm; overall textured pattern; holograms slightly raised; very smooth on inked artwork; hard to score
Brixton*	Smooth as though coated; heavier than 80gsm; overall textured pattern; holograms, foil, and embossing around denomination; hard to score

* = same paper stock

The inclusion of urls and QR codes on the notes marks them as hypertextual and has further benefits, as they allow for efficient and semiotically discreet communication about what the currency is and how it works. This is necessary because of the novelty of the currency. Even people near to an area may not be aware that the currency exists or how it should be used.

Finally, the paper on which the notes are printed is important both in terms of security and in terms of moneyness. As Lemon notes, "Currency is a sensual substance" (1998, p. 29). Thus, paper money needs to have a distinctive feel for identification by touch and also to prevent counterfeiting. Describing the feel of paper (see Table 7.3), however, is not straightforward (cf. Djonov & Van Leeuwen, 2011). Here, I invoke Djonov and Van Leeuwen's suggestion that, "The best way of studying semiotic perceptions, therefore, is subjective and comparative, bringing to consciousness the sensations that accompany the human act of feeling textural qualities" (2011, p. 548) and compare community currency with sterling. It is worth noting at the outset that none of the notes are polymer. They are all some kind of paper (with the addition of foil, holograms, and embossing).

All notes, except for Stroud, have areas of embossing and texture from holograms. The Brixton and Totnes notes appear to have the same paper stock, as the same consistent watermark is visible, and both have a slight but discernible texture from this weave. The Bristol notes use the same paper as Brixton and Totnes, but because of the heavy inking, this texture is not as discernible.

The two notes which have little or no discernible surface relief (Lewes and Stroud) have dense patterning (Djonov & Van Leeuwen, 2011, p. 553). The Stroud pounds represent stonework and the obverse contains a very dense image with great depth of field (see Figure 7.1.a). The Lewes pounds have a guilloche, off centre and laid behind the elements presented (see Figure 7.1.c). These visual elements suggest texture in the absence of variation in relation to its tactile qualities.

Overall, they feel smoother, thicker, and more 'papery' than sterling (which is made from a mix of cotton and linen). They don't feel exactly like sterling, but because of the finish and the varying texture, they also don't feel like the other paper one might accumulate in one's wallet or pocket. Yet, they are much thicker, smoother, and more textured than receipts and are not like the card stock on which loyalty cards and business cards are printed. They feel like money.

For the name, symbols, denominations, security features, and the paper of these notes, a clear referencing of traditional national and indeed international semiotic techniques around money is evident. There are good reasons for this. First, users (both individuals and businesses) will have the necessary literacies to interpret the signs, security features, and denominations. Second, as community currency is in fact marginal, it needs to draw on the cultural and symbolic capital of existing money systems. Finally, the security features in particular are connected to available and affordable printing technology.

5. Locally Imagined and Authoritatively Modern

While some choices made clearly reference existing conventions of money, other choices mark the notes as much more local and modern. Research on the design of legal tender and national currency demonstrates that the imagery on money creates a visual national identity available to both citizens and to outsiders. For nation-states, such design matters, as it can construct and maintain ideologies about and trust in the nation, community, and money itself (see Borcuch, 2015; Gilbert, 2005; Hymans, 2010; Lauer, 2008; Penrose, 2011; Penrose & Cumming, 2011; Sørensen, 2014). It is important to remember that the imagined community that this money seeks to index is both created and communicated by the choices made.

As Penrose argues: "Banknotes are one material effect of the idea of the state and one of the countless mechanisms deployed to reify it as something more substantive" (2011, p. 434). The designs also have to maintain trust and communicate reliability (Sørensen, 2014, p. 3). This is crucial for community currency, but it is also true of fiat money, as Hymans notes: "the need for legitimacy is particularly great in the case of national fiat money, whose functional value is utterly dependent on its ability to command high levels of trust" (2010, p. 97).

Balancing all these communicative goals and ensuring that uptake is positive is not easy. The choices that are made in community currency clearly orient to those usually made by designers of legal tender. One finds representations of people, places, buildings, and inventions. But rather than indexing a national identity, community currency constructs a more local imaginary. Community currency also breaks with some of the conventions followed in the design of sterling. As Blaazer notes, sterling tends to avoid 'controversial figures' (1999, p. 51) and will not depict living people. But this is not a constraint followed by community currency with living people being depicted and the individuals' connections to place being the most important consideration.

Generally, what is represented projects a local understanding of the local area. Brixton notes are oriented to the urban, including abstracted elements of the built environment as well as famous local people. Lewes is much more concerned with the natural environment and place in geographic terms, with the inclusion of maps and art portraying historical events. Stroud draws on a historical repertoire similar to that of national currency but with a distinctly local (and more recent) perspective, including local flora, fauna, and inventions. In short, the notes create, assert, and communicate a vision of a local area. Significantly, this imagined community is not connected only to the past, as is often the case with national currency. Rather, the inclusion of living people, modern buildings, and contemporary activities means the notes reflect the present and project a future. Moreover, the very existence of this community currency is an important symbol of place, identity and community.

What is depicted, however, may be less interesting than how people and place are represented and where on the note they appear. The notes clearly divide space, demarcating, for example, left and right (Figure 7.1.a), top and bottom (Figure 7.1.e). For example, famous residents are depicted in both the *given*[11] (the left-hand side) and *new* portions (the right-hand side) of the obverse (Totnes and Brixton and Lewes, respectively) and the new portion of the reverse (Stroud). As entities in the *given* slot are generally things known to the reader and those in the *new* are information the reader does not have, there is a balance between what is presented as known and familiar and what might be new and educational (Kress & Van Leeuwen, 2006, p. 57).

The people are generally at *intimate distance* and tend not to look at the viewer. They are to be observed rather than to be interacted with, making the viewer "an invisible onlooker" (Kress & Van Leeuwen, 2006, p. 119). They are generally at eye-level, suggesting equality and vary between *involvement* (frontal angle) and *detachment* (oblique angle). These features are typical of *analytical images*, with a general *absence of vectors* (Kress & Van Leeuwen, 2006, p. 89) and *compositional symmetry*, and are unmarked but in this context are also assertive.[12] The images are comprised of a *carrier* (participant) and a *symbolic suggestive process*. These processes "represent meaning and identity as coming from within, as deriving from qualities of the Carrier themselves" (Kress & Van Leeuwen, 2006, p. 106). These images show "not a specific moment but a generalised essence" (Kress & Van Leeuwen, 2006, p. 106). In this context, they are particularly potent carriers of symbolically local meaning.

Analytical images can also have an interactional purpose, especially if the carrier's gaze is directed towards the reader (Kress & Van Leeuwen, 2006, p. 89). This is the case with Paine, on the Lewes note (Figure 7.1.c) whose gaze addresses the viewer, while the text beneath invites readers to 'build the world anew' (see Figure 7.1.c).

The authority constructed in the semiotic choices of images continues in the typefaces used (Van Leeuwen, 2005, 2006). The choice of typeface is key in establishing a 'voice', a presence, and performing a textual identity. Van Leeuwen (2006) outlines some of the distinctive features that can be considered in relation to typefaces. These include: weight (whether bold or regular), expansion along the horizontal axis, slope (whether the typeface slopes or is vertical), curvature (angular vs. curved), connectivity, orientation (to the vertical or horizontal, and hence stretched up or out), and regularity (of individual letters and their parts) (2006, pp. 148–150).

In almost every detail of all the notes, the typefaces used are San Serif (e.g., Arial). They are square, apparently not condensed, and, if anything, sometimes slightly expanded. They are regular and vary from having only some weight (Totnes) to rather a lot (Stroud). There is no slope at all (with the exception of Paine's offer), no curvature nor any connectivity (with the exception of the signatures and some other elements). They are entirely regular. Together, these typographic features suggest solidity, something grounded and immovable, a voice that simply needs to state information rather than persuade the viewer or invoke anything other than the neutral position of asserting facts (Van Leeuwen, 2006, p. 143). The typefaces, being regular and solid, connote legitimacy (Van Leeuwen, 2005, p. 139), but they also suggest modernity (in contrast to the typefaces that dominate sterling). The general contrast can be seen in the exceptions as, for example, in the signatures on the notes.

The signatures differ from the other typefaces used. The signatures are connected, curved, irregular, and seem to be real signatures, if not of real people (Stroud), then of a real hand (Bristol). Legal tender also often includes the signature or distinctive mark of the issuing body (Penrose & Cummings, 2011, p. 835). These work to underpin the assertion, to sign the speech act in a unique and yet reproducible way (Derrida, 1988). The only other exception not yet mentioned is a line on the Lewes 21-pound note that is also in an italic, freehand cursive script. It can be considered part of the image and reads 'Lest we forget' in memory of the Lewes martyrs (Lewes pound, n.d). While such a typeface is routine on sterling, it is much less used on community currency. A typeface similar to that now used on sterling for 'Bank of England' has been used (albeit not continuously) since the 19th century (Bank of England Museum, 2007). It is thus clearly linked with tradition and the past.

6. Hyperreality

The final area to address in relation to what is depicted on the notes is the hyperreal. In Baudrillard's (1993) terms, the hyperreal is that which has no referent. The hyperreal is linked to late capitalism and a general crisis of signification. The hyperreal "effaces the contradiction between the real and the imaginary" (ibid, p. 72). As such, it is perhaps the ideal term with which to consider money. The semiotic production of hyperreality here depends on the use of colour, the use of holograms, abstracted images, and the hypertextual links already mentioned.

In one sense, the use of colour in community currency is straightforward. The colours serve to identify individual notes in a series. They thus constitute a colour scheme, which can be modelled as a semiotic system (Van Leeuwen, 2011, p. 57). This is common for national currencies (Garcia-Lamont, 2012, p. 9652). Generally, the notes also make use of the familiar convention of a single hue in various saturations on each note (usually green, blue, pink/fuchsia, and orange/yellow). But the effect of the colour modulation and saturation on the modality of what is presented is important.

Variation on the notes is generally due to colour modulation and saturation rather than colour differentiation. High 'saturation' is a high intensity of colour with low saturation tending towards chromatic grey; modulation refers to different shades and tints; differentiation describes the use of different hues (Van Leeuwen, 2011, pp. 60–64). Elements of the templates, including security features and local icons (the Totnes Turret or the Lewes icon) do not conform to the consistent use of colour, but as the elements are consistent across notes this can be attributed to a template rather than to the design of individual notes. Brixton and Bristol are exceptions to this use of a dominant single colour, although the template does follow the general convention.

The colours used are at the extreme ends of saturation and modulation with very little colour differentiation (except for Brixton and the artwork in Bristol notes) but great brightness and illumination (Kress & Van Leeuwen, 2006, p. 160). This has the effect of depicting people, places, and objects in a non-naturalistic modality. While photographic full-colour representations would normally be considered of high modality, this mode is generally not found in either community currency or fiat money. Indeed, the difference between successive issues of community currency notes from Totnes (see Transition Network, n.d) demonstrates visually the move from high to low modality. The use of colour in this way serves to collapse the distinction between the real and the imaginary, the iconic and the symbolic, real people and their representations on paper money. The people and buildings depicted are clearly real. They exist(ed). But their image is not mimetic here; it serves rather as a symbol for the local imaginary. They are decontextualised and abstracted (Kress & Van Leeuwen, 2006, pp. 163–164), parts of buildings are modified to serve more as design elements than as iconic representations.

This hyperreal is further bolstered by the use of holograms and foil elements. Together with the colour choices there is a general move away from a realistic modality constructing what is depicted as both icon and symbol (in Peirce's terms) at the same time. While it is possible to identify the various people, places and things, because they are abstracted and presented in hyperreal colours they are transformed into symbols of the local imagined community. For money, reality is not relevant. The appropriate modality is the hyperreal.

7. The Semiotics of Money

> What, then, is moneyness? What gives paper the "elusive characteristic of valuableness"?
>
> (North, 2010, p. 36)

In terms of community currency, and currency more generally, moneyness is clearly connected to the look and feel of money objects. Money should have a distinctive feel, and the paper on which it is printed should have a distinctive tactile or visual texture (either over the whole note, or in parts). The specific semiotic choices have to communicate value. In both community currency and legal tender, this is achieved through the use of a consistent but complex template, distinctive colours, and representations that nevertheless complement each other. Community currency conventions of colour, template design, security features, and even the kinds of things depicted all draw on existing repertoires associated with legal tender. But the specific choices in community currency—who is depicted, what is deemed worthy of attention, how the template is constructed—all orient to something modern and local rather than to a national imaginary of place and identity which is generally rooted in the past. This serves to distinguish community currency from legal currencies circulated in national and global economies.

The money object is also usually part of a system of notes. This is true for both community currency and legal tender. It is routine to have more than one denomination and these should be mutually identifiable but distinct. The size of community currency notes is comparable to that of legal tender and generally a symbol of some kind to represent the money unit will be used, one that both resembles and modifies that seen on legal tender. It also seems common for all paper money to move away from conventionally naturalistic modalities, especially in terms of colour and the way people and things are represented. They function as both icons and symbols; they are both real and rooted in the world, but also highly conventional and symbolic. This parallels nicely what money is.

In simple terms, money is both the money system and the money objects that index it. Trust in both is crucial as money allows us to do and buy real things. Fundamentally, however, it indexes a series of relationships. As such, it depends on trust. But as Keane asks, "Why should anyone trust an abstraction?" (2008, p. 32). If community currencies are trusted, it must be because they successfully create and communicate a shared 'social imaginary' (ibid., p. 32) that is connected to place and local identity. Indeed, the very existence of the notes changes the local money system. For example, choosing to use Totnes pounds rather than sterling in a store that accepts Totnes pounds sends a message, "I am like you, we are part of the same thing" (cf. Graugaard, 2012).

Of course, this only works locally. But the existence of this local money usurps the national link to money (Scott Cato & Suárez, 2012, p. 113). This usurpation can be seen in the local, modern choices made on the notes and in the signatures that authorise them. The origin of this money is not national, nor global—it is local. Moreover, their origin is their destination. It is designed to be returned to its sending community. This only succeeds, however, if the community trust the money and, more importantly, if they trust each other. "Both money's fluidity and its limits—including the extent to which people trust it—are functions of" the ideas that people have about "why and how money is valuable" (Keane, 2001, p. 76). Community currency presents an invitation to think about these ideas and reminds us that even national fiat money rests on a collective (inter)national belief that it is valuable.[13]

While money is thought to destroy, or at least make irrelevant, social bonds (Keane, 2008, p. 28), serving as an invisible veil making any exchange both possible and impersonal, this can never be entirely true: "Money, we might conclude, certainly *changes* social relations—but it does not simply *abolish* them" (2008, p. 29). Community currency foregrounds social relations and makes them local. National currency, the prototype of money, makes a promise to pay. It asks the citizen to trust the state. But this is not really how money functions. Money works because we trust each other. Community currency thus returns money to its sender (the citizen) in its real, inverted form (Lacan & Mehlman, 1972, p. 72): an index of a system of mutual trust and recognition and a community of people.

Money does indeed talk. But in order to find out what it is saying and to whom it is speaking, it is necessary to look at it closely. Van Leeuwen's work is valuable not only because of the particular features it allows one to analyse, but also in the way the underlying theories are coherent across domains. Moreover, in considering the human interpretative work involved in constructing and reading texts, Van Leeuwen's approach compels us to consider what objects, texts, and practices mean for people living together in the world.

Notes

1 Versions of this chapter were presented at the University of Southern Denmark and the University of Reading in February and March 2016. The feedback from these audiences was incredibly valuable for development of the analysis. Permission to reproduce the images was kindly given by all community currency creators.

2 Historically, this was also a challenge for national currency (Lauer, 2008).

3 www.samskara-design.com

4 www.thisaintrocknroll.com/
5 http://brixtonpound.org/blog/2016/04/11/cash-machine/
It is unusual in that it looks more like a vending machine than an ATM. This is so the money is visible rather than hidden from view (conversation with Brixton pound at Utopia Fair, 25th June 2016 Somerset House, London).
6 "Bristol is the cultural and economic hub of the South-West. There is a diversity of businesses across many sectors and yet a strong sense of identity and civic pride in the city. In a 2010 survey of Britain, Bristol was ranked as the top city in the UK for quality of life; clearly, many people love living here and have a lot to give to the place where they live. Many aspects of the region's economy are a product of the people who live here and we think that wealth and well-being created by the people of the region can be better put to use if it re-circulates within the city where it is generated" (Bristol pound).
7 LETS are also a kind of community currency, usually not backed by legal tender and denominated in various ways (e.g., hours).
8 The second edition of Brixton notes placed a capital B before the £ sign, extending the crossbar of the pound sign to join the crossbar of the B (http://brixtonpound.org/showmemoney). The symbol described here and found in Image 5 is new.
9 North notes that the 21-pound note in Lewes "symbolises the fact that 5 percent of all Lewes Pounds issues—i.e. one point of every twenty—would be donated to a community fund, the Live Lewes fund, to support local projects" (2010, p. 165). In Totnes, "Frances Northrop, manager of Transition Town Totnes remarks, 'In the Economic Blueprint we identified the huge opportunity for a massive cash injection into our local economy through a 10% shift in spending, which could bring £2m through food sales alone. By offering a 5% incentive on £21 notes the Totnes Pound is using our very own version of Quantitative Easing to inspire residents to make that 10% shift'" (Totnes Pound, 2014).
10 Demurrage for the Stroud pound was initially set at 2p every six months, with revenue generated going to a fund to serve local projects (Booth, 2009).
11 For terminologies of visual analysis (italics) please refer to Kress & Van Leeuwen (2006).
12 There are people on the Totnes notes who carry out activities as described by the writing on the texts. They seem to function as human placeholders to indicate action rather than significant in their individual identity. These are also non-transactional, but they do include narrative, or material, processes.
13 See Scott Cato and Suárez, who describe people's "absence of any understanding of how money works" (2012, p. 112).

References

Anderson, B. R. (1983). *Imagined communities*. London: Verso.

Bank of England Museum (2007). *Security by design: A closer look at Bank of England notes*. Retrieved from www.bankofengland.co.uk/archive/Documents/archive docs/freshfields/securitybydesign.pdf

Baudrillard, J. (1993) *Symbolic Exchange and Death*. London: Sage.

Blaazer, D. (1999). Reading the notes: Thoughts on the meanings of British paper money. *Humanities Research*, *1*, 39–53.

Booth, P. (2009). Guide to Stroud Local Currency. Retrieved from http://ruscombegreen.blogspot.com.au/2009/05/guide-to-stroud-local-currency.html

Borcuch, A. (2015). Money and design. *Journal of Economics and Business Research*, *21*(1), 171–181.

Bristol Pound. Retrieved from http://bristolpound.org

Brixton Pound. Retrieved from http://brixtonpound.org/

Cooke-Black, S. (2015, June 29). Meeting to discuss possible relaunch of Stroud Pound. *Stroud News and Journal*. Retrieved from http://www.stroudnewsandjournal.co.uk/news/13358845.Meeting_to_discuss_possible_relaunch_of_Stroud_Pound/.

Derrida, J. (1988). Signature event context. In J. Derrida (Ed.), *Limited Inc* (pp. 1–24). Evanston, IL: Northwestern University Press.

Djonov, E., & Van Leeuwen, T. (2011). The semiotics of texture: From tactile to visual. *Visual Communication*, *10*(4), 541–564.

García-Lamont, F., Cervantes, J., & López, A. (2012). Recognition of Mexican banknotes via their color and texture features. *Expert Systems with Applications*, *39*(10), 9651–9660.

Gilbert, E. (2005). Common cents: Situating money in time and place. *Economy and Society*, *34*(3), 357–388.

Godschalk, H. (2011). Why "demurrage"? In *International Conference on Community and Complementary Currencies 2011*. Retrieved from http://sdocument.ish-lyon.cnrs.fr/cc-conf/conferences.ish-lyon.cnrs.fr/index.php/cc-conf/2011/paper/viewFile/48/52.pdf

Granger, R. C., Wringe, J., & Andrews, P. (2010). LETS as alternative, post-capitalist economic spaces? Learning lessons from the Totnes 'Acorn'. *Local Economy*, *25*(7), 573–585.

Graugaard, J. D. (2012). A tool for building community resilience? A case study of the Lewes Pound. *Local Environment: The International Journal of Justice and Sustainability*, *17*(2), 243–260.

Hymans, J. E. (2010). East is east, and west is west? Currency iconography as nation-branding in the wider Europe. *Political Geography*, *29*(2), 97–108.

Keane, W. (2001). Money is no object: Materiality, desire and modernity in an Indonesian society. In F. R. Myers (Ed.), *The empire of things: Regimes of value and material culture* (pp. 65–90). Oxford: James Currey Publishers.

Keane, W. (2008). Market, materiality and moral metalanguage. *Anthropological Theory*, *8*(1), 27–42.

Kress, G., & Van Leeuwen, T. (2006). *Reading images: The grammar of visual design* (2nd ed.). Oxford: Routledge.

Lacan, J., & Mehlman, J. (1972). Seminar on "The Purloined Letter". *Yale French Studies*, *48*, 39–72.

Lauer, J. (2008). Money as mass communication: US paper currency and the iconography of nationalism. *The Communication Review*, *11*(2), 109–132.

Lemon, A. (1998). "Your eyes are green like dollars": Counterfeit cash, national substance, and currency apartheid in 1990s Russia. *Cultural Anthropology*, *13*(1), 22–55.

Lewes Pound. Retrieved from www.thelewespound.org/

Longhurst, N. (2010). The first transition currency: The Totnes Pound. In P. North (Ed.), *Local money: How to make it happen in your community* (pp. 147–160). Totnes: Green books.

Longhurst, N. (2012). The Totnes Pound: A grassroots technological niche. In A. Davies (Ed.), *Enterprising communities: Grassroots sustainability innovations* (pp. 163–188). Bingley: Emerald.

Longhurst, N., & Seyfang, G. (Eds.). (2011). Special issue complementary currencies: State of the art. *International Journal of Community Currency Research*, *15*.

Murray, P. (2015). *An electronic version of the Lewes Pound?* Retrieved from www.thelewespound.org/2015/05/01/an-electronic-version-of-the-lewes-pound/

Naqvi, M., & Southgate, J. (2013). Banknotes, local currencies and central bank objectives. *Bank of England Quarterly Bulletin*, *Q4*, 317–325.

New Economics Foundation (2015). *People powered money*. Retrieved from http://b.3cdn.net/nefoundation/0dba46d13aa81f0fe3_zhm62ipns.pdf

North, P. (2010). Local money: How to make it happen in your community. Totnes: Green Books.

Penrose, J. (2011). Designing the nation: Banknotes, banal nationalism and alternative conceptions of the state. *Political Geography*, *30*(8), 429–440.

Penrose, J., & Cumming, C. (2011). Money talks: Banknote iconography and symbolic constructions of Scotland. *Nations and Nationalism*, *17*(4), 821–842.

Ryan-Collins, J. (2010). Not so mickey mouse: Lessons in the nature of modern money from complementary monetary innovations. *Economic Sociology European Electronic Newsletter*, *12*(1), 58–67.

Scott Cato, M. (2010). The Stroud Pound Co-op: A local currency for the Five Valleys. In P. North (Ed.), *Local money: How to make it happen in your community* (pp. 173–182). Totnes: Green Books.

Scott Cato, M., & Suárez, M. (2012). Stroud pounds: A local currency to map, measure and strengthen the local economy. *International Journal of Community Currency Research*, *16*(D), 106–115.

Sørensen, A. R. (2014). "Too weird for banknotes": Legitimacy and identity in the production of Danish banknotes 1947–2007. *Journal of Historical Sociology*. doi:10.1111/johs.12077

Sunderland, C. (2014). *The story of the Bristol Pound*. Retrieved http://bristolpound.org/blog/2014/02/11/the-story-of-the-bristol-pound/

Totnes Pound (2014, May 20). *Totnes Pound launches new notes*. Retrieved from www.totnespound.org/events?id=1

Totnes Pound. Retrieved from http://totnespound.org/

Transition Culture (2009, September 14). *The Stroud Pound hits the tills*. Retrieved from http://transitionculture.org/2009/09/14/the-stroud-pound-hits-the-tills

Transition Network (n.d.). *Totnes*. Retrieved from www.transitionnetwork.org/projects/totnes-pound

Van Leeuwen, T. (1999). *Speech, music, sound*. Basingstoke: Palgrave.

Van Leeuwen, T. (2005). Typographic meaning. *Visual Communication*, *4*(2), 137–143.

Van Leeuwen, T. (2006). Towards a semiotics of typography. *Information Design Journal*, *14*(2), 139–155.

Van Leeuwen, T. (2009). The world according to Playmobil. *Semiotica*, *173*, 299–315.

Van Leeuwen, T. (2011). *The language of colour: An introduction*. Oxford: Routledge.

8 A Sound Semiotic Investigation of How Subjective Experiences Are Signified in *Ex Machina* (2014)

Gilbert Gabriel

1. Introduction

This chapter deploys Van Leeuwen's sound semiotic techniques ('what sound says') to investigate how the soundtrack of the independent science thriller *Ex Machina* (Garland, 2015) signifies characters' subjective experiences. *Ex Machina's* plot focuses around whether an inventor's (Nathan) robot called Ava can pass the Turing Test (i.e. illustrate human attributes of consciousness). Ava surpasses Nathan's expectations and outwits both him and his colleague before escaping from his complex and infiltrating human society. Following Van Leeuwen's (1999) notion of 'modality' (based on Halliday, 1978)—different degrees of truth—it examines how different configurations of sound can be used to express the characters' subjective experiences through the adjustment (reduction, increase, or neutrality) of aural parameters such as pitch, dynamic, volume, reverberation, and so on. Based on Thibault's (1991) notion of social semiotics (sound semiotics being a branch of social semiotics), it attempts to explain meaning-making in a social context by using analysis, transcription, sound theory, as well as practitioners' discussion of the film and its soundtrack.

The research presented in this chapter uses sound semiotics together with film sound theory as a means to investigate how film characters' subjective experience of love, intoxication, memories, and terror are signified. The chapter first discusses Van Leeuwen's (1999) premise that the boundary between music and noise has blurred with the advent of synchronised film sound in the early 20th century, and the ways in which science fiction films utilise new electronic instruments and recording techniques for soundtracks. It then traces the evolution of artificial intelligence, which provides a contextual background for the narrative trajectory of *Ex Machina*. Next, it uses Van Leeuwen's (1999) sound semiotic theory to investigate how the experiential meaning potential of soundtracks and the provenance value of songs can help to engender meaning in films. In particular, it shows how Van Leeuwen's conceptualisation of voice quality and timbre help to reveal the ways in which the android Ava uses her female wiles to deceive the male characters around her. Lastly, the chapter deploys sound semiotic practice to locate how the subjective experience of characters is signified by speech, music, and sound.

2. The Integrated Soundtrack: Speech, Music, and Sound

Van Leeuwen (1999, p. 1) argues that it is important to explore the common ground between speech, music, and sound rather than separating each into categories, with speech only being discussed by linguists, music by musicologists, and sound rarely being discussed. He points out that the voice was a musical instrument in the Middle Ages and the Renaissance where "music was embedded in everyday life", and some cultures still had songs for harvesting crops, constructing houses, political comment and so on (Merriam, 1964 quoted in Van Leeuwen, 1999, p. 1). Van Leeuwen explains how recording technology weakened the boundaries between speech, music and other sounds in the 20th century "through muzak, the transistor radio, the car stereo [and] the Walkman" (1999, p. 2), and how composers, early pioneers, and sound theorists in the 20th century changed their view of what constituted music or noise. His examples of this trend include Russolo's inclusion of typewriters, car horns, and city sounds into his 'noise orchestra' and Balaz's (1970) suggestion that the role of sound film is to let the " 'significant sounds of life' such as the 'muttering of the sea' or roar of machinery' reveal 'our acoustic environment' on the cinema screen" (p. 197).

3. Electronic Instrumentation and Science Fiction Soundtracks

Science fiction films have a legacy of adopting the latest available technology as a means to realise their visions of near/far futures or planets. From the inception of sound in the 1920s to 2016, there have been enormous changes in how films have been produced, experienced, and consumed as technologies have transformed the cinema. Van Leeuwen (1999) points out how in the 20th century it became commonplace to hear electronic beeps, clicks, buzzes, and ringtones emitting from automated doors, lifts, computers, mobile phones, and so on, it was not always that way before the advent of electricity, loudspeakers, etc.

Donnelly (2013) points out how after the advent of synchronised sound, "one of the first significant science fiction films to build an image of the future was the British film *Things to Come* (Menzies, 1936)" (p. 1932). Donnelly argues that Arthur Bliss's score for the film didn't construct an idea of the future itself but used a contemporaneous idiom. He suggests that John William's orchestral style with its distinctive sound is reminiscent of the classical Hollywood scores that were used in several mainstream science fiction films in the 1970s and 1980s. These include the *Star Wars* trilogy (Lucas, 1977), *Close Encounters of The Third Kind* (Spielberg, 1977), and *E.T the Extra-terrestria*l (Spielberg, 1982).

In the 1950s, science fiction films began to incorporate electronic instruments as they became available. Examples of this include *The Day the Earth Stood Still* (Wise, 1951) and *Forbidden Planet* (Fr Wilcox, 1956), which used the eerie and unworldly sounds of the theremin, an early electronic instrument. Consequently, the distinction between music and sound effects became less predetermined and harder to distinguish. The move away from the conventions of the Hollywood classical model of scoring continued into the 1960s, with directors deploying pre-composed popular music and songs in their films. For example, Stanley Kubrick used pre-composed music and songs as a way of constructing narrative and giving provenance value to sci-fi films such as *2001 A Space Odyssey* (Kubrick, 1969) *and A Clockwork Orange* (Kubrick, 1971).

Donnelly (2013) notes the proliferation of synthesizer scores in the 1980s with Brad Friedels's score for *Terminator* (Cameron, 1984), Vangelis's score for *Blade Runner* (Scott, 1982), as well as John Carpenter and Ennio Morricone's work. Kathryn Kalinak (1992) points to the additional timbres offered by synthesizers and suggests that "synthesizers . . . are often exploited in sci-fi and futuristic genres to create an otherworldly effect" (p. 188). Recent examples of 21st-century sci-fi films that rely heavily on electronic synthesizer scores include *Solaris* (Soderbergh, 2002), *Moon* (Jones, 2009), and *Gravity* (Cuaron, 2013). Cliff Martinez's score for *Solaris* (Soderbergh, 2002) *c*ombines electronic and acoustic instruments in a hybrid minimalistic fashion, while *Gravity* (Cuaron, 2013) foregrounds cutting-edge visual effects as well as Dolby Atmos 3D sound.

Whittington (2007, p. 5) argues that science fiction both informs and is informed by our world as it prepares us for a future that embraces undreamt technological possibilities. He observes that the soundtrack is one of "the most aggressively manipulated areas of film art" (p. 3) where teams of sound recordists, editors, and mixers work together to create it. Their work involves the recording, editing, smoothing, and sometimes even re-recording or modifying of sounds in inventive and imaginative ways.

4. Artificial Intelligence and Terminal Identity

The idea of man-made humans threatening human existence was the focus of Shelley's novel *Frankenstein* (1818), in which a scientist created a creature from a deceased person's body parts. Martin Ford, in *The Rise of The Rob*ots (2015) shows how humans will become redundant in the future when education, travel, healthcare, industries, and even computer programs themselves are operated by humanoids. Technology is now central to everyday life with the advent of driverless cars, automated phone-answering systems, robot workers, and so on. Artificial intelligence and 'technological singularity' (the concept that intelligent computers and robots are capable of creating their own programs to solve problems) have taken another step in 2016 with a new virtual assistant called *Viv. Viv* supersedes the iPhone assistant *Siri*, as it uses dynamic programming generation to solve complex natural-language requests. The manufacturing car giant Ford has also recently announced that it will be mass-producing autonomous vehicles without steering wheels in 2020.

Cultural theorist Bukatman writes in *Terminal Identity: The Virtual Subject in Postmodern Science Fiction* (1993) that the nature of human identity has been redefined in the 'Information Age'. He argues that the use of advanced electronic technologies in Western culture has resulted in humans experiencing an existential crisis with their sense of 'self' becoming inextricably immersed with computers, cyberpunk, and science fiction concepts. The concept of artificial intelligence lies at the centre of the film *Ex Machina* narrative, where a female android called Ava, is tested to see if her 'intelligence' (consciousness) matches human intelligence. At the end of the film, Ava demonstrates that she has superior intelligence and social skills to her human creator and manages to outwit him. She becomes a potential threat to mankind as she escapes to New York City. As *Ex Machina* relies on intensive dialogue to inform its audience of the complex philosophical and moral issues of intelligent androids in a human world, it was necessary to have minimalistic score that helps to mark out key dramatic moments but does not interrupt or overwhelm the film's narrative.

5. *Ex Machina*: A New Sound Grammar

The notion of robots with artificial intelligence posing a potential threat to mankind's survival has been central to sci-fi films with films such as *Metropolis* (Lange, 1927), *2001: A Space Odyssey* (Kubrick, 1968), and *Blade Runner* (Scott, 1982). Chapman and Cull (2013) argue that these films have a recurring theme of "individual liberty and freedom of thought" being suppressed by technology in a dehumanised and dystopian future. Ava in *Ex Machina* is the female equivalent of Hal in *2001: A Space Odyssey*, a computer system that sees its agenda more important than that of human and as a result causes their demise. Ava not only has a superior intelligence but also occupies the body of an android 'femme fatale' who easily seduces and outwits her human counterparts.

The director's (Garland) decision to break away from visual and sonic clichés of science fiction led to his choice of electronic composers Geoff Barrow (Portishead) and Ben Salisbury (documentary scores), creating a minimalist and subversive sounding soundtrack that echoed their left-of-field electronic sound aesthetics. Their soundtrack, reflecting a broad range of emotions such as love, fear and anger, helps the audience navigate the intensive and thought provoking dialogues concerning the impacts of artificial intelligence on humanity in the future. For example, the main motif for Ava is a childlike melody played on a xylophone sound, that reflects her vulnerability. In a scene that portraits her brutal killing of her creator, the sound design is at first suspenseful and marauding before erupting into an outpouring of dissonant electronics.

Sound Modality

Van Leeuwen adopts a social semiotic approach to sound analysis. He writes that "social semioticians have extended the linguistic concept of modality beyond language, pointing to the importance of non-verbal communication in expressing modality" (1999, p. 158). He cites Hodge and Kress (1988) and Kress and Van Leeuwen (1990, 1996) as social semioticians who have applied the notion of modality in theorising the 'meaning' of images. For Van Leeuwen, sound modality can be approached along the same lines:

> Modality judgments cued by the *degree* to which a number of different parameters are used in the articulation of the sounds . . . the coding orientation used in that context, determines the modality value of a particular sound . . . and more specifically the *coding orientation* used in that context, determines the modality value of a particular sound—the *degree* and *kind* of truth we will assign to it.
>
> (Van Leeuwen, 1999, p. 170)

Van Leeuwen's idea is that modality judgements can be made about conventional musical resources such as pitch, timbre, dynamic, rhythm or perspective depth, fluctuation, friction, absorption range, and directionality. Van Leeuwen (1999) links coding orientation to the context of how a sound event signifies meaning. He suggests that a 'sensory'coding involves sound events being dramatised, whereas a naturalistic sound coding is one in which a sense of neutrality is maintained. Examples of naturalistic coding can be found in documentaries and certain genres of feature films, such as neo-realist films. Examples of sensory coding can be found in seductive advertisements, and in horror films, where the directors deliberately heighten the emotive impact of soundtrack and visuals. Van Leeuwen's sound modality system provides a powerful tool for identifying how characters' subjective modalities are signified by film soundtracks, as it shows how the aural parameters of speech, music and sound may be amplified, decreased or left neutral in order to signify either 'altered' states or 'reality'.

Cinema and Aural Realism

Van Leeuwen argues that different degrees and kinds of aural realism are dependent on how articulatory parameters (pitch, volume, and texture) are amplified or reduced to signify a particular event. He suggests that "mixed coding orientations are common in high art practices which questions definitions of truth and reality" (Van Leeuwen, 1999, p. 182). As cinematic sound invariably involves artifice and the intervention from those that record it and edit it, Whittington's (2007) suggestion that it is best to qualify the term 'realism' in cinema as a 'cinematic realism' seems a reasonable notion here. The cinema audience is not governed by their expectations and perceptions of 'the real world' but the 'cinematic worlds'. Film is a technically and socially constructed medium that presents and represents directors' ideas of narrative, which in turn shape audiences' expectations. This takes place through various configurations of multimodal resources and the use of technical devices such as ellipsis, montage, and camera angles as well as the spatial placement of sounds, including speech, music and sound design. Van Leeuwen (1999) asserts that it is preferable to approach music representation in the same way sound designers approach film soundtracks.

> When conceiving a sound effect, Serafine will first analyse the physical nature of its source; is it delicate, is it awkward, does it fly? Next, he will attempt to pinpoint its affects; can it frighten, is it calming, must it astonish you?
>
> (Mancini, 1985, p. 362)

Whereas Foley sounds (props, clothes and movement, and so on) are used to help anchor the protagonists of *Ex Machina* in 'reality', electronic music and sound design are often used as 'sensory coding' to help signify characters' subjective experience. The electronic heartbeat motif that accompanies Ava's appearances signifies her mood via its rises and falls in dynamic as well as tempo.

The Female Voice in Ex Machina

Van Leeuwen's (1999) discussion of voice quality and timbre shows how a person's voice pitch, volume, timbre, and vibrato ('fluctuation') help to convey their mood or manner. He suggests that it is not just one aspect of a person's voice qualities that portrays their mood or manner, but the combination of them. For him, it is necessary not only to describe a person as having a low voice but also to indicate if their voice is rough, tense, breathy, etc. He shows, for instance, that the tensing of the throat muscles often results in a voice that sounds higher, sharper, and brighter, as lower overtones are reduced. The opposite happens when a person relaxes their throat muscle, as their voices become lower, mellower, and laxer.

In contrast to many sci-fi films in the 1950s and 1960s that featured robots with male voices, *Ex Machina* features a female android. Although her mechanical body shows that she is clearly not human, her voice sounds soft and feminine with its breathy quality making her appear vulnerable and harmless. The soundtrack of the film also features several other automated female voices announcing door opening, power cuts, and the activation of various technologies.

Van Leeuwen (1999) suggests that breathy and soft voices are frequently associated with 'intimacy' and cites how advertisers use these voices to give their message a sensual and erotic quality. As the plot of *Ex Machina* centres on Ava's capability of exhibiting human characteristics (both emotionally and intellectually), her subjective experience is conveyed through her actions and sounds. Some of these sounds are crafted as non-diegetic music and sound design via a naïve and simplistic xylophone leitmotif and an electronic pulse that conjures the idea of her having an electronic heart. Table 8.1 contains a transcription which examines how the soundtrack is used to signify Ava's identity as an android through non-diegetic sounds and her speech.

Table 8.1 Transcription: Ava Session 1

Screenshot	*Action*	*Dialogue*	*Sfx*	*Music*
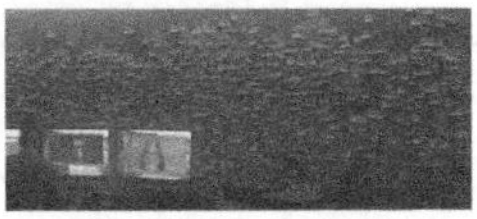	Nathan is seen observing Caleb entering a room on his monitor		Bleep of electronic activated door opening	Hypnotic repetitive mechanistic music
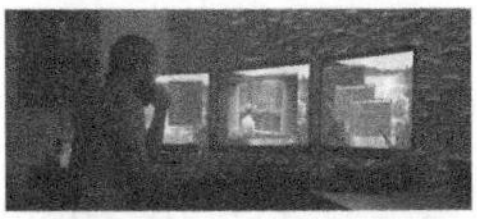	Close-up of Nathan looking at his monitors			Synthesizer filter opens and sound crescendos
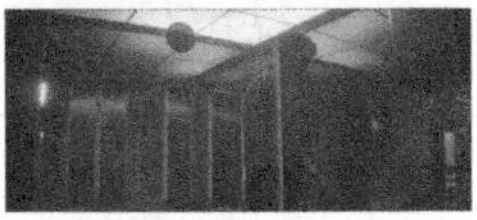	Caleb knocking on a glass window		Sound of Caleb knocking on a glass window	Sustained synthesizer chord
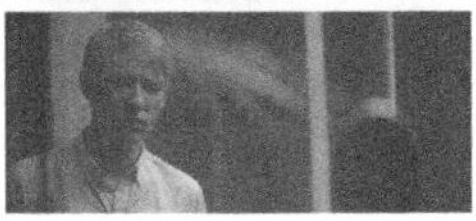	Close-up of Caleb staring intently into a room			Sustained electronic synthesizer chord. Arpeggiated synthesizer (Activation)
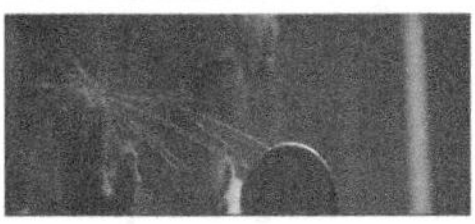	Caleb touches smashed area of glass			Held synthesizer chord. Higher synthesizer tone signals danger
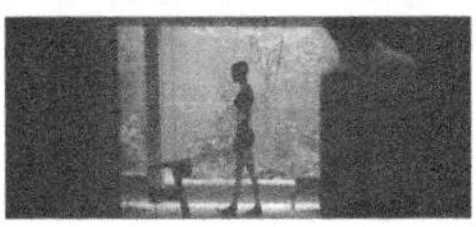	Caleb stares intently at Ava who is behind a large glass window			Held synthesizer chord. Childlike xylophone melody begins.
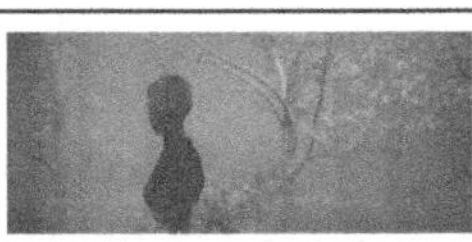	A mid-shot of Ava turning and looking Caleb			Held synthesizer chord. xylophone melody
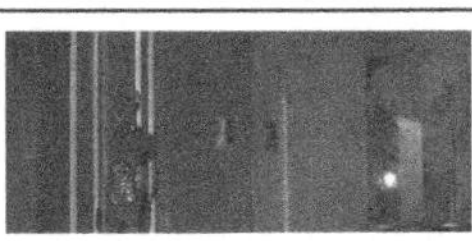	Long shot of Ava revealing her android body	Ava: Hello (clear and soft).		Held synthesizer chord. Xylophone sustained note. Pulsing low bass note.

(*Continued*)

Table 8.1 (Continued)

Screenshot	*Action*	*Dialogue*	*Sfx*	*Music*
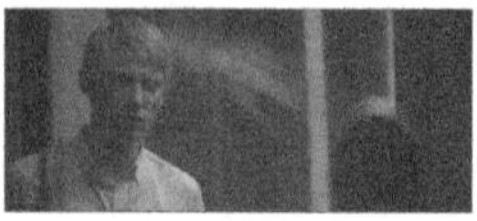	Caleb looking awestruck	Caleb: Hi. I'm Caleb.		Synthesizer chord. Xylophone melody. Pulsing low bass note
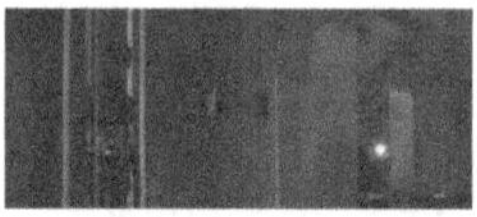	Mid-shot of Ava	Ava: Hello Caleb.		Synthesizer chord. Pulsing low bass note
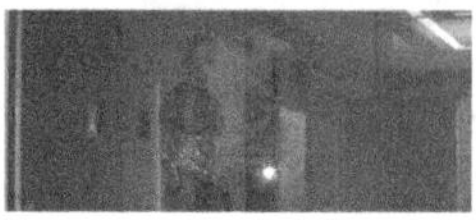	Long- shot of Ava	Ava: Yes. Caleb (off-screen). Pleased to meet you Ava		Pulsing low bass note. Slightly grainy synthesizer noise

The transcription above illustrates how music and speech signify Caleb's (a programmer who requested by Nathan to administrate Ava's Turing Test in the film) first meeting with Ava, when he decides whether she could pass the test. It shows how their subjective experiences are signified by the soundtracks speech, sound, and music. Specifically, it illustrates how pitch range, dynamic range, rhythm, duration, and so on signify what the characters are experiencing. The scene's slow pace, absence of dialogue as well as the subtle nuances of pitch and volume help the audience to understand Caleb's subjective perspective as he observes Ava during the Turing Test. At 00:11:34, the mid-range held synthesizer chord and higher-pitched synthesizer tone signify the potential danger as Caleb presses his fingers onto an area with broken glass.

When Ava first appears she is accompanied by the sound of a xylophone leitmotif and an electronic heartbeat that signifies her non-human status. At 00:12:27, when Ava greets Caleb, her voice is low, soft, and confident in contrast to Caleb's voice, which portrays his shyness. By sounding demure and subservient, Ava is able to use her feminine charms to trick and manipulate Caleb so that she can escape from the scientific compound where she was created. In a Telegraph review of *Ex Machina*, Collin (2015) describes Ava as a female android that does not intend to be scary but "only wants to get inside" our heads. He considers her "sharp blue eyes . . . even and inquisitive voice and a skin so clear that it seems to soften the air around it" as her feminine wiles (Collin, 2015).

In the following transcription (see Table 8.2.), Nathan's (the mastermind behind the android complex) drunkenness is signified by his unsteady gait

Table 8.2 Transcription: The subjective modality of intoxication

Timecode	*Image*	*Dialogue*	*Sfx*	*Music*
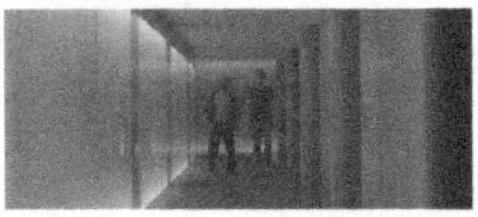	Nathan and Caleb walking down a corridor.	Nathan: Ah		
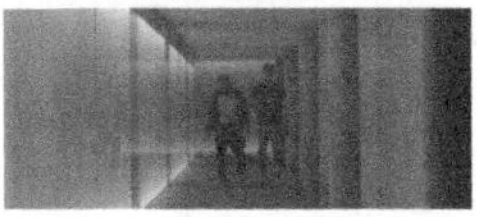	Nathan has trouble walking as he is drunk			
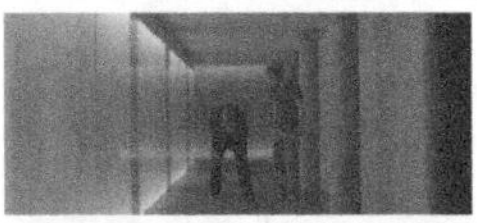	Nathan stops and bends over	Nathan: Uh		
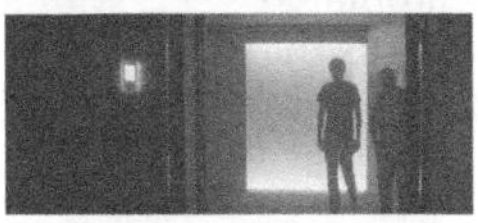	Nathan and Caleb walk towards a door		Low sound of white noise	
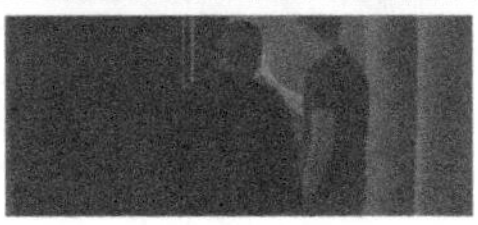	Nathan bends down to pick up his keycard from the floor, which he has dropped	Nathan: uhhh		
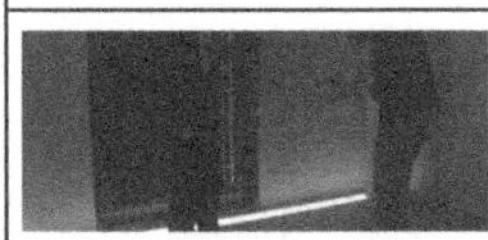	Nathan stands upright with his keycard in his hand	Nathan: Ahh everything is spinning		
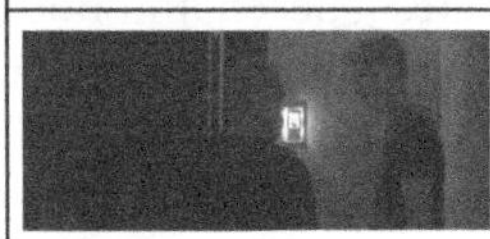	Caleb opens Nathan's bedroom door with his keycard	Caleb: That's because you are drunk		
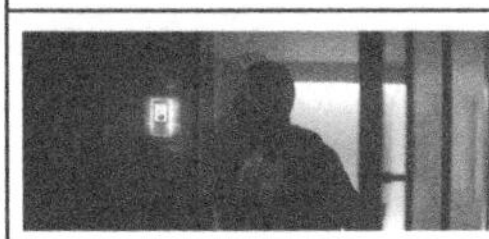	Nathan confronts Caleb	Nathan: no it's called relativity Nathan—everything is spinning. Just being drunk makes it worse		

(*Continued*)

Table 8.2 (Continued)

Timecode	*Image*	*Dialogue*	*Sfx*	*Music*
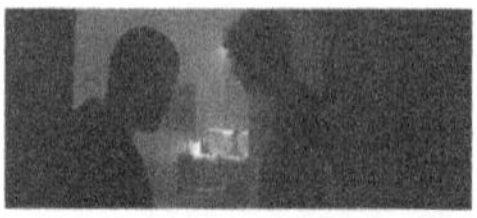	Mid-shot of Nathan and Caleb	Nathan: Am I going in there	Foley sounds of Nathan's movements	
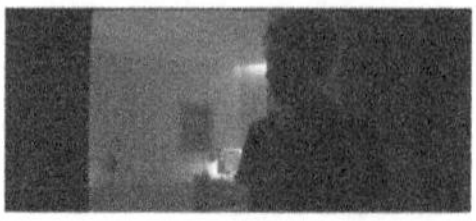	Nathan goes into his bedroom	Sounds of him breathing heavily	Foley sounds of Nathan's movements	
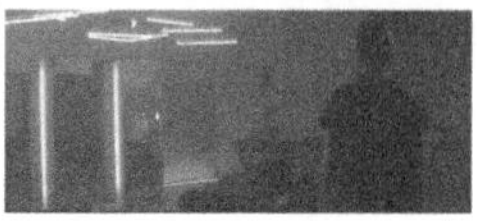	Nathan falls flat onto his bed	Nathan: muttering	Foley sounds of Nathan's movements	
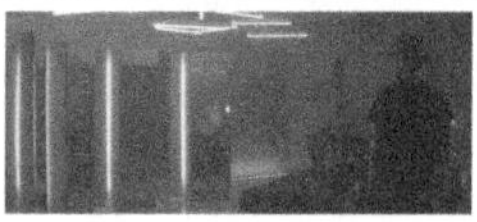 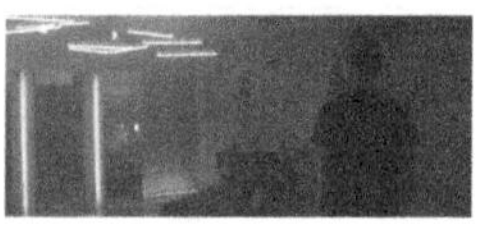	Nathan lying on his bed	Nathan: lights	Automated beep as the lights go off	

and his verbal and non-verbal utterances. Unlike the preceding scene, where the soundtrack is dominated by *Get down Saturday Night*, this scene is a 'sonic close-up', zooming on all the sounds Nathan makes (speech and body movements). This helps tune the audience into Nathan's drunken perception of the reality and subjective modality as he freely associates how he feels with 'relativity theory' before staggering into his bedroom and falling fast asleep.

Nathan's drunkenness is signified by his non-verbal utterances as he attempts to find his bedroom and ends up dropping his keycard on the floor. As Nathan is drunk, his speech, breathing, and motor skills are impaired as he staggers towards his bed, and, at 00:57:26, he awkwardly goes into his room.

Source Music: Provenance Value of Songs and Music

Whittington (2007) shows how popular music infiltrated film scores in the 1960s and "navigated the boundaries between source music and score, to create new associates and intents, such as nostalgia, irony, or intertextual references" (p. 42) in films such as *The Graduate* (Nicholas, 1967).

He describes how sci-fi films began to blur the lines further by 'weaving source music' into their narrative action and themes as part of the film's diegesis. Whittington points out how the recycling of *Singing in the Rain* in Kubrick's *A Clockwork Orange* (1971) turns its Hollywood cheerfulness is used to construct a dark and ironic comment on a rape scene. In *Ex Machina*, the use of "Get Down Saturday Night" helps to 'humanise' a scene where a drunken Nathan decides to relax and dance to a retro dance track of the 1980s. This scene is a comical respite from the philosophical debate on the possibilities of artificial intelligence. Up to this moment, the main protagonists in the film (Nathan, Caleb, and Ava) have focused on serious conversations about the consequences of artificial intelligence for mankind. In this scene they are seen dancing in a mechanical and ridiculous fashion.

The metronomic groove and soulful lead vocals of "Get Down Saturday Night" encourage listeners to relax and escape from the daily grind of the working week. Its increased tempo contrasts well with the slower paced crescendos and decrescendos of the synthesizer score. The comical synchronised choreography movements of Nathan and his mute robot, Kyoto, provide an almost surreal reference to the of 1970s dance culture. Although Nathan and Kyoto's movements are energetic and aerobic, they serve no functional purpose other than entertainment, as Van Leeuwen notes:

> According to Tagg (1984, p. 32), the regular beat of "disco" music thus "represents a high degree of affective acceptance of and identification with clock time, digitally exact rhythm and hence with the system in which time sense dominates".
>
> (Van Leeuwen,1999, p. 38)

In *Ex Machina*, the robotic nature of Nathan's and Kyoto's dance moves creates a playful atmosphere which provides a moment of levity in an otherwise dark film.

Experiential Meaning Potential

Van Leeuwen (1999) defines "the experiential meaning potential of sound" as what we physically have to do to produce a particular sound, he explains that by "tensing our articulatory musculature" (p. 205), we can create tense sounds. For him tense sounds are associated with aggression, repression, nervousness, and excitement. Machin (2010) cites John Lydon's 'closed throat' vocal sound on the punk song *Anarchy in the Uk* as an example of how pent-up tension and aggression can be signified by human voices. He also explains how "the meaning of sound quality" may also derive from associations with real world events such as the way thunder can frighten us with its loud volume and booming low pitch. Similarly, Donnelly (2005) emphasises the importance of material effects and cultural background in the research of media (including film) soundtracks. He writes:

> It is possible to make—perhaps a temporary, contingent and heuristic distinction between film music that works primarily through conscious and semi-conscious linguistic codes (and thus can be simply decoded by the analyst using semiotics, and film music that is premised upon having a material effect as sound volume and the action of sound waves on the listeners.
>
> (Donnelly, 2005, p. 94)

The transcription in Table 8.3 shows how the deployment of sound semiotic resources including voice quality, timbre, pitch, dynamic, and fluctuation signify Nathan's subjective experience of terror as he tries to first pacify and then fight Ava, who intends to kill him.

As the transcription shows, the soundtrack becomes more ominous and dissonant as a battle between the human and the android ensues. From 01:24:25 to 01:24:44, the soundtrack signifies Ava's presence and her interest in the proto-type robot masks hanging like artworks on a wall.

Table 8.3 Transcription: The subjective modality of terror

Timecode	*Image*	*Dialogue*	*Sfx*	*Music*
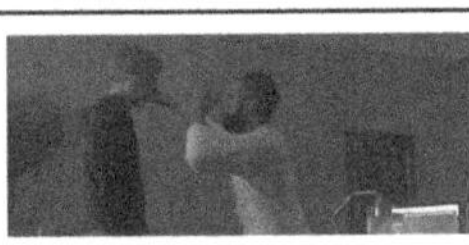	Nathan punches Caleb, who falls to the floor.			Pulsing low bass note ('Activation')
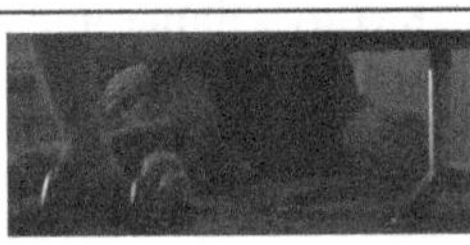	Nathan reaches for part of his weight lifting equipment		Clanging sound as Nathan picks his weights up.	Synthesizer square tooth waveform
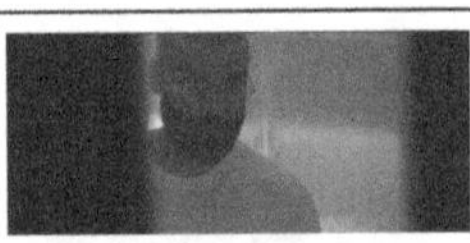	Close-up of Nathan's furious expression.		Clanging sound	Synthesizer square-tooth waveform
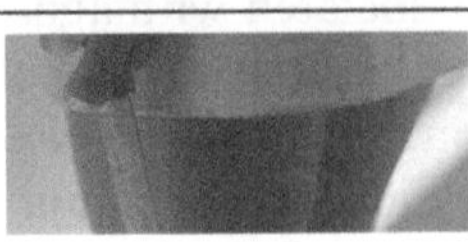	Close-up of Kyoto's hand that wields a long, sharp knife			Synthesizer chord crescendos

Timecode	*Image*	*Dialogue*	*Sfx*	*Music*
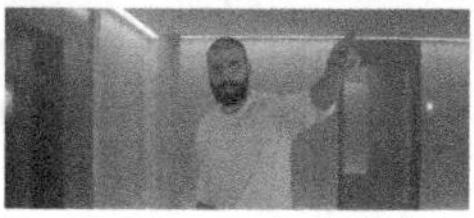	Mid-shot of Nathan gesticu-lating to Ava	Nathan: Go back to your room		Low drone sound
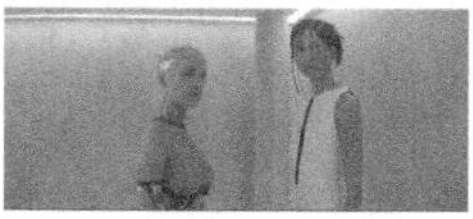	Ava and Kyoto	Ava: If I do are you ever going to let me out?		Synthesizer pulses ('Activation') Electronic heartbeat
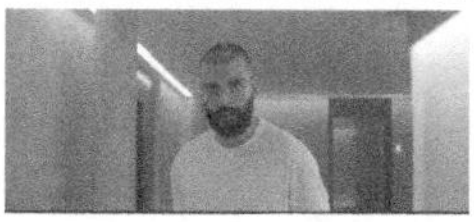	Mid-shot of Nathan	Nathan: Yes		Low volume synthesizer chord
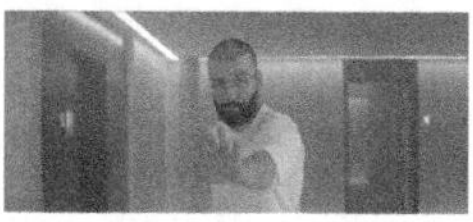				
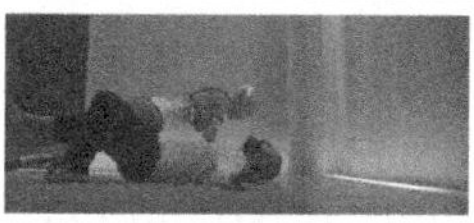	Ava knocks Nathan to the ground	Nathan: Oh whoa whoa		Reversed sound crescendos in synchr-onisation with Ava's action
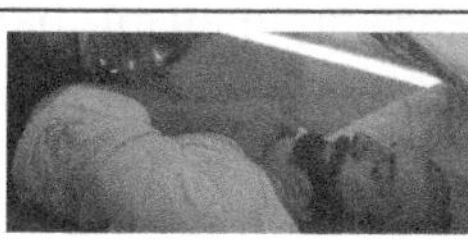	Nathan struggling to push Ava off him	Nathan: What are you doing?	Sounds of struggle	Ominous low dissonant synthesizer pad and slow pulsing sound
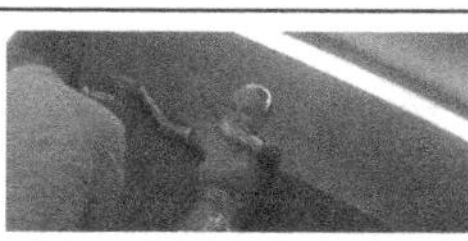	He hacks one of her arms off		Slicing of her metal arms off	
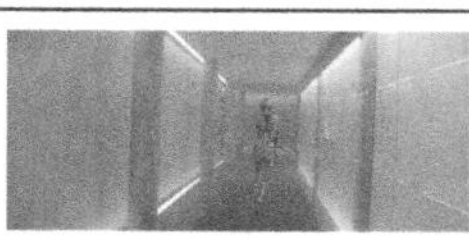				

Her status as an android is signified by electronic heartbeat sounds and a simple xylophone motif that can be heard when she first appears on the screen. At 01:24:57, the dissonant sounds of Nathan falling to the ground create a sense of tension, while the synthesizer crescendo signals Nathan's anger as he prepares to confront Ava. At 01:25:42, when Nathan orders Ava to go back to her room, a low, ominous drone is used to signify her non-human status.

Nathan's voice rises in pitch and volume at 01:26:09 as he orders Ava to stop running towards him. The intensity of the situation is amplified by the crackling distortion of the soundtrack, that signals Ava's frantic behaviour as she disobeys Nathan and hurtles towards him. At 01:26:20, the impact sounds of Ava knocking Nathan to the ground are heard, with a slow electronic pulse sound adding to the sensory nature of the event as he tries to push her off.

6. Conclusion

This chapter has used Van Leeuwen's (1999) sound semiotic theory to investigate the ways in which various subjective experiences of the characters' in *Ex Machina* are signaled by different configurations of sound resources such as pitch, dynamic, volume, reverberation, and so on. It considers how pre-existing music and songs help to 'humanise' a film centred around computers and artificial intelligence. By examining how speech, music, and sound signify characters' subjective experiences, this study reveals the 'new grammar' that the composers of the film attempt to deploy. That is, they tend to use synthesizer sounds as 'sound design' rather than orchestration in order to mark out dramatic moments and the beliefs, feelings and actions of the characters. The 'new grammar' is their left-of-field aesthetic, which owes more to the minimalistic band sound of Portishead with its guitar riffs and electronic soundscapes that drift and hover.

In keeping with the tenets of social semiotics theory this study has attempted to examine 'meaning-making' by including practitioners' discussion alongside analysis, transcription and the use of sound theory. Such an approach has helped to contextualise the historical and cultural contexts in which science fiction films, technology and soundtracks have co-evolved. This chapter also showcases Donnelly's (2005) idea that since new electronic instruments emerged they have provided a valuable and easily recognisable departure from more traditional modes of orchestration. The proliferation of personal computers, recording technology and playback devices and the integration of artificial intelligence into everyday life in the 21st century mean that science fictions have become 'science-fact'. As our modern environment embraces a new 'sound language' far removed from sounds of the natural world, it is important to consider where sounds come from (their provenance value) and what their experiential meaning potential is (i.e. what we physically have to do to produce them).

Filmography

A Clock Work Orange (Stanley Kubrick, 1972)
Blade Runner (Ridley Scott, 1982)
Close Encounters of the Third Kind (Steven Spielberg, 1977)
Dark Star (John Carpenter, 1974)
E.T the Extra-Terrestrial (Stephen Spielberg, 1982)
Ex Machina (Alex Garland, 2015)
Forbidden planet (Fred M Wilcox, 1956)
The Graduate (Michael Nicholas, 1967)
Gravity (Alfonso Cuaron, 2013)
Metropolis (Fitz Lange, 1927)
Moon (Duncan Jones, 2009)
Terminator (James Cameron, 1991)
Things to Come (William Cameron Menzies, 1936)
2001: A Space Odyssey (Stanley Kubrick, 1969)
Star Wars (George Lucas, 1977)
The Day the Earth Stood Still (Robert Wise, 1951)
The Stepford Wives (Frank Oz, 1975)
Solaris (Steven Soderbergh, 2002)
Westworld (Michael Crichton, 1973)
Dr Who (Gordon Fleming, 1965)

References

Balazs, B. (1970). *Theory of the film: Character and growth of a new art* (1945–48) (E. Bone, Trans.). New York: Dover Publications.
Bukatman, S. (1993). *Terminal identity: The virtual subject in postmodern science fiction*. Durham, NC: Duke University Press.
Bukatman, S. (1997). *Blade runner*. London: British Film Institute.
Collin, R. (2015). *Ex-Machina*. Retrieved February 19, 2015, from www.telegraph.co.uk/film/ex-machina/review/
Donnelly, K. J. (2005). *The spectre of sound: Music in film and television*. London: BFI.
Donnelly, K. J., & Hapward, P. (Eds.). (2013). *Music in Science Fiction Television – tuned to the future*. London/New York: Routledge.
Ford, M. (2015). *The rise of the robots: Technology and the threat of mass unemployment*. London: Oneworld productions.
Halliday, M. A. K. (1978). *Language as social semiotic*. London: Arnold.
Hodge, R., & Kress, G. (1988). *Social semiotics*. Cambridge: Polity.
Kalinak, K. (1992). *Settling the score music and the classical Hollywood film*. Madison, WI: University of Wisconsin Press.
Kress, G., & Van Leeuwen, T. (1996). *Reading Images-The Grammar of Visual Design*.London: Routledge.
Machin, D. (2010). *Analysing popular music: Image, sound, text*. New York: Sage.

Mancini, M. (1985). 'The Sound Designer'. In E. Weis & J. Belton (Eds.), op. cit.
Shelley, M. (1818). *Frankenstein*. London: Lackington, Hughes, Harding.
Tagg,P. *Understanding Musical Time Sense*. Retrieved February, 2015 from http://tagg.org/articles/timesens.html
Telotte, J. (2001). *Science fiction film*. Cambridge: Cambridge University Press.
Thibault, P. J. (1991). *Social semiotics: Text, meaning and Nabaokov's Ada*. Minneapolis, MN: University of Minnesota Press.
Van Leeuwen, T. (1999). *Speech, music, sound*. London: Macmillan.
Whittington, W. (2007). *Sound design and science fiction*. Austin, TX: University of Texas.

9 Unravelling the Myth of Multiple Endings and the Narrative Labyrinth in *Mr. Nobody* (2010)

Chiao-I Tseng

1. Introduction

The main goal of this chapter is to elucidate just how the comprehensive analytical frameworks developed by social semioticians to date, including Van Leeuwen and others (cf. Van Leeuwen, 2005; Bateman, 2007; Tseng, 2013a), can be employed to effectively deal with significant empirical issues, such as narrative complexity, genre, and transmedial comparisons, which have been the subject of perennial debate in studies of narrative and the moving image. In particular, this chapter will focus on the issue of multiple endings in fiction films.

The feature of multiple endings is a narrative device often employed in complex narratives in film and literature. In recent decades, a considerable body of research has endeavoured to unravel just how non-linear fictional narratives trigger puzzling effects in readers/viewers and lead them to adopt interpretation paths distinct from those for conventional linear fiction. Particularly in film analysis, multiple endings/open endings are often targeted as a phenomenon that could help develop tools for analysing complex narratives, including the complexity of puzzle films with multiple plot lines, non-linear narratives, and the mechanism of multiple endings (cf. Buckland, 2009, 2014).

The mechanism, its cognitive impact, and ideological power are most thoroughly discussed in the recent work by Cova and Garcia (2015). Although the authors do not provide a definitive answer as to why multiple endings are rare, the way they investigate the uses and functions of multiple endings confuse several issues at distinct analytical levels. This highlights the need to broaden the theoretical grounds of the discussion as well as to situate this issue of multiple ending in a framework clearly distinguishing between the concepts of *textuality*, *media*, and *genre*.

Most importantly, this chapter will show how addressing the issue of multiple endings drawing on systematic multi-level analysis suggests effective strategies for unravelling puzzle films in general: these non-linear, unconventional narrative films can be most effectively unpacked using a multidimensional discourse framework. In the following sections, I will elucidate precisely how the multi-dimensionality can be achieved on the basis of the methods proposed by Theo van Leeuwen and other social semiotic research on film discourse (cf. Van Leeuwen, 2005; Bateman, 2007; Tseng, 2013a). The contention will be empirically supported through a social semiotic analysis of the well-known puzzle film with multiple endings, *Mr. Nobody* (van Dormael, 2010).

2. Problems Raised by Multiple Endings in Fictional Narratives

In addressing multiple endings as unnatural, non-immersive, and an incoherent design of story events in fiction, Cova and Garcia (2015) compare multiple endings of fiction to open endings of serial comic books and TV series. Despite the fact that very often each issue of a comic book series or each episode of a TV series is open-ended, and readers/viewers need to wait for days until the story continues in the next issue/episode, comic books, and TV series remain popular and readers/viewers don't seem to be disturbed by the incomplete and incoherent story events in each issue/episode. Yet, multiple endings, which also violate the conventional and natural single-ended, close-ended fiction structure, are rare (p. 108–109).

This comparison immediately brings to the fore the issue of the audience's top-down expectation of media genres. Specifically, a reader/viewer's understanding and evaluation of story events is substantially supported by several devices mobilised in the surrounding context within a novel, a film, a TV show or a comic book, as well as in the cultural context outside the work being read or viewed, including expectations of genre and media.[1] It is fairly unlikely for a long-time comic book reader or TV series viewer to be taken by surprise when seeing 'to be continued' at the end of each issue or episode. In other words, readers/viewers expect an open-ended story structure in these media genres.

In addition, there is a paradox in Cova and Garcia's discussion of the effects of open endings in comic books and TV series: Even if it is true that open endings undermine immersion and make an appreciator uncomfortable about having to wait for the next issue/episode, that must also indicate that the story events within the present episode/issue are well presented, highly coherent, and the viewers/readers are immersed until the last minute, until realising the issue/episode is not an immediate resolution of the story. This paradox brings to light another fundamental difference between multiple endings in fiction and open endings in serialised media genres. That is, they deal with different levels of textual structures.

Here it is necessary to take into account the social semiotic concept of meaning strata and textual coherence, particularly the cohesive mechanisms between textual units and how text structure is related to genre. Several conceptual frameworks have been developed by text linguistics over recent decades, for instance, SFL and Rhetorical Structure Theory.[2] More recently,

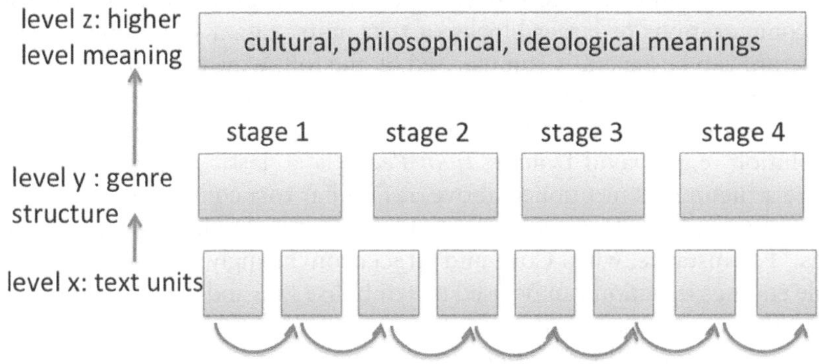

Figure 9.1 Meaning strata—a multi-level meaning structure of text

Note: The curved arrows between textual units at level x are cohesive ties, which make a text a meaningful unity and which guide the reader/viewer to understand a coherent narrative. The straight arrow between level x, y, and z refers to the process of realisation of meaning strata, a construct and mechanism much used in linguistics

these frameworks have also been applied to the analysis of non-verbal and multimodal texts, such as visual images, films, comic books, printed documents, etc.[3]

Figure 9.1 illustrates the concept of *stratification*, a construct and mechanism much discussed in linguistics, particularly within social semiotic theory (Halliday & Matthiessen, 2004). The strata are inter-related through *realisation*. In Figure 9.1, the lowest level x refers to units within a text. The coherent co-patterning of these units realise the stratum at a higher level, such as a genre structure widely recognised within a cultural context. Different conventional genre structures then realise and reflect certain ideologies and cultural interpretations at the highest level.

At level x in Figure 9.1, the curved arrows between the units at the level x are cohesive ties that give the necessary cues for the recipient to interpret a text as a meaningful whole. Within SFL, several analytical tools have been developed to describe this kind of cohesive tie (Halliday & Hasan, 1976). The present chapter makes significant use of the tool of logical relations, as it considers whether the paragraphs and chapters of a novel or scenes and the shots of a film are related spatially, temporally, causally, etc. can be analysed using this tool.

Conventionally, the storylines in each issue/episode of serial comic books and TV series are presented linearly and temporally and thus coherently. Although sometimes in a comic book, "fictional characters are referencing events that happened in a previous issue" (Cova & Garcia, 2015, p. 108), often enough cohesive ties, e.g., cohesive reference links (Tseng, 2012), are mobilised to avoid disorientation in the comprehension of a narrative.

Level y in Figure 9.1 refers to genre structure. A genre structure is realised by configurations of larger blocks of text units, e.g., a well-known drama structure can be generally summarised by the following stage blocks: beginning—complications—crisis—climax—resolution—ending. In serial comic books or TV series, the storyline in an issue or episode might end before the resolution (e.g., David Lynch's *Twin Peaks* is a classic example), and this genre structure, as mentioned above, is familiar to a competent audience.

Finally, configurations of levels x and y realise higher-level abstract meanings.[4] For instance, when Cova and Gracia convincingly point out that multiple endings in fiction can be used to symbolise fate and determinism in our lives, they are addressing abstract themes, namely, level z in our framework, which is supported by the coherent deployment of lower-level textual features. In Figure 9.1, the straight arrows between levels x, y, and z, refer exactly to this kind of meaning realisation across strata.

Drawing on this stratified theoretical framework, we can uncover several myths of the puzzling phenomenon discussed by Cova and Gracia. First of all, one should not assume that multiple endings are a phenomenon exerting a specific kind of effect, because, analysed on the basis of the textual stratum (level x in the figure), multiple endings could be realised in different textual forms and lead to very different narrative evaluations and interpretations. For instance, Kieslowski's film *Blind Chance* (1987), mentioned by Cova and Gracia, presents three separate storylines and three different outcomes in succession. Nevertheless, each storyline is shown in a conventional temporal narrative structure. In the beginning of the second and the third storylines, clear visual repetitions function to signal the re-telling of the characters' story. That means this film, although with multiple endings, is presented in a straightforward, coherent textual form. We can compare *Blind Chance* to another film with multiple endings, *Mr. Nobody* (2010). This film also shows the different storylines and outcomes of a character's life. However, these storylines are interwoven throughout the film rather than separately told. This kind of complex narrative structure with complicated spatial, temporal and causal relations between the scenes and shots challenges the viewers' inferences of story events and guides them to a very different narrative interpretation process from that in *Blind Chance*. In later sections, I will show just how the narrative complexity of *Mr. Nobody* can be effectively unravelled, drawing on the multi-levelled analytical frameworks of social semiotics.

Another example of multiple endings of fiction is the novel *Hopscotch* (Spanish: *Rayuela*) by the Argentine writer Julio Cortazar. The novel can be read in two ways: either linearly, from Chapters 1 to 56, or by 'hopscotching' through the entire book of 155 chapters according to a 'Table of Instructions' provided by the author. In the author's table of instructions, the last 99 chapters are inserted among the first 56 chapters and function as filling information gaps and at some point also solving some questions in the main storyline. This means that in the second route of reading, the cohesive ties between the chapters are re-configured into a different and more complex set of logical relations.

To sum up, according to the stratified framework presented here, the frequency of multiple endings is simply a matter of choice-making: Multiple endings is a narrative choice. It can be realised in various forms of textual configuration with very different degrees of coherence and thus lead to different narrative evaluations and interpretations. Along the same lines, the philosophical meaning of determinism is also a thematic choice and multiple endings is one possible textual choice to realise this ideological meaning. The degree of rarity of multiple endings is probably comparable to that of other unconventional textual choices, such as reversing the temporal order of storylines (e.g., the films *Memento* (2000), *Irreversible* (2002), and Harold Pinter's play *Betrayal* (1978)), which could be used to stress the meanings of causation, despair in life, etc. Furthermore, comparing multiple endings in fiction to serial comic books/TV series is not theoretically plausible. As Figure 9.1 suggests, multiple endings are realised by the employment of textual units at level x, while storylines with open endings in comic books and TV series are conventional genre structures at level y.

Furthermore, Cova and Gracia also compare multiple endings in traditional fiction to interactive fiction, where the user always plays a role and can reach different endings depending on different choices along the narrative routes. They consider why multiple routes are feasible and welcomed in interactive fiction, while multiple endings in traditional fiction are rare. In this context, one philosophical concept they refer to is the theory of *make-believe* proposed by Kendall Walton (1990). In Walton's theory, our engagement with fiction should be understood on the model of games of make-believe. Briefly speaking, the readers/viewers are convinced that they are witnessing story events personally. On the basis of this philosophical theory, Cova and Garcia (2015) contend that if Walton's theory were true, multiple endings should have thrived in traditional fiction because having multiple endings available to freely choose from, and being able to select a preferred one, should increase our enjoyment and engagement with fiction, because this process is similar to the 'make-believe' effect in interactive role-playing games. In the course of their discussion, the authors finally admit that "It seems very likely that our engagement with traditional forms of fictions rests on very different psychological bases than our engagement with interactive fictions" (p. 113).

Precise comparisons between the engagement with interactive fiction and traditional fiction require more empirical investigations. However, there have been empirical studies of the fundamental differences between an appreciator's ongoing perceptual reaction in the traditional versus interactive media genres, particularly in film studies.[5] While in interactive games, a user actively participates in the development of story events, empirical evidence shows that a viewer of a traditional fiction film always keeps a certain perceptual distance from the screen (Zacks, 2015). No matter how immersive a film seems, viewers remain to some degree distanced and fully conscious of their outsider role in the story events. In other words, it is unlikely that a viewer really believes he or she can participate in the story events. That means, in the context of traditional fiction, the philosophical theories about immersion and games of 'make-believe' are metaphorical descriptions rather than cognitive explanations. Based on the fundamental difference in perceptual distances, the textual form of multiple-endings in traditional fiction is unlikely to provide a cognitive response similar to the active participation in story development in interactive media.

I will end this section by pointing out that Cova and Gracia's stimulating discussion can definitely be seen as opening several lines of discussion and there are still many empirical discussions in the offing regarding traditional and interactive media genres; nevertheless, probing into the uses and functions of features of fiction could be more effective and theoretically better grounded if one applied a broader and fine-grained conceptual framework as suggested above. This contention will be exemplified through the analysis of *Mr. Nobody* presented in the following section.

3. Untangling the Labyrinth of Multiple Endings in *Mr. Nobody* (2010)

This section analyses the narrative complexity of *Mr. Nobody* on the basis of the multi-level social semiotic framework delineated in Figure 9.1. This film is well known for its ideological theme of *choices in life*. Most discussion of this thematic revolves around the interpretations at the level of cultural, philosophical or ideological meanings (see level z in Figure 9.1). The following sections will elucidate just how this abstract thematic can be reflected and supported by functional structures, patterns of textual mechanisms at the analytical levels x and y. Figure 9.2 maps out the three tools used throughout this section: 1. **schematic structures**, namely, Van Leeuwen's concept of multimodal genre structures (Van Leeuwen, 2005), 2. **cohesion** (Tseng, 2013a), and 3. **character development** (Tseng, forthcoming). This figure also shows how these tools are related back to levels x and y in Figure 9.1. In particular, different from the problem-solving approach taken

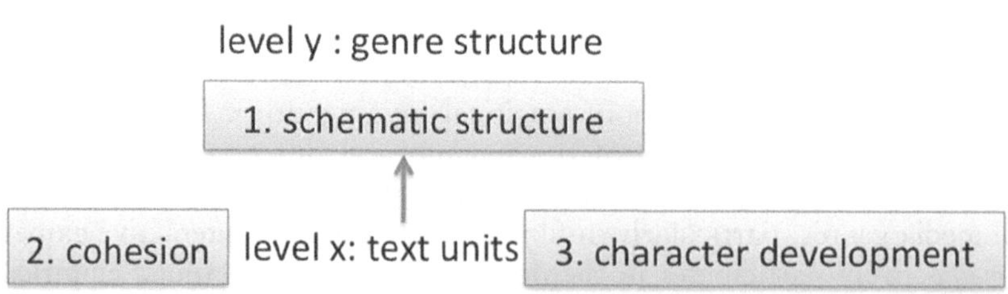

Figure 9.2 Three analytical tools used in this section

by several fabula/suzhet-based descriptive schemes (cf. Bordwell, 1985), the social semiotic analysis presented in this chapter shows how meaning patterns combine bottom-up construction of and top-down constraints on discourse and can more effectively unpack how a non-linear film guides its viewers to coherent narratives.

In brief, through employing these three tools, this section will show how the narrative strands in this film are intertwined yet equipped with certain discourse devices for guiding the viewer's interpretation.

3.1 Schematic Structure

This section maps out the overall functional structure of the entire story in *Mr. Nobody*, namely, the meaning structure at level y in Figure 9.1, by employing Van Leeuwen's (2005) concept of genre as a staged and multimodal process. The key characteristics of Van Leeuwen's multimodal genre analysis, drawing on social semiotic theory (Eggins, 1994; Martin, 1992), rest on the construction of a series of stages. The sequence of stages as a whole, also referred to as a schematic structure, realises a particular strategy for achieving an overall communicative goal—in this case, to present the film story. In other words, applying Van Leeuwen's multimodal genre structure to a film can be seen as a more functionally oriented analysis of plot and story structure.

The schematic structure of *Mr. Nobody*, consisting of five stages, is shown in Figure 9.3. The story of *Mr. Nobody* starts with **stage 1: prologue**, composed of fragmented scenes of the main character, Nemo. The bits and pieces of sequences of Nemo in unspecified time and space immediately function to 'anchor bias', namely, to frame and direct the viewer's inferences to a rather demanding, non-linear narrative structure (Bateman & Tseng, 2013).

The prologue is followed by **stage 2: beginning of the story**, which functions to present the background of the main storyline and the identity and traits of the main character. This stage is realised in a longer scene set in the year 2092, where the character Nemo Nobody is first specifically introduced—he is the last mortal man on earth. For some reason, the 118-year-old man Nemo Nobody never had telomerisation treatments that granted immortality to everyone else on Earth. Nemo was probably too old to benefit from them when they were first introduced, and he simply

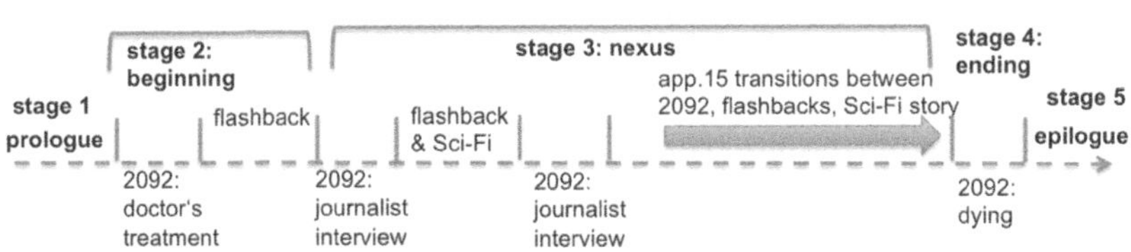

Figure 9.3 Overall schematic structures of *Mr. Nobody* with five stages

outlived everyone else from his generation. As the viewers first see him, he is staying at a hospital in a very frail state and under constant supervision. Being the last man to die of old age, he is in all the headlines, and his death is promised to be televised for the masses. Everyone wants to know the story of Nemo Nobody. The only problem is that Nemo's memory is vague and fading. Therefore, his doctor helps him put together his memories by using hypnosis. Following the hypnosis, Nemo starts to remember his childhood and hallucinate some jumbled images from his life with different women and children.

The next stage, **stage 3: nexus**, functions to map out the connection between several choices and their possible results in Nemo's life. This stage starts with a scene depicting a young journalist slipping into Nemo's room to interview him. The film then unfolds, following Nemo's non-linear flashbacks and descriptions of several tangled lines of his life stories picked up from his fragmented memories. Some memory strands are often contradictory—for instance, in some flashbacks, he dies, and in others, he is paralysed after a motorbike accident.

The clearest strands involve the adult Nemo with three different women: Anna, the love of his life, although fate keeps getting in their way; Elise, his depressed wife, whom he loves hopelessly; and Jeanne, the wife Nemo never loved. The permutations of these love stories with the three women, seemingly unfolding at the same time, leads the viewers across the entire film. These fragmented narrative strands around the three different women all trace back to the film's central point, at which Nemo's life branches out and splinters into a myriad of possible realities. This focal point is a scene in which the nine-year-old Nemo Nobody finds himself at a train station in the early 1980s, as his divorced parents go their separate ways. His mother will leave for North America, while his father will stay in England. Nemo has to decide whether or not to get on that train, which will dramatically alter the course of his life.

These sometimes converging yet jumbled narrative strands across Nemo's life are also intercut with the interview scenes in 2092, in which the 118-year-old Nemo is never sure which of the lives he actually lived and which he could have lived. Furthermore, some scenes in this stage also show the story contents of a science fiction story about a group of people travelling to Mars, written by the 15-year-old Nemo when he was living with his father. These complex intercuts repeat approximately 15 times in this stage and present a highly complex, non-linear narrative structure with jumbled scenes across different times and spaces in Nemo's life and his imagined science fiction story. Nevertheless, as the next two sections will show, despite its demanding spatio-temporal structure, this stage actually consists of a well-mapped goal-oriented causal plan cued to the viewers through well-mobilised cohesive mechanisms. These dimensions can only be effectively unpacked by using other discourse analytical methods.

This stage is followed by **stage 4: ending.** This stage functions to explicitly point out the overall theme of the film—while the young journalist finishes recording the interview and is fully frustrated by not knowing which story is the right story, Mr. Nobody states the motif of the story by quoting Tennessee Williams: Every path is the right path, and "everything could have been anything else and it would have just as much meaning".

Before his death, Mr. Nobody tells the journalist that neither of them exist. They are figments in the mind of the nine-year-old Nemo at the train station, as he was forced to make an impossible choice. The young boy tries to find the correct decision, following each choice to its conclusion. In this stage, a scene shows another possible outcome of his life, when the boy takes a third option. He leaves both parents and runs away towards an unknown future.

The final stage, **stage 5: epilogue**, functions to wrap up the theme by a symbolic sequence, in which the expansion of the universe comes to a halt and time begins to reverse. The 118-year-old man springs back from his deathbed into awareness, cackling triumphally with the realisation that he is now able to freely return to any path in life and to reunite with Anna.

The mapping of the overall generic structure shows that *Mr. Nobody* is actually similar to some other complex, non-linear films, such as Wong Kar-Wai's *2046*. In particular, Tseng's (2012) exhaustive analysis of scene transitions in *2046* shows a precise similarity of genre structures between the two rather demanding puzzle films: *2046* also starts with an unspecified sequence, followed by a main chronological narrative strand, cross-cut with several fragmented sequences of the main character's flashbacks and contents of a science-fiction story written by the main character. Furthermore, another possible inter-textual reference between *Mr. Nobody* and *2046* is the use of the same soundtrack, an aria from Bellini's opera *Norma*, as in *2046*, when the scene transitions into the sequences of the science-fiction world are cued to the viewers.

In sum, despite the non-chronological nature of the scenes in these two films, one main linear narrative strand is nevertheless identifiable and coherently presented as the main schematic structure with a chronological progression of functional stages. The coherent construction of a schematic structure is supported by the configurations of several lower-level discourse dimensions analysed in the following subsections.

3.2 Cohesive Devices in Scene Transitions

This and the following sections show how several dimensions at level x in Figure 9.1, the stratum of discourse and textuality, can be systematically analysed on the basis of social semiotic frameworks.

In several non-linear puzzle films, one main set of discourse mechanisms that hold together an interpretable narrative path is *cohesion* (cf. Bateman & Tseng, 2013; Tseng & Bateman, 2012; Tseng, 2012;

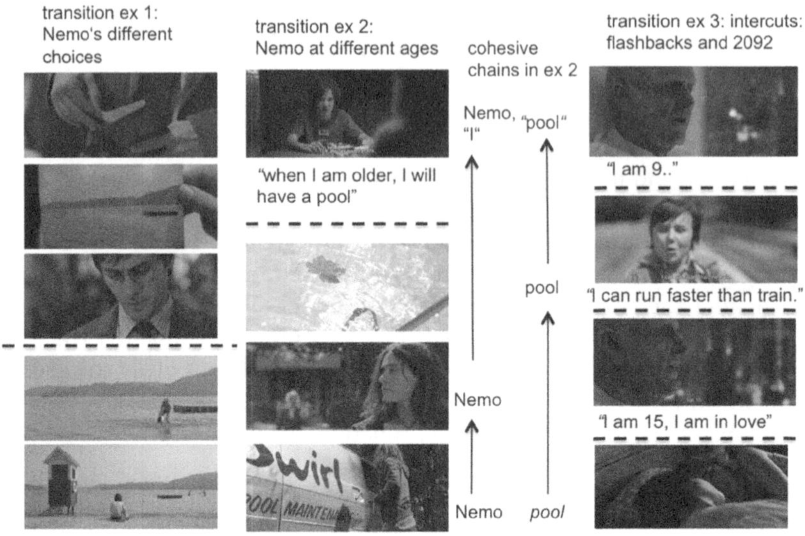

Figure 9.4 Three examples of the hook: cohesive mechanisms of scene transitions and intercuts across different narrative strands

Note: The dotted lines indicate transitions of scenes and settings.

Tseng & Bateman, 2010). In *Mr. Nobody*, the cohesive devices are also well mobilised to guide the viewers across the jumbled scenes and shots of the entire film. As described in the last section, this film intercuts scenes at two levels: It intercuts the main chronological strand of 2092 with Mr. Nobody's memories; and within his memories, the film also intercuts across the different narrative lines following Nemo's multiple choices, the science fiction novel Nemo is writing and another artificial world full of argyle patterns in which Mr. Nobody seems to be trapped sometimes during his navigation across different parts of memories. These intercuts and scene transitions are, nevertheless, mostly cohesively *hooked* together (cf. Tseng, 2012) by devices such as explicit repetition of the same characters, their actions, and their settings. Figure 9.4 includes three examples of such cohesive devices at work in the non-linear transitions of scenes and intercuts in this film.

The first example is a transition between Nemo's two different choices of reactions to and relations with Anna: In his first choice, 15-year-old Nemo, although secretly in love with Anna, deliberately insults her friends and rejects her invitation to swim at the beach for fear of revealing that he cannot swim. Anna then walks away and never comes back. Nemo regrets this choice ever since. He bumps into Anna with her kids one day in front of the train station. The first three images in Figure 9.4 show that Nemo takes out a picture from his wallet after Anna and her kids leave.

He stares with regret at the picture of the exact beach where Anna walked away from him. This is then cut to Nemo's second choice, in which he admits to Anna that he cannot swim, and Anna stays with him. Across the scene transition, the picture of the beach in Nemo's hand is hooked to the reappearance of the same beach, shown in the fourth and fifth images in Figure 9.4. The same identity of the setting and the repetition of Nemo's and Anna's actions (e.g., Nemo sitting at the beach, Anna running to him and asking him to swim) are robust devices signalling the cohesive ties between Nemo's two different choices. Throughout the film, a focal point, from which every choice splits in another branch, is explicitly signalled by this kind of cohesive strategy.

The second example in Figure 9.4 shows how the repeated motifs of this film, such as pools, swimming, and drowning, are often used as hooks across different scenes. This example uses 'pool' to hook together two stages in Nemo's life. The first image shows the last scene of the strand following young Nemo's second choice described above—he falls in love with Anna, whose father has an affair with Nemo's mother. Anna and Nemo develop a close relationship. However, it is forcefully broken when Nemo's mother and Anna's father separate. This image shows Nemo full of anger, telling his mother that she never understands him and he actually would like to have a pool. "When I am older, I will have a pool", Nemo says. This image is cut to the next scene, beginning with a pool and panning to the adult Nemo as a pool cleaner, suggested by his van labelled 'Pool Maintenance'.

The two scenes are tied by at least two cross-modal cohesive chains, displayed next to the screenshots in Figure 9.4. The cohesive chain of Nemo is linked across the two scenes with the visual and spoken element 'I' in the first image when he refers to himself. The motif of the film, pool, is also realised cross-modally: in Nemo's spoken text, in the visual track shown in the second screenshot, and in the printed text on the van in the fourth screenshot. Analysing such cross-modal cohesion chains effectively highlights just how cohesive mechanisms are mobilised and the same identities of people, places and settings throughout a film are cohesively tracked (Tseng, 2013a).

The third example in Figure 9.4 is a rapid intercut between the three different flashback strands of the 118-year-old Mr. Nobody, and the nine- and 15-year-old Nemos. Apart from the repetition of the same identity, the cohesive ties are simultaneously established by using the same action patterns cross-modally (Tseng, 2013b). In the first image, the 118-year-old Mr. Nobody says: "I am 9". This is then cut to the nine-year-old Nemo running next to a train, while the old man's voice continues to describe the same action "I can run faster than a train". This is cut back to the old Mr. Nobody, continuing to say: "I am 15 and I am in love". This is followed by a transition to the next scene in his flashback, cohesively hooked back to the action of 'being in love' by showing Nemo lying in bed with her.

In sum, sufficient cohesive mechanisms for cuing and tracking the reappearances of the same identities, settings, and actions dominantly function to hook together the jumbled shots, scenes, and rapid intercuts across the multiple, non-linearly structured narrative strands throughout the film.

3.3 Character Development and Event Progression

The cross-cutting of the multiple layers of storylines following Nemo's multiple choices within and across three different women are the most intertwining and demanding narrative designs of the entire film. However, the complex labyrinth of Nemo's different choices and their consequent outcomes can be effectively unpacked by applying the tool of character development (Tseng, forthcoming) through mapping out goal- and motivation-oriented causal relations across the progression of events the main character experiences.

This tool is developed on the basis of combining the social semiotic framework of event and action patterns (Tseng, 2013b) with the tools developed by Trabasso and his colleagues (cf. Trabasso, van den Broek, & Suh, 1989; Trabasso & Nickels, 1992), particularly their framework for causal network discourse analysis originally designed for examining children's understanding of coherent verbal narrations of events and narrative goals. Causal logical relations in a filmic text have been investigated in several social semiotic studies (cf. Van Leeuwen, 1991; Bateman, 2007; Wildfeuer, 2014). These studies all suggest systematic methods for constructing fine-grained analyses of discourse relations across meaningful units in moving images. In the present paper, the analysis of character development focuses on another dimension of causal relations in film narratives—this discourse dimension examines how the main characters experience main events in the narrative lines and achieve their goals throughout a film. The discourse analysis builds on a series of event progressions. With the discourse method proposed in this section, event progression can be systematically analysed through examining how the narrative events of the main characters are motivated, enabled, and psychologically or physically triggered.

Figure 9.5 maps out the complex plan of the event progression and character developments of Nemo across the ages of nine, 15, and 35. Nemo's different choices at the age of nine at the station enable different branches of further choices. His choice to stay with his father enables him to meet Elise. This then triggers two possible paths: dating and marrying Elise, or being abandoned by Elise and then dating and marrying Jeanne. Each path leads to further event progressions logically and causally built and developed toward the end of the story: for instance, marrying Elise enables two types of event progressions: Nemo and Elise happily go on a honeymoon trip, which then leads to a car accident. Elise dies in the accident, or Elise suffers depression from their marriage and eventually leaves Nemo.

The choice of Nemo to leave with his mother enables his encounter with Anna. This then enables their relationship, which also branches out to different types of event progressions and outcomes. For example, Anna's leaving

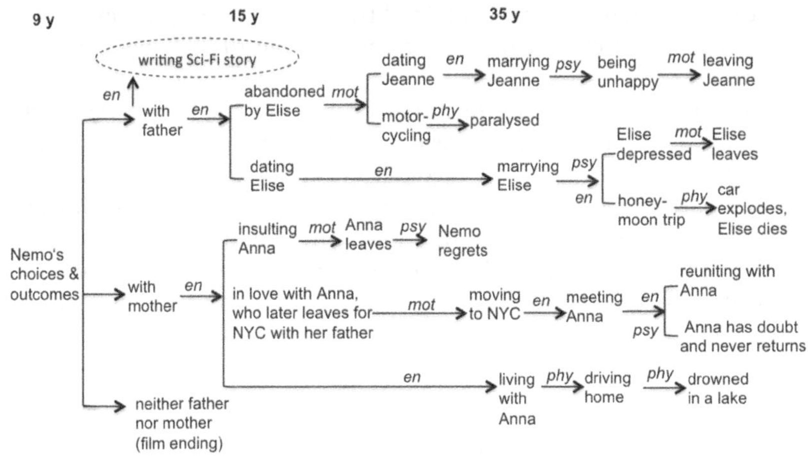

Figure 9.5 Goal plan and event progression of Nemo's choices and outcomes (en = enabling, psy = psychologically trigger, phy = physical trigger, mot = motivating)

for New York motivates Nemo to move to New York, with the goal of meeting her some day. This enables him to bump into Anna coincidentally.

In sum, despite the seemingly loose connections between bits and pieces within and across multiple layers of Nemo's story lines, a clear event progression concerning Nemo's goals and character development are nevertheless coherently constructed and tightly planned.

4. Conclusion

Targeting the narrative device of multiple endings, this chapter combined Van Leeuwen's (2005) method of multimodal schematic structure analysis with Tseng's (2013a, forthcoming) methods of multimodal cohesion and character development to highlight just how a highly demanding film with a non-linear structure and multiple endings can be systematically anatomised to see just which underlying discourse mechanisms function as robust cues for the viewers' narrative interpretation.

Through analysing the well-known puzzle film *Mr. Nobody*, this chapter showed that the film's schematic structure carries a straightforward, chronological narrative strand similar to the main scaffolding of other puzzle films, such as *2046*, and the cohesive strategies work well to hook the jumbled transitions and cross-cuts and often to function as motifs linking different paths of the character's life. In this chapter, I also presented the hypothesis that the most complex yet narratively significant dimension of the film for the audience is to make sense of Nemo's multiple choices and their consequent paths. Nevertheless, as the results of the analysis of Nemo's character development reveal, the discourse dimension of character development is equipped with a highly compact and tightly planned event progression with identifiable, goal-oriented causal relations between the events experienced by Nemo.

In sum, this chapter has demonstrated that a multiple-level framework is needed in order to avoid the confusion of different concepts such as media materiality, genre expectations, ideological interpretations, textual coherence, and narrative impact. In particular, it has presented one such framework, which draws on the work of Van Leeuwen and linguists working in the social semiotic realm and illustrated how it can be employed to untangle the narrative complexity of puzzle narratives such as fiction films with multiple endings.

Notes

1 See, for example, the empirical study on genre prediction of fiction films by Magliano et al. (1996).
2 See Martin (1992); Mann and Thompson (1988).
3 For recent developments applying the functional linguistic analysis of text coherence to multimodal text, see, for example, Bateman (2008) for the analysis of printed documents, Van Leeuwen (1991); Bateman (2007) for logical relations in film, Tseng (2013a), for cohesive reference in film, and Bateman and Wildfeuer (2015) for text coherence in comics.
4 See Halliday (1978) for the original idea of meaning realisation across strata in SFL.
5 For more comparisons and discussions of narrative interpretation in interactive media, traditional films, and fictional films with computer-generated materials, see Tseng (2016).

References

Bateman, J. A. (2007). Towards a grande paradigmatique of film: Christian Metz reloaded. *Semiotica*, *167*(1/4), 13–64.

Bateman, J. A. (2008). *Multimodality and genre: A foundation for the systematic analysis of multimodal documents*. London: Palgrave Macmillan.

Bateman, J. A., & Tseng, C-I. (2013). The establishment of interpretative expectations in film. *Review of Cognitive Linguistics*, *11*(2), 353–368. [Special issue on Multimodality and Cognitive Linguistics, edited by Maria Jesus Pinar Sanz].

Bateman, J. A., & Wildfeuer, J. (2015). Defining units of analysis for the systematic analysis of comics: A discourse-based approach. *Studies in Comics*, *5*, 373–403.

Bordwell, D. (1985). *Narration in fiction films*. Madison, WI: University of Wisconsin Press.

Buckland, W. (Ed.). (2009). *Puzzle films: Complex storytelling in contemporary cinema*. Chichester: Wiley-Blackwell.

Buckland, W. (Ed.). (2014). *Hollywood puzzle films*. New York/Oxon, UK: Routledge.

Cova, F., & Garcia, A. (2015). The puzzle of multiple endings. *The Journal of Aesthetics and Art Criticism*, *73*, 105–114.

Eggins, S. (1994). *An introduction to systemic functional linguistics*. London: Pinter Publishers.

Halliday, M. A. K. (1978). *Language as social semiotic*. London: Edward Arnold.
Halliday, M. A. K., & Hasan, R. (1976). *Cohesion in English*. London: Longman.
Halliday, M. A. K., & Matthiessen, C. M. I. M. (2004). *An introduction to functional grammar* (3rd ed.). London: Edward Arnold.
Magliano, J. P., Dijkstra, K., & Zwaan, R. A. (1996). Generating predictive inferences while viewing a movie. *Discourse Processes*, *22*, 199–224.
Mann, W. C., & Thompson, S. A. (1988). Rhetorical structure theory: Toward a functional theory of text organisation. *Text*, *8*(3), 243–281.
Martin, J. R. (1992). *English text: Systems and structure*. Amsterdam: Benjamins.
Trabasso, T., & Nickels, M. (1992). The development of goal plans of action in the narration of a picture story. *Discourse Processes*, *15*, 249–275.
Trabasso, T., van den Broek, P., & Suh, S. Y. (1989). Logical necessity and transitivity of causal relations in stories. *Discourse Processes*, *12*, 1–25.
Tseng, C-I. (2012). Audiovisual texture in scene transition. *Semiotica*, *192*, 123–160.
Tseng, C-I. (2013a). *Cohesion in film: Tracking film elements*. Basingstoke: Palgrave Macmillan.
Tseng, C-I. (2013b). Analyzing characters' actions in filmic text: A functional-semiotic approach. *Social Semiotics*, *23*(5), 587–605.
Tseng, C-I. (2016). Revisiting dynamic space in film from a semiotic perspective. *Semiotica*, *210*, 129–149.
Tseng, C-I., & Bateman, J. A. (2010). Chain and choice in filmic narrative: An analysis of multimodal narrative construction in The Fountain. In C. Hoffmann (Ed.), *Narrative revisited: Telling a story in the age of new media, pragmatics and beyond* (pp. 213–244). Amsterdam: John Benjamins.
Tseng, C-I., & Bateman, J. A. (2012). Multimodal narrative construction in Christopher Nolan's *Memento*: A description of method. *Visual Communication*, *11*(1), 91–119.
Tseng, C-I. (2017). The role of genre in shaping our narrative knowledge: Analysing narrative events and characters' motivations beyond the media boundaries. *Discourse, Context and Media*. Online: https://doi.org/10.1016/j.dcm.2017.05.001
van Dormael, J. (2010). *Mr. Nobody*. Pan Europeenne.
Van Leeuwen, T. (1991). Conjunctive structure in documentary film and television. *Continuum: Journal of Media and Cultural Studies*, *5*(1), 76–114.
Van Leeuwen, T. (2005). *Introducing social semiotics*. London: Routledge.
Wildfeuer, J. (2014). *Film discourse interpretation: Towards a new paradigm for multimodal film analysis*. London: Routledge.
Walton, K. L. (1990). *Mimesis as make-believe: On the foundations of the representational arts*. Cambridge, MA: Harvard University Press.
Zacks, J. (2015). *Flickrs. Your brain on movies*. Oxford University Press.

10 New Codifications, New Practices

The Multimodal Communication of CrossFit

Per Ledin and David Machin

1. Introduction

At the time of writing, the fitness phenomena called CrossFit, originally founded in the US in 2000, was emerging as a hugely successful international brand. CrossFit gyms were appearing in cities around the world, with national and international competitions taking place where scoring was facilitated through online databases. CrossFit differed in many ways from traditional commercial gyms or fitness studios. This was a new kind of 'functional fitness' where the body is seen as a system, emphasising power but also balance, accuracy, stamina, and endurance (Glassman, 2002, p. 1). The CrossFit slogan is 'forging elite fitness' which reflects this idea of a perfect natural powerful body derived by complete devotion and effort. Those who follow CrossFit often also take on specific 'caveman' diets which emphasise natural proteins from ecological meat as opposed to carbohydrates from pasta or bread which come from agricultural processes. Unlike the plush commercial gym, the setting is ideally a basement in a building formerly used for industrial or other commercial purposes.

In our previous work using Multimodal CDA, we have argued that the nature of wide-ranging forms of communication in contemporary society can be usefully understood by combining Fairclough's (1992) concept of 'technologisation' and Van Leeuwen's (2008) concept of 'New Writing'. We showed that performance management documents, strategy diagrams, design in news, and even IKEA kitchens are characterised by increased codification and regulation of semiotic resources (Ledin & Machin, 2016a, 2016b, 2017). This is a process whereby social practices are stripped down to number of symbols and indexical meanings where things like causalities, coherence, and agency are represented through increasing levels of abstraction and symbolism.

In this chapter, we show that the notions of New Writing and technologisation can also help us to understand much about CrossFit. Here, too, we find a drive to construe a system of interlocking parts which relies on the basic qualities of New Writing and the logics and causalities which it permits, which we will explain shortly. We argue that what we find relates strongly to the stripped back representations of space and causalities found in management steering documents and corporate flowcharts. And as with these steering documents the codification of CrossFit relies on neoliberal ideas, values, and forms of social relations.

2. CrossFit, Commodification, and Neoliberalism

CrossFit has begun to attract the attention of scholars, particularly in the field of sport sociology. Interest has for the most part been in the idea of the designed body which has been explained in relation to consumer society, where particularly for women there has been a trend in media images of muscular, yet also slim, torsos (Cohen & Colino, 2014). Elliot (2013) places contemporary fitness regimes in the context of the way that consumerism always requires the 'new', 'the latest thing', and creating a culture of reinvention. The body here has become one key site for such reinvention.

Other scholars have been struck by the voluntary institutionalisation which CrossFit involved, where members commit to a strict system of rules as a means to identity change (Scott, 2011, p. 234). In existing commercial gyms, members are able to train at their own pace; they occupy machines which can allow them a private sort of space. In CrossFit, a member trains as a team to a strictly regulated schedule where their performance is closely monitored and where the meaning of what they do is clearly defined and highly scripted. This led Dawson (2015) to call CrossFit a 'reinventive institution'. He argues that whereas traditional institutions control behavior by coercion, in these new kinds of institutions, we come ourselves to seek out subservience to regulations. Yet this is experienced not as any kind of surrendering of agency but rather as positive as regards the "overall goal of self-improvement" (Scott, 2011, p. 242). It comes as no surprise that CrossFit has been called an "ideal neoliberal body practice" (Heywood, 2015, p. 32). As Dawson (2015, p. 8) observes there is a "manifest agency", which is "expressed as volition or desire to improve oneself" and continuously increase outputs and fitness.

In this chapter, however, we show that we can understand CrossFit in a different way. Indeed, at the heart of CrossFit are the core ideas, values, identities, and social relations required by neoliberalism. But more than this, we show that we can think about CrossFit in regards to broader shifts in how we communicate multimodally across different domains and the kinds of priorities, identities, and social relations that this has been used to foster and naturalise.

3. The New Writing

The New Writing, we argue, can be understood as part of what Fairclough (1992) called the 'technologisation of discourse', which is the creeping codification of all semiotic discourses for the purposes of more systematic control over communication. This is also aligned with processes of commodification and marketisation which sit at the heart of neoliberalism.

It is easy to see that texts have become increasingly multimodal, in documents, books, brochures, and other media (cf. Kress & Van Leeuwen, 2001). This involves a fundamental shift in the use of language, including the demise of running text. The overall coherence no longer comes from what linguists call 'cohesion', for example, by conjunction that codes the relations between sentences and ideas with devices such as 'because', 'on the other hand', 'consequently', or 'thus'. Nor does the New Writing rely on rhetorical composition, on an overall structure and reading order where different sections are placed after each other. Instead, the overall coherence comes from a visual design where different semiotic resources are deployed such as alignment, spacing, color coordination, iconographic representations, graphic shapes, etc., and the reading order does not have to be top-down and left-right but might well be bottom-up (Ledin & Machin, 2016a).

Documents and media design characterised by the New Writing are visually stimulating, where, rather than banks of running text, we find bulleted lists, flowcharts, images, and graphics (Van Leeuwen, 2008). The difference can be seen comparing two lifestyle magazines from 1990 and 2016 or school text books and learning software over the same period, where not only text, images, and graphic elements become more integrated, but a shift has taken place in how basic things like causalities and categorisations are communicated—where text can appear more as smaller units in lists or even 'floating' words, which work alongside other visual fragments in a way that appears highly functional.

The New Writing enables texts and semiotic materials to take on new relations, to be connected to each other in specific ways where different documents are circulated and related to databases. In this way, systems of performance management that ensure accountability can be set up in, for example, public institutions such as universities (Ledin & Machin, 2016b). Each document will then get its meaning from the interrelated documents and the interlocking system will specify and monitor 'quality' and demand higher outputs. A mission statement dense with buzzwords and promotional, highly symbolic photos will be related to a strategy document mostly using language in bullet points which get its meaning specified in a document with numerical performance indicators, and from this system it is possible to manufacture templates in the form of 'activity tables' where each subject leader becomes accountable and must report according to the 'quality standards' of the system.

Here we can see that the New Writing transforms social practices and in fact creates new ones, such as a new public management or a new fitness regime like CrossFit. In IKEA catalogues, we have pointed to how the social practices in kitchens have been transformed (Ledin & Machin, 2017). While the kitchen in the 1970s was a place for cooking and eating, it has become a creative space where you can manage and find solutions to specifically formulated life challenges and have quality time with children or engage with colleagues. What we find over time is not least an increased coding of space and materiality based around neoliberal values of 'flexibility' and 'self-management', where the persons who inhabit these spaces are part of the coding. The logics and causalities of these ideas and processes are never fully articulated but are represented through forms of naturalism, symbolism and indexical and affective meanings. They also take place across interrelated and mutually independent domains of representation.

That space is used for communicating neoliberal meanings and shapes social practice is also highlighted by Roderick (2016), who shows that contemporary office workspaces are now technologised with a shift away from rows of desks to be replaced by flexible, dynamic designs, which communicate the move away from stable, fixed jobs to impermanence and the role of the team and newer forms of monitoring. He argues that contemporary office furniture transforms social practice and "communicates and materialises how work has been reconstituted under neoliberalism" (p. 276). Aiello and Dickinson (2014) in their analysis of the redesign and global aesthetic of Starbucks stores were interested in the use of materiality and texture to a new and much more local sense of 'authenticity'. Different materials were used in the redesigned stores to signal provenance, and consumer-citizens were construed as part of a local community, for example through large communal tables made of old and irregularly shaped wood planks from a nearby area, a design strategy that made each store stand out as seemingly unique. Here, 'uniqueness' and 'locality' are communicated through a limited repertoire of symbols which can be bolted into to an overall global template.

What is clear from this research is that physical and social space interact in semiosis and function in many ways to regulate social behaviour and perform social status (cf. Thurlow & Jaworski, 2012). There is an interplay between the actual material properties of a certain locality and the construction of it in communication, and this also enables new practices to take form. This is important for our analysis of CrossFit, which we see as a neoliberal practice codified by the New Writing and based on technologies that foster a system of performance monitoring.

4. Theory and Methods

In what follows, we present an analysis of one specific CrossFit location in Stockholm called CrossFit Solid, which, when it was founded in 2010, became one of the first 'boxes' (as the CrossFit gyms are called) in Sweden. We obtained permission to follow the WODs ('workout of the day') for one week, where we took photographs and made field notes. In this chapter, we use data from one of the WODs. To show how CrossFit constitutes a system, a highly regulated semiotics, we depart from three main aspects presenting our analysis: the box as the space where training takes place, the language that is found in the CrossFit location, and, finally, the WOD or the actual training program itself. One of the authors trained CrossFit for two years, and the analysis partly relies on this background knowledge. We are not critical of CrossFit per se; rather, the analysis is to be taken as a critical discussion of how the New Writing reshapes social practice in line with a neoliberal order.

Theoretically, the analysis draws on the principles of social semiotics (Van Leeuwen, 2005) and Multimodal CDA (Machin & Mayr, 2012). Social semiotics is interested in the use of semiotic resources, such as in language, visual and material design, space, etc., to achieve particular goals. It also seeks to describe the resources available to communicators. This involves identifying the choices available to people as regards things like language, visual and material design, etc., upon which they can draw.

All semiotic resources and their canons of use will carry traces of the socio-political contexts in with they were formed (Bezemer & Kress, 2010) and therefore reflect the dominant ideologies of those contexts, which is the basis for our critical approach. Here, discourse is an important instrument of power and one way by which ideologies are disseminated, legitimised and naturalised. Our analysis is designed to reveal such ideologies. Specifically, two forms of semiotic resources deployed for communicating the discourse of CrossFit run through the chapter: framing and texture. As we will show, these resources are interwoven and part and parcel of the New Writing.

The model for analysing framing departs from Van Leeuwen (2005) (cf. Roderick, 2016; Ledin & Machin, 2017). Framing is about how spaces are comprised of interrelated elements which can form frames or be framed in terms of degrees of connectedness and disconnectedness. We use the following categories:

> *Separation.* This is how 'open' or 'closed off' different spaces are—by walls, curtains, or being distant in space from each other. Spaces may not be sealed off but run into each other. We can talk about 'integration', for example, when a kitchen opens up into a living room or entrance space. When a room is closed off from the surrounding space, we can talk about 'segregation'.
>
> *Permeability.* This is the degree to which framing elements afford interaction be it visual, auditory, or both. Permeability can limit or allow specific kinds of interactions.
>
> *Permanence.* This is the degree to which framing is dynamic. For example, curtains and doors can be opened, and furniture can be designed to be easily moved or changed according to the task to be carried out.

Texture relates to a further level of materiality, objects that can be touched. This allows us to combine the visual with the haptic, with seeing and touching, and also to point to how the experience of materiality is linked to the provenance of materials, where we make assumptions about its physical and cultural sources. Djonov and Van Leeuwen (2011) and Abousnnouga and Machin (2013) point to some basic categories of texture upon which we draw:

> *Rigidity*. Surfaces may be resistant, or they can give to the touch. This can be to different degrees such as a soft sponge or a car dashboard. The meaning of this can relate to durability, stability, or submissiveness.
>
> *Liquidity*. Surfaces may be more or less wet or dry, which can relate to life and vitality or to rot and decay. But dryness can also communicate comfort.
>
> *Relief*. Part of surfaces can extend below or above a horizontal plane, which can point to what is manufactured vs. what is more organic and shaped by time. We can contrast a glossy kitchen surface to the shape of a tree bark.
>
> *Regularity*. Regular textures are predictable and can mean homogenous, lack of surprise, and consistency. Irregularity can mean less predictable, the whimsical, the heterogeneous, or the natural.
>
> *Roughness*. Rough can mean natural; it can suggest wear and tear and the lack of comfort. Smoothness can suggest well maintained, processed, or refined, as in silk, and as opposed to a rough-knit sweater.

As regards both framing and texture, the notion of *rhyming* is particularly important in our analysis. Rhyme refers to how elements or features are connected through the use of common qualities such as colour, shape, texture, or construction material. Rhyming is an important semiotic feature, since it unites elements and gives them coherence. This is a crucial aspect of the New Writing, where parts of representations that formerly would have been linked by the coherence in running text are now linked and differentiated by different kinds of semiotic materials. This allows for new kinds of connections and distinctions to be made and new kinds of coherent wholes to be signified.

5. The CrossFit Setting: The Box

The CrossFit training space is called 'the box'. The box of CrossFit Solid is located in central Stockholm in a basement which is entered through a steel door from the underground parking lot. The box has two floors. In Figure 10.1 we look down to the lower floor and the workout area. As regards the nature of the space and its framing we can see that the box is a confined basement space, segregated from the outer world. This contrasts with other kinds of commercial gyms which are on the ground floor and favour extensive windows and use of glass, which gives a sense of permeability to its boundaries. In the case of CrossFit, this suggests an environment which is stripped back, with a minimum of artifice. This simplification, typical for the New Writing and representing the core details and processes, has become highly important in the shift to functionality. It enables the elements which are represented as forming the system to work as a coherent whole.

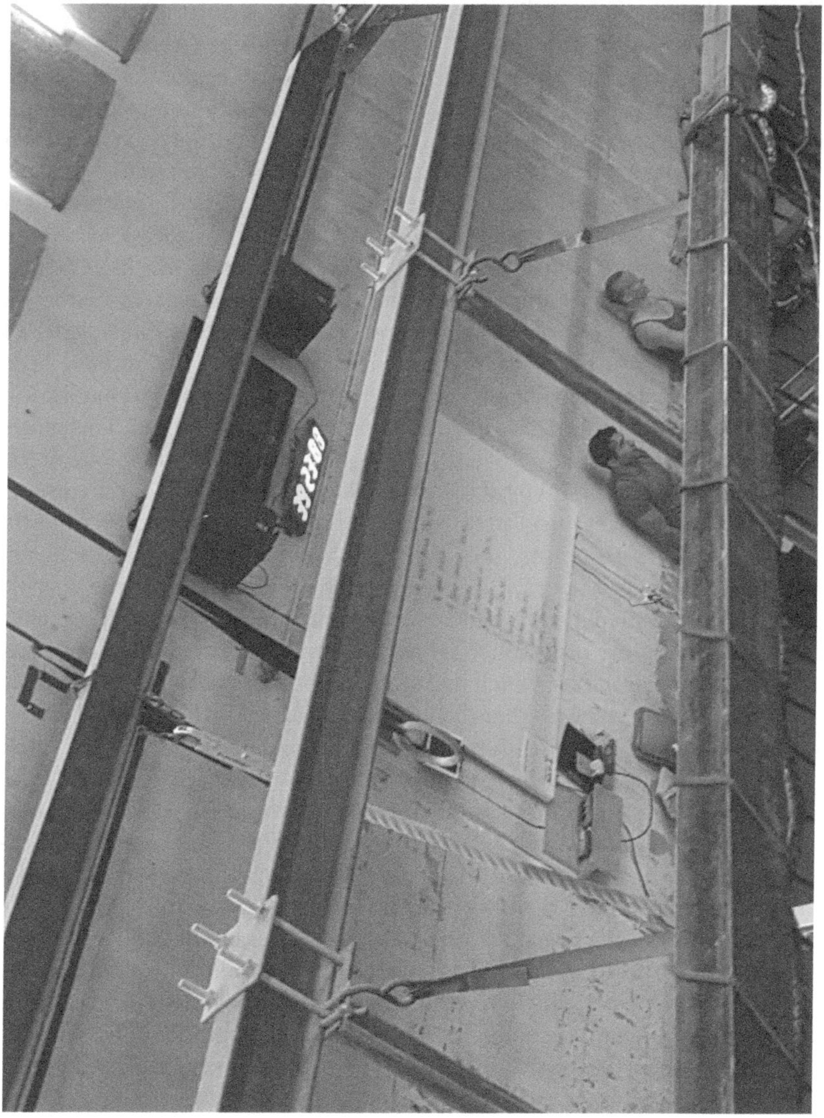

Figure 10.1 The workout area shot from above

Continuing with framing, we also see the recurring angularity of the shapes formed by the girders and equipment. This creates rhyming across the overall internal space again creating coherence. This rhyming is also created by the bleached industrial color scheme using greys and off-white. This kind of regularity can mean homogenous, lack of surprise, consistency. And certainly, this is one core message that the box communicates. Members follow a tight, functional system. They simply do not, as in most commercial gyms, work at their own pace, to their own routine.

There is also an affective dimension in this revealing of structures that can be related to seeing or revealing of internal mechanisms (Abousnnouga & Machin, 2013). The revealing of bare components is an important part if the affective bond CrossFit creates, indicating moral certainty and commitment. One observation we have made about New Writing and the ways it is used to represent social practices is that we must be increasingly prepared to leave aside our own beliefs to organise ourselves in a kind of performativity as a response to evaluations, targets, and goals, where, in the process, we find a comprehensive suppression of history and context (Ledin & Machin, 2016b).

We also find one other important form of rhyming as regards texture in the box. The surfaces of iron, steel, and concrete tend to have some degree of relief. The surfaces of the walls are uneven, where layers of paint have been torn off over time as seen in Figure 10.2. The iron girders tend to be oxidised in some places but not others. These are all typical of CrossFit boxes. This unites elements by communicating provenance and authenticity. We find none of the flat, polished surfaces of a typical commercial gym, nor the use of mirrors.

The uneven surfaces suggest something organic and shaped by time. In trendy inner-city restaurants, too, it is common to find this use of 'lived' surfaces on walls and floors, even where they are installed for the specific look. CrossFit systematically chooses premises which were formerly used for other manufacture or commercial purposes. This particular building was formerly a coal warehouse which had stood empty for many years. What we begin to see here is the way that the box as a space creates a sense of coherence of parts through rhyme in texture and framing.

The photo in Figure 10.3 is taken from the workout area, looking in to the section where the equipment is stored and where some box members train individually or stretch. Even if the framing of the box completely segregates it from the outer world, the inside has an open-plan solution and a consequent permeability that afford interaction. A CrossFitter is on display and the possibility for visual, verbal, and aural interaction is always there. This space and the equipment are designed for flexibility, for using equipment in variety of ways, where new exercises can be introduced. This is different to equipment in commercial gyms where machines are for specific, fixed purposes. In the box, the barbell, for example, or simply a bumper plate, as in Figure 10.2, is used for many different exercises with varying weights and combined with gymnastic and other exercises.

Roderick (2016) discusses the meaning of the shift in office designs from more fixed spaces with individual work desks which may be segregated, to flexible, open-plan spaces created for adaptability and social interaction, rather than carrying out private work tasks. He relates this to the neoliberal ideas of flexible, adapting worker, the value of the small team and also to the decline of individual roles. Neoliberal offices tend to be oriented around ideas of 'innovation', 'creativity', and teamwork.

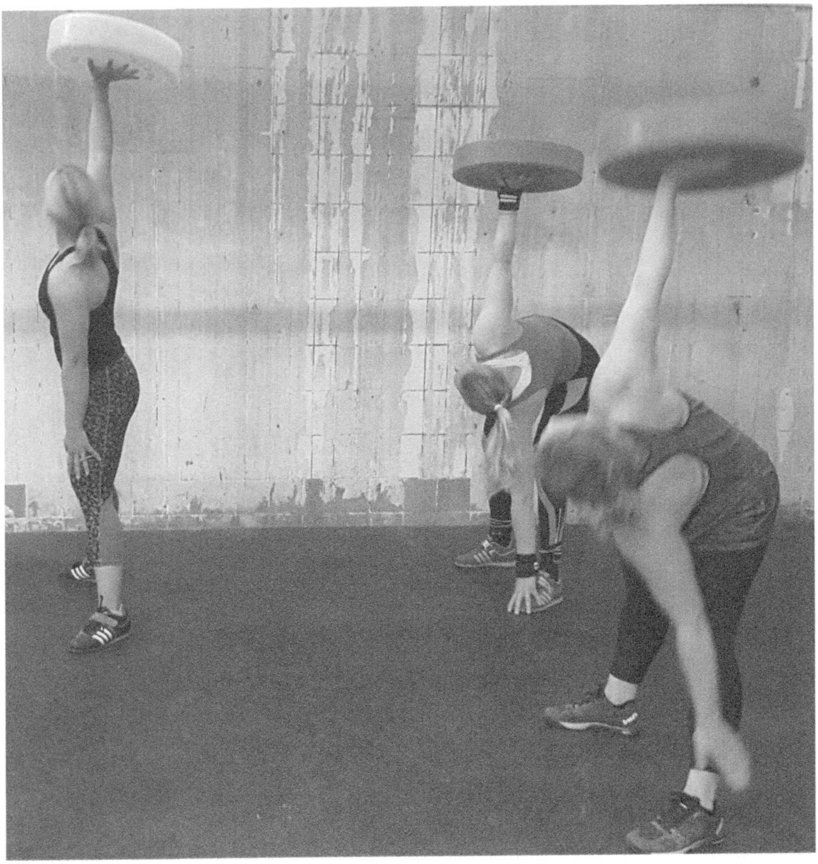

Figure 10.2 Warm up with bumper plates against the rough concrete wall in the workout area

The functionality of the box is also seen in the sorting of the equipment in Figure 10.3. The barbells, dumbbells, and kettlebells are in separate racks, the rowing machines are folded and thoroughly placed against the wall. Hanging under the ceiling we see carefully sorted T-shirts from other boxes around the world, signifying the CrossFit community, once again an obligatory furnishing of boxes. On the wall in the equipment area in Figure 10.3, we see red letters which are part of the slogan also typical for every box, in this case, WORK HARD & BE NICE TO PEOPLE, in itself a summary of CrossFit, where stamina and camaraderie should go hand in hand.

In the nature of the equipment, we also find the affective communicated through texture. While the equipment in commercial gyms may have comfort rubber-foam grips and be placed on soft matting, we find none of these

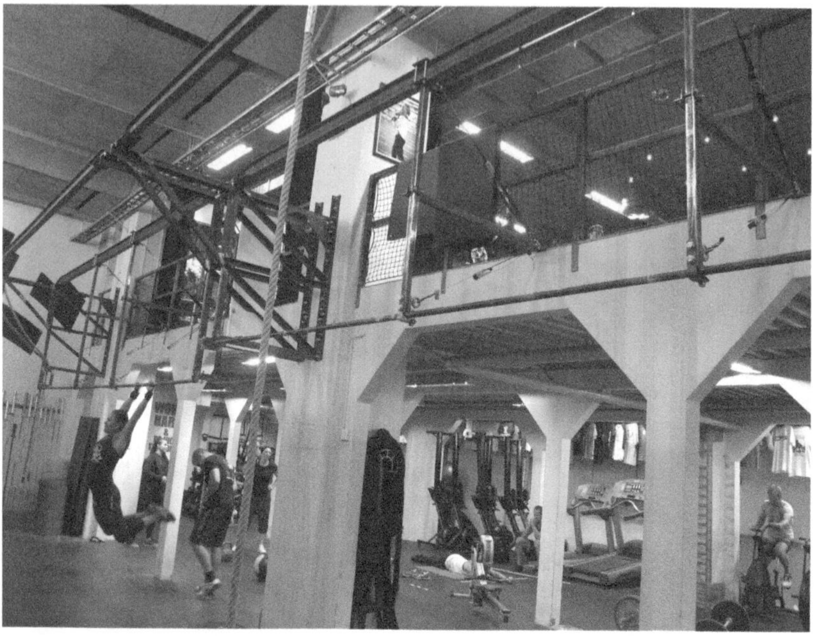

Figure 10.3 Looking into the equipment area from the workout area

textures in the box. None of the surfaces in the box give when they are touched to suggest 'accommodation' or 'submissive'. The functional system is rigid and unyielding. There is flexibility but only within the functional system of the box. Overall, the texture brings a feeling of the box being not only durable and resistant in relation to most other places, but almost indestructible, the kind of closed-off space you will be safe in during a hurricane, thunderstorm, or possibly even a terrorist attack.

In sum we can understand the box through its symbolic naturalism, the striped back and highly codified use of space, in which elements can form coherence based on the rules of New Writing. As happens with New Writing, we find the decoupling from context and history where the former industrial space becomes a symbolic element in the design, alluding, as in the case of the same use by art galleries and cafes, to authenticity and provenance. This is a space which communicates flexibility but only within a tight functionality.

6. Language Found in the Box

Looking at Figure 10.3, we can see that writing is not prominent in the box. Yet it regularly appears in two important places: on the whiteboard, as seen in Figure 10.4, and on Tee-shirts, as seen in Figure 10.5. These also carry language, all in English, and are important for communicating the shared values of the international CrossFit community.

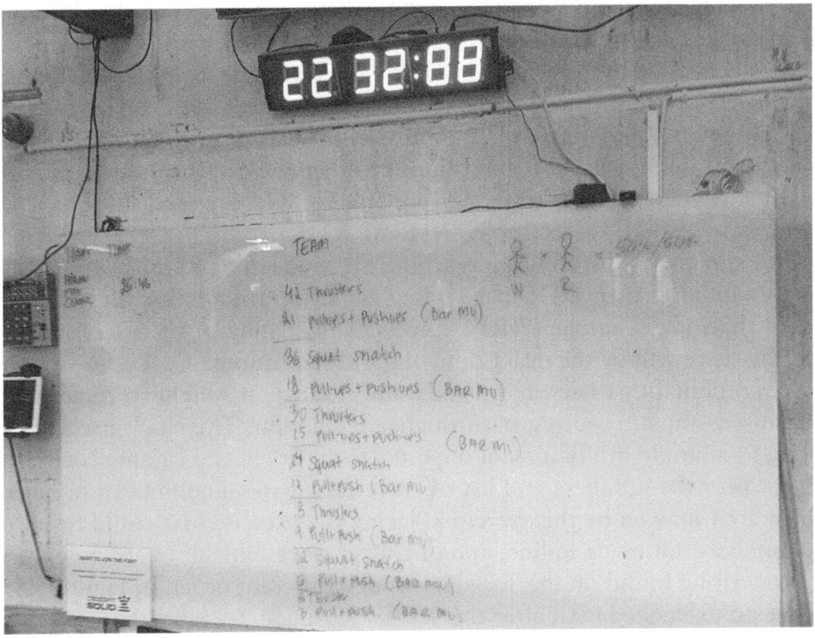

Figure 10.4 The WOD noted on the whiteboard, and above it, the digital clock

The whiteboard in the workout area, displayed in Figure 10.4, is an obligatory object in all CrossFit boxes. Everyday a new WOD is written on it, using a specialised language that clearly separates insiders, the CrossFit community, from outsiders and non-CrossFitters. The WOD is performed in what is called a 'class' to which you have to register.

This daily WOD prescribes exercises with barbells ('Thrusters', 'Squat snatch'), gymnastics ('Bar MU', 'Pullups'), and body weight ('Pushups'). It is of importance here that we find a standardised language which is in English. In a commercial gym in Sweden, you would do 'armhävning' and 'ryck', whereas in CrossFit, you do 'pushup' and 'snatch'. This kind of linguistic colonisation is related to the basic regulation and codification of CrossFit. The movements and the language are standardised as a kind of law.

There are numbers connected to each exercise. On the whiteboard in Figure 10.4, we see that there is a falling number of repetitions ("46–31", "36–18", etc.) that should be done as quickly as possible against the digital clock positioned above the whiteboard. This WOD is performed in pairs, and the symbols to the top right of the whiteboard, separated from the listed exercises, say that both the weight (W) and number of repetitions (R) should be equal in each pair. To the top left, also separated from the exercises, a score is noted from an earlier WOD to indicate previous levels of performance.

Clearly, acronyms are abundant in CrossFit language, just as they are in performance management systems, where they connote a specialised technical language, and where they can also be coordinated with other elements in ways permitted by New Writing. The daily routine is a WOD. MU stands for 'muscle-ups' done on the bar. During the warm up seen in Figure 10.2, the participants did GTO or 'ground-to-overhead', lifting bumper plates. This can be done using different kinds of objects. WODs can have the format of AMRAP, 'as many rounds as possible', and in this case, the time is set beforehand so that, for example, 'AMRAP 12 min' would start the writing, and the clock would stop when reaching the time limit and the rounds done were counted. Other WODs are based on RFT, 'rounds for time', which means that, for example, '7 RFT' precedes the listing of the exercises and that the score will be the exact time of the seven rounds.

The combination of acronyms and numbers suggest a highly technical and specialised system ensuring performance regulation. The clock itself, measuring to a hundredth of a second, points to accuracy and rigour. The framing used for the numbers and list of exercises creates a column of numbers which are followed by the exercise. Placing the exercise first could result in the numbers not being in line, and of course more difficult to see quickly.

The writing found on the Tee-shirts is of a different order. In Figure 10.5, we see an exhausted man after the WOD wearing a Tee-shirt that says:

constantly
varied
high
intensity
functional
movement
CrossFit

This is a dense nominal group where the head noun 'movement' is preceded by five modifiers that point to central notions of CrossFit: It is 'functional' (it mimics the natural movements of everyday life and is about the natural functional movements of the body as a system rather than the more artificial muscle development of body building), 'constantly varied' (the WODs are never the same), and with 'high intensity' (it maximises work in short periods of time). This is in fact the definition of CrossFit on the official website.

In sum what we meet here is a technologised language. There are lots of acronyms, lots of specialised definitions (also of movement standards), and dense nominal groups. Importantly, this is the same type of grammar that we have met in performance management language (Ledin & Machin, 2016a, 2016b). There are clear similarities as to how data and numbers are used to monitor and regulate performance.

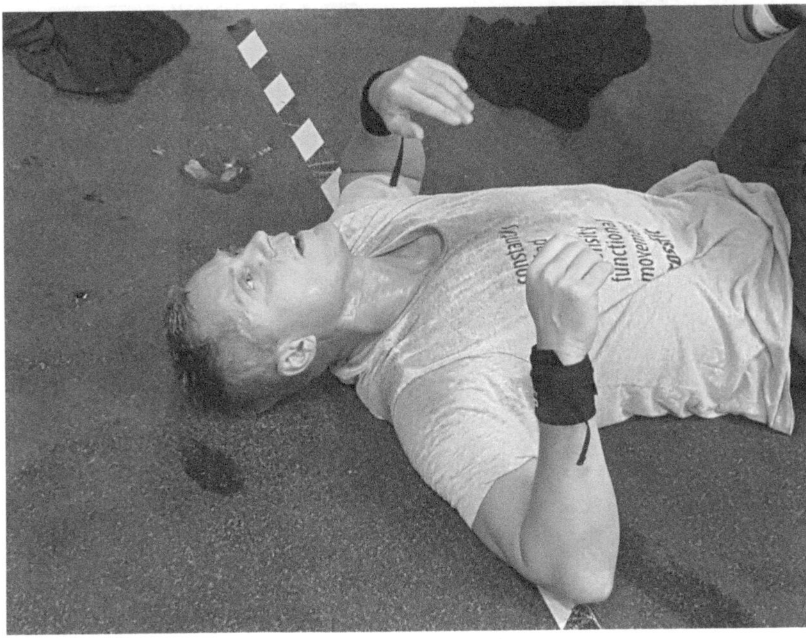

Figure 10.5 Exhausted man after the WOD wearing a Tee-shirt with writing

7. The Training Routine: The WOD

A CrossFit class lasts for one hour and has a principled structure. It starts with a warm up that the coach is free to plan. The warm up is given special meaning. One CrossFit slogan, often carried on Tee-shirts is "our warm up is your workout". This comparison to other fitness regimes appears clearly appropriate in the era of self-promotion and branding. Skills or strength work often follow, and then the obligatory WOD takes place, and it can, as explained above, be designed in many ways, not only for movements and exercises but also for time. Cool down and stretching end the class.

In Figures 10.6 and 10.7, we see the WOD as it is taking place. We see a cluttered space. The class is scattered, and some of the pairs have to use the equipment area due to shortage of space. The different spaces where each exercise takes place can blend and shift. Negotiation and courtesy are important between the members in the class. There is some differentiation of space, such as the area for working with the barbells and area for working on the frames.

But while we find order and functionality in overall design and framing, we find relative disorder at this level. If we look at posture and gaze, there is huge variation, and different (inter)actions are going on. What is evident

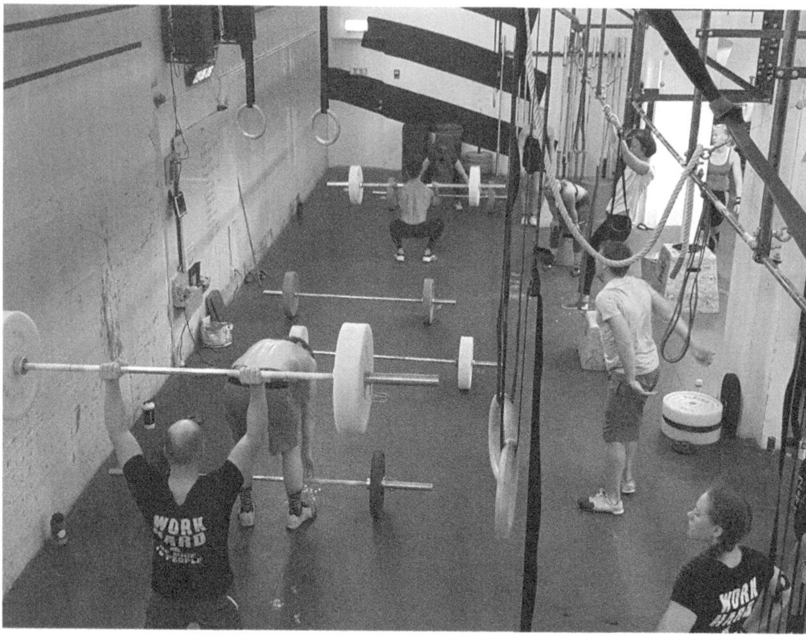

Figure 10.6 During the WOD

here is that CrossFit on the one hand codes the functional and the highly regulated system, and on the other hand the dynamic and the flexible. While the CrossFitters are required to subject themselves to the system, it is also one which relies on self-management.

In Figures 10.6 and 10.7, we also see the kind of clothing worn by members. We can sense a resistance to the artifice of branding culture and to the idea of surface gloss, and the shabby clothing also rhymes with the wall covering. We do not find men with tops designed to show muscles, as we might in a body-building gym. We also see that men will often train topless, which would be considered inappropriate in many other fitness contexts. Women can train in sports bras, which would also appear excessively revealing in a commercial gym. This nudity corresponds with the naturalism represented in the textures, the symbolism of the setting and to the caveman diet. And the naturalism transfers to a kind of moral affective idea of how this kind of commitment is to be seen and felt. As the workout approaches the body as a system, developing it in a natural functional way, so the setting communicates this naturalism as do the stripped and sweaty bodies.

In sum, we see how New Writing tends to offer tightly coded and regulated systems within which, at least within the bounds of this system,

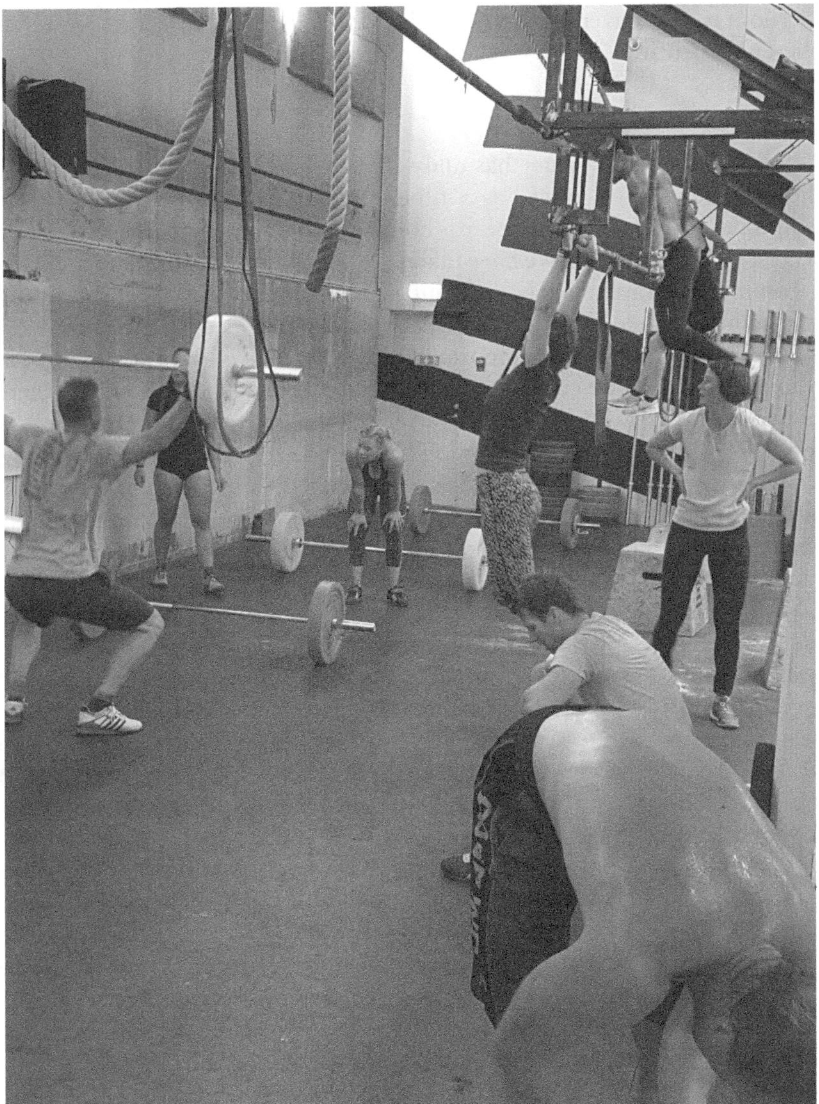

Figure 10.7 During the WOD

flexible kinds of activities can take place. They are realised through a training program which describes and codes the body as part of a regulated system. The meanings of the affective commitment to the system is seen in the naked bodies, the unyielding surfaces, and the provenance of the peeling walls. In systems of performance management, individuals must in similar ways be innovative and compete. This is an important part of the value of self-management, where there are good and bad choices to be made. Yet, this room to maneuver is strictly regulated within a system whose logic and coherence is entirely at the level of the New Writing.

8. Conclusion

The analysis in this chapter has allowed us to make a contribution to the scholarly view that CrossFit is a fitness regime suited to its times where we find neoliberal values as regards competition and self-management. The social semiotic approach we have taken, drawing attention to smaller details of communication through different semiotic materials, has, we would argue, allowed us to reveal some finer level analytical details as regards how CrossFit works. But, more importantly, this analysis allowed us to look at an important shift in communication across domains, what we call here the rise of the New Writing. This is a process whereby social practices are stripped down to number of symbols and indexical meanings where things like causalities, coherence and agency are represented through increasing levels of abstraction. It is a process where the kinds of coherence formerly provided by running text had been lost, where it had become replaced by graphics, symbols, and more fragmented uses of text.

What is striking is the loss of context and of history and of actual individual difference. All this must be subsumed to the creeping codification, symbolism and abstraction. And all is coupled with commodification and marketisation. It is, on the one hand, truly fascinating to see the way that leisure activities such as CrossFit, drinking a coffee in Starbucks, buying an IKEA kitchen or planning a child's learning targets at school are governed by an underlying set of principles. But on the other hand, it is exactly what we should expect. As Hall (1984) argued, we should expect forms of power and the forms of social relations, values, and identities that they require for their maintenance to be found diffused across all kinds of social forms and cultural activities. In this paper, we can see that such social forms would be found not only in official settings but also in leisure and entertainment. And as we were completing this very paper, one author received a letter to say that his children's kindergarten would now be introducing a database system where the development of every child could be followed as regards specific categories of progress.

Acknowledgements

We wish to thank CrossFit Solid for granting us access and accommodating us in a very supportive way. We are specifically grateful to the fantastic staff Karl Dyall, Felix Ledin, and Mikaela Dyall and to the participants who agreed to be photographed.

References

Abousnnouga, G., & Machin, D. (2013). *The language of war monuments*. London: Bloomsbury.

Aiello, G., & Dickinson, G. (2014). Beyond authenticity: A visual-material analysis of locality in the global redesign of Starbucks stores. *Visual Communication*, *13*(3), 303–321.

Bezemer, J., & Kress, G. (2010). Changing text: A social semiotic analysis of textbooks. *Designs for Learning*, *3*(1–2), 10–29.

Cohen, J., & Colino, S. (2014). *Strong is the new skinny: How to eat, live and move to maximise your power*. New York: Harmony.

Dawson, M. C. (2015, June 30). CrossFit: Fitness cult or reinventive institution? *International Review for the Sociology of Sport*, 1–19.

Djonov, E., & Van Leeuwen, T. (2011). The semiotics of texture: From tactile to visual. *Visual Communication*, *10*(3), 541–564.

Elliot, A. (2013). *Reinvention* (Shortcuts—little books on big issues). Oxford: Routledge.

Fairclough, N. (1992). *Discourse and social change*. Cambridge: Polity Press.

Glassman, G. (2002). Foundations. *The CrossFit Journal*, 1–8. Retrieved September 5, 2016, from http://library.crossfit.com/free/pdf/Foundations.pdf.

Hall, S. (1984). Cultural studies and the centre: Some problematics. In S. Hall, D. Hobson, A. Lowe, & P. Willis (Eds.), *Culture, media, language* (pp. 117–121). London: Hutchinson.

Heywood, L. (2015). "Strange borrowing": Affective neuroscience, neoliberalism and the "cruelly optimistic" gendered bodies of CrossFit. In C. Nally & A. Smith (Eds.), *Twentyfirst century feminism: Forming and performing femininity* (pp. 17–40). London: Palgrave Macmillan.

Kress, G., & Van Leeuwen, T. (2001). *Multimodal discourse*. London: Bloomsbury.

Ledin, P., & Machin, D. (2016a). The evolution of performance management discourse in corporate strategy diagrams for public institutions. *Discourse, Context and Media*, *13*(B), 122–131.

Ledin, P., & Machin, D. (2016b). Performance management discourse and the shift to an administrative logic of operation: A multimodal critical discourse analytical approach. *Text & Talk*, *36*(4), 445–467.

Ledin, P., & Machin, D. (2017). IKEA kitchens and the rise of a neoliberal control of domestic space. *Visual Communication*.

Machin, D., & Mayr, A. (2012). *How to do critical discourse analysis: A multimodal introduction*. London: Sage.

Roderick, I. (2016). The politics of office design: Translating neoliberalism into furnishing. *Journal of Language and Politics*, *15*(3), 274–287.

Scott, S. (2011). *Total institutions and reinvented identities*. Basingstroke: Palgrave Macmillan.

Thurlow, C., & Jaworski, A. (2012). Elite mobilities: The semiotic landscapes of luxury and privilege. *Social Semiotics*, *22*(5), 487–516.

Van Leeuwen, T. (2005). *Introducing social semiotics*. London: Routledge.

Van Leeuwen, T. (2008). New forms of writing, new visual competencies. *Visual Studies*, *23*(2), 130–135.

11 The 'Semiotics of Value' in Upcycling

Arlene Archer and Anders Björkvall

1. Introduction

The work of Theo van Leeuwen has influenced and inspired researchers in a number of disciplines on a global scale. One of the reasons is that Van Leeuwen manages to connect 'grand theories' from the social sciences in general and from sociology in particular to the often critical analysis of the material artefacts, texts, colours, and sounds which are formed by, and form, human life. In other words, Van Leeuwen's way of presenting his ideas and transforming them into ways of understanding specific aspects of the social and material world has made his research relevant far beyond the realm of, for instance, multimodality and discourse studies. This chapter draws on a number of key concepts in Van Leeuwen's studies, including recontextualisation (2008) and semiotic change (2005), to address the issue of value adding in 'upcycled' artefacts. It combines these notions with theories of the social control of 'value' in social practices.

The last 20 years have seen the rise of various consumer movements that critique overconsumption. The focus is on the whole life of an artefact and on how consumer products can be both designed and used in an environmentally friendly way. A key aspect of these movements is the re-use of artefacts and materials. Traditional 'recycling' involves converting materials from one product to create another one, such as when glass from light bulbs is recycled into bottle glass. New value is not necessarily added in such processes, even though recycling may be said to have an intrinsic value of being 'sustainable', 'environmentally friendly', and even 'economically rational'. In 'upcycling', on the other hand, value is always added when wasted, used, thrown-out, found and repurposed artefacts and materials are transformed into new ones for different markets. Such upcycled products tend to gain not only economic, aesthetic, and functional value in the upcycling process, but also ethical value through being created out of, for instance, a responsibility for the environment and resistance toward mass consumerism.

In a developing country like South Africa, upcycling is often driven by high-priced unprocessed raw materials and the need to find an income. Numerous small-scale poverty prevention projects have emerged in order to

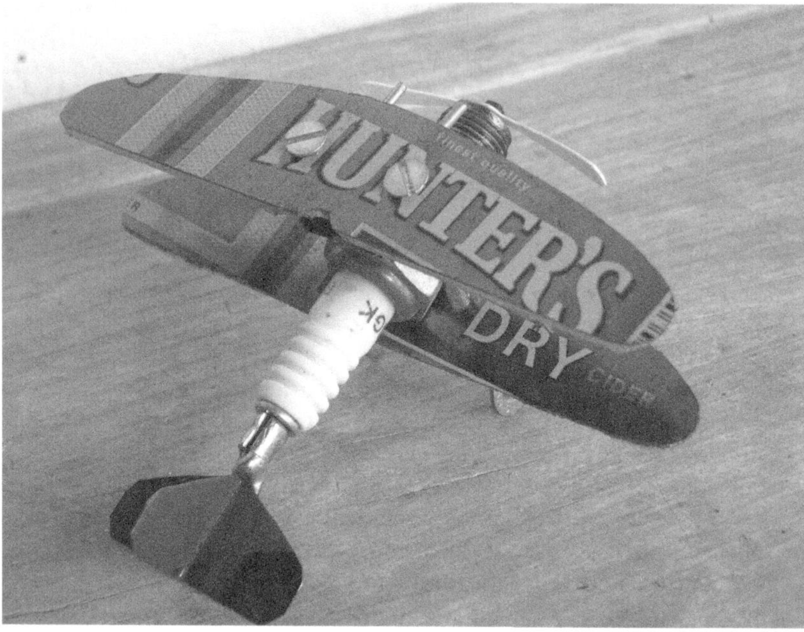

Figure 11.1 Upcycled tin aeroplane

create upcycled accessories and homeware items out of waste. Objects that previously had another defined purpose are turned into more 'arty' objects, for instance, upcycled tin cans are converted into consumer products such as toy cars, handbags, radios, or hold-all containers. Such products are then often exported globally, either through the regular global chains of distribution or through tourists that buy the products and carry them home. Thus, these types of products are sold on competitive markets, and, accordingly, need to be branded in some way, for instance as 'handmade in the developing world' or 'African', but potentially also as 'ethical', 'sustainable', and 'socially responsible'. Some of the upcycled artefacts are branded in a directly observable way: the brands of the primary products are made highly visible on the upcycled artefacts. For instance, the logo and colour of a brand of South African cider is salient on the upcycled tin aeroplane in Figure 11.1. This type of re-use of trademarks has become a significant feature, a brand in itself, for many upcycled artefacts made in the developing world.

Whereas a lot of academic research on upcycling focuses on economic viability (Albinsson & Yasanthi Perera, 2012), environmental benefits, or sustainability of design (Crabbe, 2012; McDonough & Braungart, 2002, 2013), we focus on 'value adding' in upcycling as semiotic practice. More specifically, we look at upcycled artefacts from a social semiotic perspective

(Van Leeuwen, 2005; Archer, 2008; Björkvall, 2014; Björkvall & Karlsson, 2011), using South Africa and Sweden as our specific sites of study. The data consist of a collection of approximately 50 upcycled artefacts that either have moved or have the potential to move between Africa and Europe, primarily toys, jewellery, ornaments, and interior design or household items. They were collected from street retailers and shops in Cape Town and in Stockholm during 2014 and 2015.

The artefacts to be examined in this paper are household items: coasters, plastic curtains, and wire bowls. Our aim is to explore how value is added in upcycled artefacts through recontextualisation, broadly defined as the iterative semiotic process when language, logos, shapes, materials, and colours move between contexts (cf. Van Leeuwen, 2008; Linell, 1998). More specifically, we identify key semiotic resources that are recontextualised and, to various degrees, recognised in upcycled artefacts. The chapter concludes with a short discussion of the implications of this type of analysis for questioning the 'ethical' and 'anti-consumerist' foundation on which much of the upcycling movement rests.

2. Upcycling as Marketing and Critical Commentary

As stated in the introduction, there are anti-consumerist movements that connect upcycling to values such as 'ethical responsibility' and 'sustainability'. Emgin (2012) describes how designers and others involved in upcycling can be "ennobled by virtue of their commitment to nature and humanity" (p. 65). Partially emanating from anti-consumerist and environmentalist movements, upcycling, rather paradoxically, now offers business opportunities. Emgin (2012) observes that

> Certain designers labelled eco-friendly are earning money through upcycling, competitions are organized around trashion, numerous websites are devoted to promoting and selling upcycled objects, and online and print resources explain how to upcycle at home. In short, there is a whole sector of upcycling now.
>
> (Emgin, 2012, p. 65)

When the possibility of earning money through the upcycling of artefacts and materials considered as rubbish by others is combined with scarce economic and material resources, new markets arise. Crabbe (2012) describes this type of upcycling.

> First, it creates work cooperatives in low-income communities that are isolated from wealth-creating opportunities. Second, it uses indigenous design-and-make skills not only to make traditional products, but also to transform local waste into secondary products, some having a value as great as the primary one.
>
> (Crabbe, 2012, p. 12)

It is in these markets for artefacts produced in Africa and other parts of the developing world that the types of upcycled and 'rebranded' products like the aeroplane in Figure 11.1 are common. Such products illustrate the iterative nature of commercial brands and the producers' and manufacturers' declining control over their uses and meanings. With regard to upcycled artefacts, brands can 'travel' beyond the point of disposal of the primary product to be reused in other, secondary artefacts with partially 'transformed' meanings and values attached to them (cf. Van Leeuwen, 2008, p. 17–21).

One way of understanding why logos and trademarks are so often highlighted in upcycled artefacts from the developing world, like the aeroplane in Figure 11.1, is to look at the brands from an aesthetic perspective (cf. Adami, 2015). Much of the waste that ends up in rubbish bins and on garbage dumps is colourfully branded with carefully shaped logos that can function as 'ready-made' resources for value adding in the process of upcycling. A much more mundane interpretation is that these types of rebranded artefacts share properties with certain household products that Chang Coupland (2005) analyses as carrying 'invisible' brands. She talks about a product that is "taken from the marketplace and now exists in the household, yet is considered mundane and blends into the household environment in an inconspicuous manner" (2005, p. 106). In other words, a product becomes so incorporated in daily household routines that it is not considered a brand any more (which in many ways is a sign of successful branding). Chang Coupland adds, "consumers do have agency, but this agency lies not just in the ability to embrace or create new brand meanings but in the capacity to forget, minimise, and overlook brands that enter the home" (2005, p. 115–116). The Hunter's brand on the aeroplane in Figure 11.1 may work similarly; when recontextualised, it may be just a colour scheme or shapes on an artefact, rather than recognised as a brand by a person receiving it as a souvenir, for example. However, as we argue below, recontextualisation of brands in upcycling often realises more specific semiotic potentials.

Further, the overt use of brands on these secondary products could be viewed as anti-consumerist branding in itself, as a type of critical commentary on consumerism. By critical commentary, we mean the ways in which the dominant discourses encapsulated by the brand are highlighted and imploded in order to critically reflect on some aspect of society. Logos in upcycled objects can often be manipulated for the purposes of critical social commentary through the use of parody. Culture jamming, for instance, inverts consumerism and remixes commercial discourses. This is Bakhtin's (1981) notion of dialogism, the recognition of the polyvocality of any sign. Reusing a logo in an upcycled artefact could be seen as a kind of ironic recontextualisation.

3. Toward a 'Semiotics of Value' in Upcycling

Social semiotics (Van Leeuwen, 2005; Halliday, 1978; Hodge & Kress, 1988) provides a way of thinking about meaning-making, in this case value adding, as a motivated, social activity in which humans always draw on the semiotic resources that they consider most relevant or apt (Kress, 2010). Upcycled artefacts, just as any text or artefact, have materiality, but as pointed out by Kress and Van Leeuwen (2001) and others (cf. Djonov & Van Leeuwen, 2011; Björkvall & Karlsson, 2011) research in linguistics and semiotics has tended to focus on the design of texts and artefacts more than on semiotic potential of materiality. However, materiality itself has semiotic potential. This insight becomes particularly important in the semiotic analysis of value adding in upcycled artefacts.

In order to avoid over-interpretation, it is pertinent to point out that not all the semiotic potential of semiotic resources is recognised by everyone at all times. Van Leeuwen (2005) states that semiotic resources have "a *theoretical* semiotic potential constituted by all their past uses and all their potential uses and an *actual* semiotic potential constituted by those past uses that are known to and considered relevant by the users of the resource" (p. 4, italics in original). Theoretical semiotic potential exists in features such as the colour, shape, texture, weight, and language of primary artefacts, and is reinforced or downplayed in the process of upcycling to varying degrees. Some aspects of this semiotic potential are actualised in the upcycled artefact, and others left untapped. And certain aspects tend only to be recognised by persons that are familiar with particular cultural contexts (like South Africa), whereas others can travel across continents and cultures and be actualised in other countries (like Sweden).

In addition to the notion of semiotic potential, 'recontextualisation' and 'transformation' are other key concepts in Van Leeuwen's approach that are relevant for our analysis. Van Leeuwen (2008, p. 12–21) describes how 'social practices' are recontextualised and how they, in that process, are transformed. Elements of social practices such as participants, happenings, and locations can, for instance, be substituted, deleted, rearranged, added, legitimised, and evaluated in the recontextualised practice. In a similar vein, we view upcycling as a social practice in which semiotic resources are recontextualised from primary products and the social practices and meanings connected to them into upcycled, re-designed, and materially transformed artefacts.

Since such recontextualisations and transformations have to result in some kind of value adding in upcycling, there is a need for a theory of the social construction of value of artefacts, and of rubbish in particular. Thompson's (1979) theory of the recursivity of rubbish, including more recent readings with regard to sustainable design, trashion, and upcycling (Frow, 2003; Hetherington, 2004; Crabbe, 2012; Emgin, 2012), offers a dynamic perspective on the value of rubbish. Thompson (1979, p. 7–12) argues that disposal is not a permanent state, as it was sometimes viewed in different stages of modernity, but disposed artefacts can always move from being rubbish to being more highly valued. The dynamic view is pertinent for an understanding of upcycling as a semiotic process of value adding: "The delightful consequence of this hypothesis is that, in order to study the social control of value, we have to study rubbish" (p. 10).

Thompson recognises three categories of values for objects and artefacts: *durable* objects, *transient* objects, and *rubbish*. Durable objects are viewed as having constant or increasing value; examples include pieces of art or other collectables. The transient status is the normal value of everyday objects in the world, with constantly decreasing value as time goes by. Food packaging, mobile phones, and clothes are examples of objects in this category. Rubbish has zero value. With regard to our interest in upcycling the main theoretical point that Thompson (1979) opens up is an understanding of the movement of objects between categories of value, including the zero value of being rubbish. Thompson explicitly points to the dynamics of rubbish: Artefacts can move into the category of rubbish but also move on into either of the other two categories. Hetherington writes that "rubbish is itself a conduit of disposal—a conduit of the disposal of value—but it acts more like a door than a rubbish bin" (2004, p. 165). Further, Thompson's (1979) theory of the recursivity of rubbish allows us to categorise different types of upcycling. First, upcycling can be a process involving the transfer of an object from the category of rubbish to that of transient value; an example would be when driftwood is used to build a simple worktable. Second, rubbish can move directly to be valued as durable—as in the case of collectables. Finally, upcycling can also be a movement between transient and durable value; an object that is in use can move upward to the status of durable, for example when a used car becomes a 'vintage' car.

When Thompson's categorisation of dynamic values of objects is complemented with a social semiotic approach to materiality and recontextualisation, a few important theoretical points become visible. Generally speaking, Thompson's (1979, p. 7) statement that "the way we act towards an object relates directly to its category membership" and that "we treasure, display, insure, and perhaps even mortgage the antique vase, but we detest and probably destroy its second-hand mate" is in line with a social semiotic view of the importance of social practices in value adding. In other words, and according to Thompson, the value of an object as rubbish, transient or durable does not primarily depend on the material properties or the design of the product as such, but on norms, practices, and power relations in social groups and communities.

However, the focus of social semiotics is directed toward the intersection of social practices and 'materiality' (Björkvall & Karlsson, 2011): materiality always matters. The durable value of an antique vase can never be viewed only in relation to how we act towards it; neither can it be viewed only in relation to its material properties or the semiotic potentials that come with them. Hetherington (2004) discusses a more materially oriented semiotic approach to disposal and claims that "when we dispose of something to hand—a material form of some kind—we do not necessarily get rid of its semiotic presence and the effects that are generated around that"

(2004, p. 159). From a social semiotic perspective, this would be described as a recontextualisation of semiotic potentials, in this case, how branded semiotic resources keep part of their theoretical semiotic potential when they move between the categories of rubbish, transient, and durable. More specifically, with reference to the recontextualisation of the green Hunter's brand in Figure 11.1, the theoretical semiotic potential of the typeface, the colour, the brand name, and the tin material of the original can of cider are partially actualised in the upcycled products. But the 'semiotic regimes' (Van Leeuwen, 2005) in the new environment of, for instance, upcycling of rubbish in Africa, transform the theoretical semiotic potentials of the resources, combining them with other semiotic potentials, perhaps aesthetic ones or those tied to sustainability.

Two processes are of interest: recognition of 'connotative provenance' and 'experiential meaning potential' (Van Leeuwen, 2005; Kress & Van Leeuwen, 2001; Djonov & Van Leeuwen, 2011). Broadly speaking, connotative provenance has to do with how different types of cultural knowledge are required for the interpretation of where a branded resource in an upcycled artefact comes from. Experiential meaning potential (which can also be described as a sub-type of provenance alongside the connotative type) has to do with our concrete experiences of the world that we inhabit: we tend to recognise tin of a certain thickness and weight as a functional material of beer, cider, and soda cans, and this experience of the material is semiotically productive when an artefact moves between categories of value in the upcycling process. An example would be when the 'cheap feel' of plastic as an extremely transient material—always close to being rubbish—is drawn upon when the process of upcycling leads to 'arty' objects.

Upcycling can thus be understood not just as a process of reuse, recontextualisation, and transformation, but also of 'recognition' of semiotic resources and semiotic potentials across different categories of value for artefacts and materials: rubbish, transient, and durable.

4. Case Studies

Three different types of upcycled products are analysed below: coasters, plastic curtains, and wire bowls. They are all made from artefacts and materials in South Africa, but whereas the coasters were bought in an art shop in Cape Town, the plastic curtain and the wire bowls were found in two separate shops in Stockholm.

Paper, Cork, and Logos: Coasters

The three pairs of coasters are shown in Figure 11.2; they were found in a South African shop in which the majority of the artefacts for sale were upcycled.

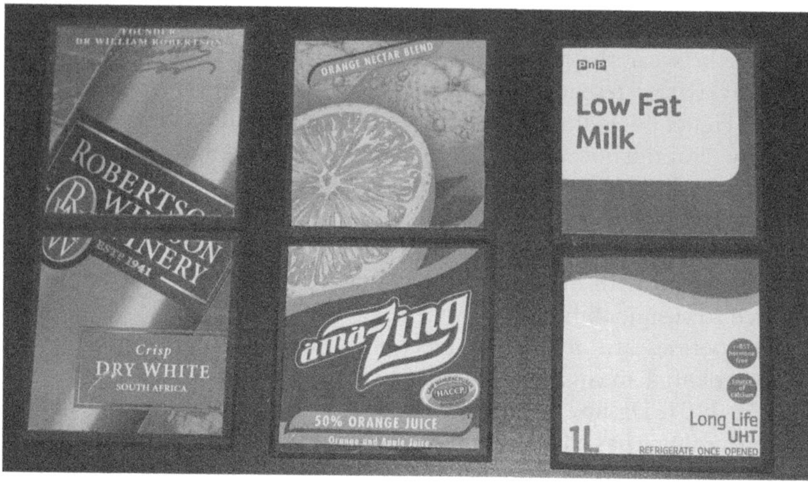

Figure 11.2 Coasters

In the coasters, there are a number of recontextualised semiotic resources with obvious connotative provenance. These are made from cheap orange juice boxes, box wine, and long-life milk containers, which connote everyday use, 'necessary but not glamorous'. The milk container resembles the look of 'no frills' basic supermarket-owned brands, which is slightly more 'everyday' than the other two containers. In all three, the colours, logos, and brand names connect the coasters to the branded original products found in South African supermarkets. African languages are drawn on in 'ama-Zing' ('ama' as a plural form indicating 'lots of zing'), as are resources of authenticity from the South African context ('UHT', 'r-BST hormone free'). In the primary products, these brands could be described as 'invisible' brands (Chang Coupland, 2005) that blend in to such an extent in South African homes that they become integral parts of daily household routines.

The colours in the coasters have a recognisable provenance. In the Ama-Zing coaster, primary colours of blue and orange and green are used. These colours are connected, more connotationally to other commercial genres and products that communicate 'tropical' and 'exotic'. The Robertson winery white wine coaster makes uses of the green colours of the primary wine box; the same colour as the grapes used. The colours of the milk coasters have less of a 'naturalistic' provenance since they use only red and white. This points to human experiences of controlled, perhaps lab-like, environments. The use of terms like 'UHT', 'r-BST hormone free' also contributes to this. In terms of experiential provenance, the coasters show signs of being torn, gluing irregularities, skew cut lines. Experientially, this type of texture points to processes of creating handmade objects out of used materials (cf. Djonov & Van Leeuwen, 2011). However, the cork of the backing is solid and seems to be brand new. This gives a 'decorative' meaning to the use of the food packaging. In addition, the artist stated that the re-use of the food packages is highly functional: the plastic coating keeps the coasters moist resistant (interview with artist, March 2013). This material functionality is thus added to the branded packaging from the primary product to the upcycled coasters.

The branding works at two distinct levels. Most directly noticeable, the coasters are branded with the recontextualised logos, brand names, and colours of the primary products, recognisable to almost any South African as 'specific', 'everyday' food and drink brands. This can be referred to as 'branding in upcycling through connotative provenance': The 'everyday' character and perhaps 'invisibility' (Chang Coupland, 2005) of the primary products are recontextualised as a semiotic potential also in the upcycled coasters. While outside of South Africa, the specific brands of the primary products and their full semiotic potentials may not be recognised, they would still be more generally identified as 'brands'. In social semiotic terms, the 'specific' semiotic potential of the brands is less likely to be actualised in this context; what remains, however, is the semiotic potential of "previously transient and branded artefacts and rubbish". The recognition of this provenance of Ama-Zing, P n P, and Robertson coasters is a key factor for connecting them to the broader, globally recognised semiotic potentials of upcycling in the developing world as 'ethically responsible' and 'sustainable'.

In terms of value adding, the upcycling process has gone from food packaging—transient objects with rapidly decreasing value—to rubbish, and then back to upcycled transient coasters. These coasters may have less rapidly decreasing use value than the primary food packages, partially due to the stabilising influence of the 'new', robust cork material to which the packaging paper is glued.

Plastic as Semiotic Potential: Curtain

The upcycled artefact in Figure 11.3 is made from cut-up plastic bottles, which are strung on twine to make a curtain to hang across a doorway. It was displayed in a shop in Stockholm, hanging against a glass wall.

Each object in the curtain comprises only one colour. From an experiential perspective, the colours are primary, gaudy, and somewhat exotic, with minimal use of white. All the objects in the curtain have been worked upon in some way; even the bottle tops have holes made in them. Only the tops and bottoms of the bottles have been used, no middle parts. There is aestheticisation (Adami, 2015) of the shapes: The bottom parts of bottles look like flowers. The pattern of the curtain reflects a kind of symmetry. Size is employed as a resource, as there is a pattern of a big bottle top followed by

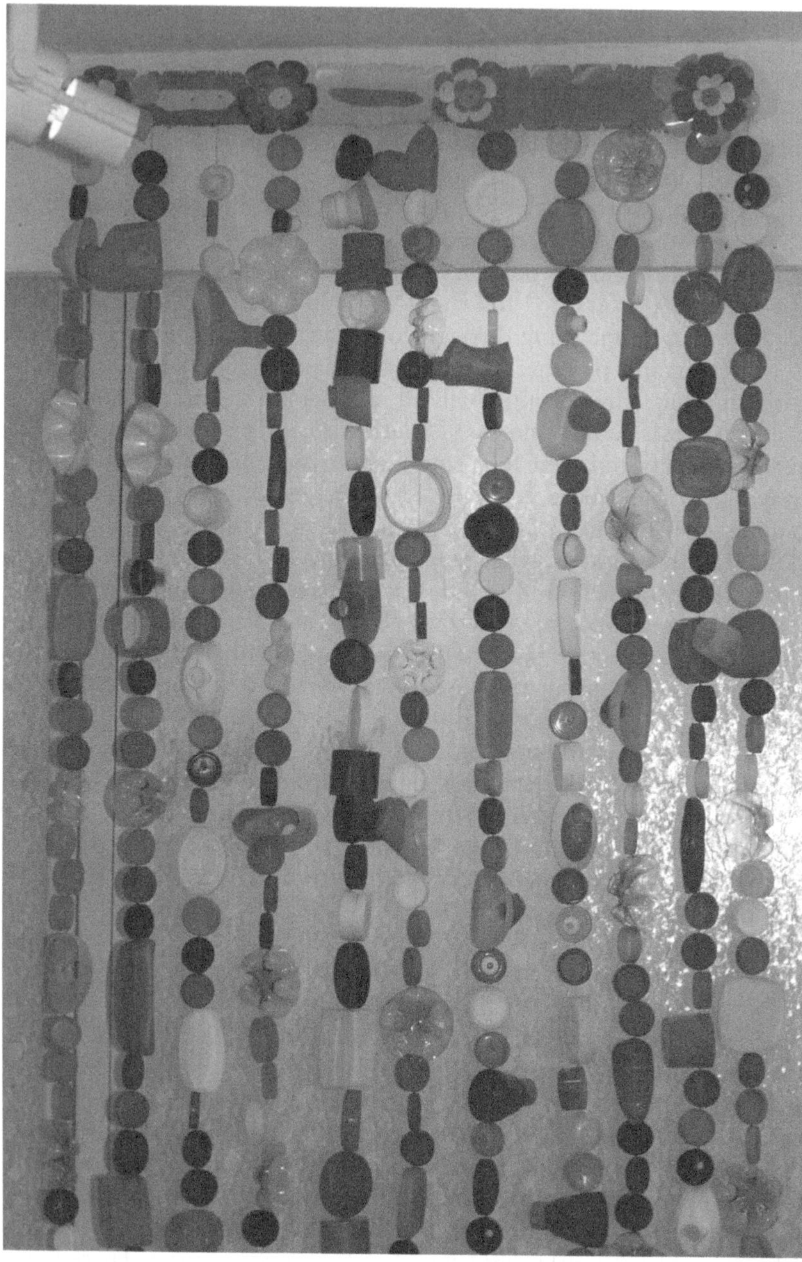

Figure 11.3 Plastic curtain

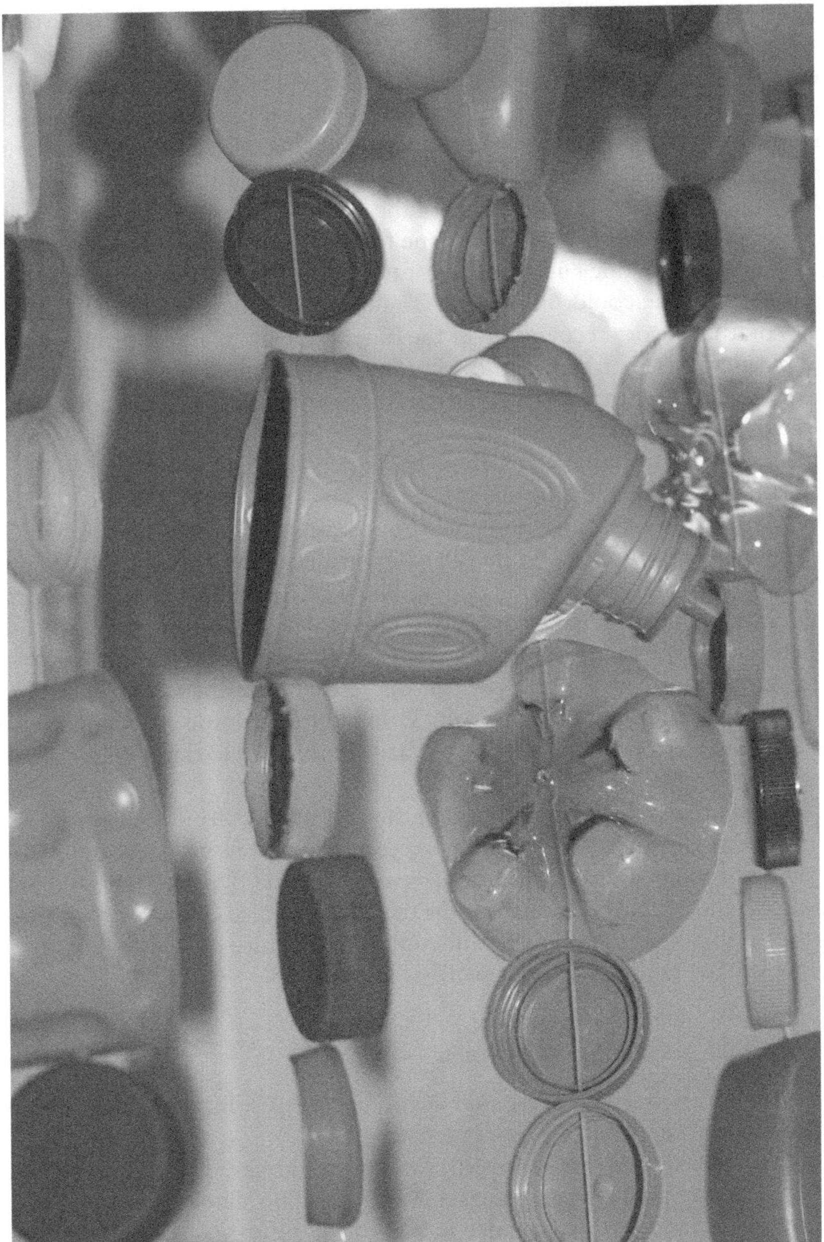

Figure 11.3 (Continued)

three small ones. Colour and shape are also resources in the pattern, with the regular repetition of the yellow bottoms of bottles.

The experiential provenance is significant for the branding of the curtain. In contrast to the objects in Figure 11.1 and Figure 11.2, the plastic bottles that form the curtain's substance have largely had their logos removed, except the bottle tops of 'Minute Maid' and 'Coca-Cola'. Instead, the branding of the curtain as an upcycled product is mostly realised through the semiotic resource of shape, the materiality of the plastic and the aesthetic use of patterning. Shapes of the fragments of the bottles remain recognisable, so we are able to discern the highly mundane function of the objects in other contexts, such as the long curved necks of the toilet cleaner bottles and the lift-up nozzles of the cooldrink bottles. The curtain's 'upcycled' branding thus relies on the sensory recognition of the functional and material properties of the plastic parts that make up the curtain. The connotative provenance of the plastic also plays a role as plastic is detrimental to the environment and is the preferred material of mass production and modernity: the material of "chemistry, not of nature" (Barthes, 1972, p. 54).

In the design of the curtain, we see a play with the provenance of the materials. We see a concoction of irony, humour, and irreverence, which encourages critical reflection on the overconsumption of plastic goods coupled with a desire to own good design. Humour lies in the choice of bottles, especially the predominance of toilet cleaners. The most down-to-earth and practical, cheap plastic objects, described by Barthes (1972, p. 54) as "at once gross and hygienic", have been upcycled for aesthetic purposes. The hand-made patterning of shapes and colour of the plastic parts could also function as a critical commentary towards mass-produced and highly transient plastic.

To sum up, the upcycling process of the curtain goes from transient mass-produced plastic objects of various shapes and functions into rubbish, which is then re-designed into a curtain of transient value. Due to the elaborate, aesthetic and humorous design of the curtain, and also due to its high price in the Stockholm shop, the curtain could also acquire durable value, to be displayed as a piece of art on a wall, as in the shop.

Intertextual Anchorage: Wire Bowls

The bowls in Figure 11.4 were sold in another Stockholm shop, and they are made from plastic-coated telephone wire.

In the bowls, there are no overt branding resources. There is no writing or any other type of typographical resources, and no shapes are directly recognisable as having a provenance in previous artefacts. However, the mixture of different colours into different patterns may point to an experiential provenance in the same type of cultural milieu that was found in the coasters and the curtain. In comparison with the two case studies above, there are no dents, marks, or scratches on the bowls. Nor is there any resemblance to

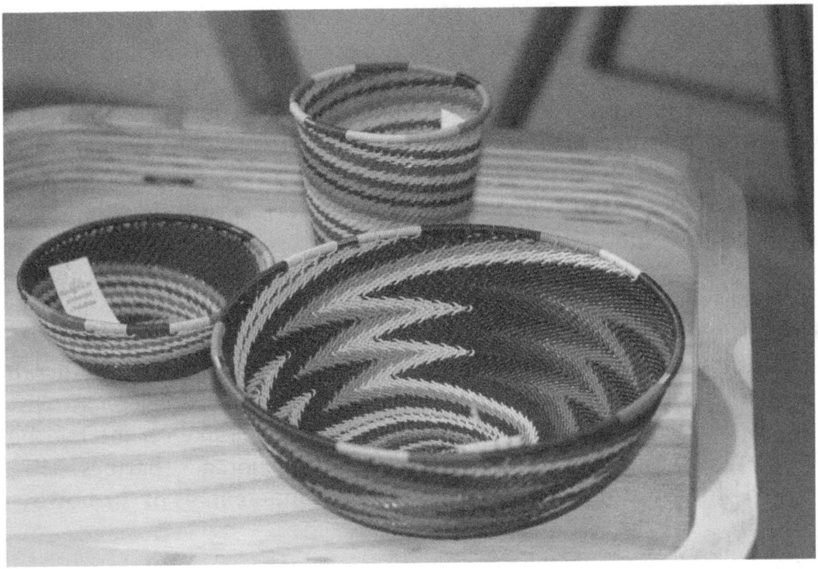

Figure 11.4 Wire bowls

the 'cheap' feel of the material that was found in the curtain. When touching the bowls, it is difficult to recognise the material as wire because of the smooth, seemingly brand-new plastic coating (cf. the semiotic potential of texture, especially of 'complexity', systematically mapped out by Djonov & Van Leeuwen, 2011). In terms of experiential provenance, the potential of the material—the telephone wire—to brand the bowls as upcycled is quite low. In other words, the bowls look so smooth that the 'sustainable', 'ethical' semiotic potential of upcycled products is at risk of being lost.

The branding of the bowls as upcycled, or at least to some extent 'sustainable', is partially to be found in the connotational provenance of the wire bowls in a South African tradition of handcraft, for example weaving and basket-making, in which traditional skills are applied using unconventional material. In terms of connotational provenance, the use of wire, often in combination with beads of different sizes and colours, is common in handmade animal figurines, toy cars, and many other objects in any street market in South Africa. However, the raw material in such objects is often 'new'; the wires and beads are bought just as any raw material to be used in the manufacturing of consumer goods.

In other words, there is connotative provenance for the bowls in an African handicraft tradition of using unconventional materials. However, here we are looking at a process in which the material of the bowls shows no signs of having gone through the stage of being de-valued into rubbish. It is therefore questionable whether the material has moved between Thompson's (1979) categories of value: The wire as a primary product is certainly to be considered as transient, and so are the wire bowls, unless they are treated as durable pieces of art. A move within the category of transient value is more of a process of recycling; a move from transient to durable value could still be considered upcycling, even if the object does not pass through the value category of rubbish.

Since the signs of upcycling may not be not evident in the wire objects themselves, the connection to the values of upcycling is instead made by a close intertextual relation between the bowls and a written tag carefully attached to them. The written tag states that the bowl is "Handmade out of telephone wire in South Africa" ('Handgjord av telefontråd i Sydafrika'), thus connecting the bowls to a physical location, South Africa, to handicraft, but also explicitly pointing out the unconventional material: telephone wire. There is no mentioning of upcycling, trashion or the like on the tag, but the message of the tag functions as a sort of 'anchorage' (Barthes, 1977, p. 38–41) for the semiotic, economic, and ethical potentials of the bowls.

5. Conclusion

Our aim has been to explore how artefacts produced in the developing world are branded with regard to upcycling as well as to gain an understanding of the process of value adding as such artefacts move between categories of value. The analysis has pointed out a few key semiotic resources for branding and value adding in upcycled artefacts. The most directly noticeable resources are writing and other typographical resources (such as typeface, shape, and logos) that are recontextualised from a primary product into the upcycled artefact. Colour is another resource that is recontextualised from earlier stages in the processes of upcycling. In addition, everyday household materials like used tin, plastic, and plastic coated paper are resources that explicitly point to the upcycled nature of an artefact. We argue that when such semiotic resources are combined and elaborately remixed in the redesign of an artefact or used materials, they become a higher-order signifier for 'upcycling' in the developing world, a sort of trademark that is generally recognised as 'ethical', 'sustainable', and 'responsible'.

Value adding in upcycling to a large extent depends on the formation of such higher order signifiers. This paper has shown how processes of value adding can be performed in at least three different ways (not excluding other possibilities): as *spatio-linguistic recontextualisation, sensory recontextualisation*, or through *intertextual anchorage as a marker of provenance*. The first refers to the manifest recontextualisation of brand names, logos, colours, and patterns from a primary artefact to an upcycled artefact, for example the use of brand names and logos such as 'P n P' and 'amaZing' on coasters (Figure 11.2). In *sensory recontextualisation*, there is a manifest recontextualisation of specific materials and shapes from a primary artefact to an upcycled artefact, as in the use of household plastic with partially maintained shapes in the curtain (Figure 11.3). In cases where the provenance of materials and resources in rubbish or, at least in less valued primary products, is not recognisable in the artefact as such, intertextual anchorage can be used as a marker of provenance. The analysed bowls are part of the same commercial culture as the other upcycled artefacts, sold in the same types of shops, and they are handmade in South Africa, just like the other products. However, with the exception of their colourful patterns, none of the semiotic resources that make up the branded remix of resources were found. Instead the bowls were intertextually connected to upcycling and its 'ethical' values through a tag with writing in Swedish.

Our approach has shown how upcycling may work as a movement of objects between at least two categories of value: from transient value, for example the value of a toilet cleaning bottle, to the value of rubbish, a toilet cleaning bottle disposed on a beach in the Western Cape, in order to end up as upcycled, transient, or, depending on its use, durable value as a curtain sold in a shop in Stockholm, Sweden. As social semioticians, we are not only interested in showing the global, iterative nature of such recontextualisation, we are also able to show how the transformation of value was traceable in the materiality and design of the artefacts.

This approach has implications for critiquing the production of ethical discourses around global upcycling practices. The analysis of meaning-making through upcycling across global contexts raises questions about how artefacts can mobilise societal and cultural difference for profit. The practice of upcycling in the developing world of the type we have analysed here is often driven by the need to sell products on any available market in order to survive. This is a practice that has different roots than the 'unconsumption' movement that prevails in many parts of the Western world (Unconsumption Blog, 2015). Although the consumption of upcycled artefacts from the developing world may both *be* and *feel* more ethical, and even though upcycled artefacts can be creative and function as means for critical comment on various issues, including mass consumerism, upcycling as consumption and production is still largely oriented towards globalised consumer markets. We provide a semiotically grounded way of looking at such processes, focusing on recontextualisation and provenance. This way of looking could be useful in the critique of artefacts, but perhaps it can also complement other critical approaches in related fields such as anthropology, sociology, and material culture.

References

Adami, E. (2015). Aesthetics in digital texts beyond writing: A social semiotic multimodal framework. In A. Archer & E. Breuer (Eds.), *Multimodality in writing: The state of the art in theory, methodology and pedagogy* (pp. 43–62). Leiden/Boston, MA: Brill.

Albinsson, P. A., & Yasanthi Perera, B. (2012). Alternative marketplaces in the 21st century: Building community through sharing events. *Journal of Consumer Behaviour*, *11*, 303–315.

Archer, A. (2008). Cultural studies meets academic literacies: Exploring students' resources through symbolic objects. *Teaching in Higher Education*, *13*(4), 383–394.

Bakhtin, M. M. 1981. *The dialogic imagination: Four essays*. Austin, TX: University of Texas Press.

Barthes, R. (1972). Toys. In *Mythologies*. London: Vintage.

Barthes, R. (1977). Rhetoric of the image. In S. Heath (Trans.), *Image music text*. London: Fontana Press.

Björkvall, A. (2014). Practical function and meaning: A case study of IKEA tables. In C. Jewitt (Ed.), *The Routledge handbook of multimodal analysis* (2nd ed., pp. 342–353). London/New York: Routledge.

Björkvall, A., & Karlsson, A.-M. (2011). The materiality of discourses and the semiotics of materials: A social perspective on the meaning potentials of written texts and furniture. *Semiotica*, *187*, 141–165.

Chang Coupland, J. (2005). Invisible brands: An ethnography of households and the brands in their kitchen pantries. *Journal of Consumer Research*, *32*, 106–119.

Crabbe, A. 2012. Three strategies for sustainable design in the developing world. *DesignIssues*, *28*(2), 6–15.

Djonov, E., & Van Leeuwen, T. (2011). The semiotics of texture: From tactile to visual. *Visual Communication*, *10*(4), 541–564.

Emgin, B. (2012). Trashion: The return of the disposed. *DesignIssues*, *28*(1), 63–71.

Frow, J. (2003). Invidious distinction: Waste, difference, and classy stuff. In G. Hawkins & S. Muecke (Eds.), *Culture and waste: The creation and destruction of value* (pp. 25–38). Lanham/Boulder, CO/New York/Oxford: Rowman & Littlefield.

Halliday, M. A. K. (1978). *Language as social semiotic: The social interpretation of language and meaning*. London: Edward Arnold.

Hetherington, K. (2004). Secondhandedness: Consumption, disposal, and absent presence. *Environment and Planning: Society and Space*, *22*, 157–173.

Hodge, R., & Kress, G. (1988). *Social semiotics*. Cambridge: Polity Press.

Interview with artist (2013, March). Cape Town, South Africa.

Kress, G. (2010). *Multimodality: A social semiotic approach to contemporary communication*. London/New York: Routledge.

Kress, G., & Van Leeuwen, T. (2001). *Multimodal discourse: The modes and media of contemporary communication*. London: Arnold.

Linell, P. (1998). *Approaching dialogue: Talk, interaction and contextx in dialogical perspectives*. Amsterdam/Philadelphia, PA: John Benjamins.

McDonough, W., & Braungart, M. (2002). *Cradle to cradle: Remaking the way we make things*. New York: North Point Press.

McDonough, W., & Braungart, M. (2013). *The upcycle: Beyond sustainability—designing for abundance*. New York: North Point Press.

Thompson, M. (1979). *Rubbish theory: The creation and destruction of value*. Oxford: Oxford University Press.

Unconsumption blog (2015, February 3). Retrieved from www.unconsumption.tumblr.com

Van Leeuwen, T. (2005). *Introducing social semiotics*. London/New York: Routledge.

Van Leeuwen, T. (2008). *Discourse and practice: New tools for critical discourse analysis*. Oxford: Oxford University Press.

12 Multimodal Recontextualisations of Images in Violent Extremist Discourse

Kay L. O'Halloran, Sabine Tan, Peter Wignell, and Rebecca Lange

1. Introduction: Multimodal Discourse Analysis and Big Data

Van Leeuwen's (2008, p. vii) view "that all [multimodal] discourses recontextualise social practices, and that all knowledge is, therefore, ultimately grounded in practice" arose from his seminal work as co-founder of critical discourse analysis and multimodal semiotics, which is concerned with the study of the interaction of language, images and other resources in texts, interactions, and events. Using Bernstein's (1990) concept of recontextualisation, Van Leeuwen (2008) develops a model of recontextualising principles to explain how changes in social practices take place recursively through multimodal discourse. The approach involves the reconfiguration of social actors, activities, and circumstantial elements across sequences of multimodal activities, which function to regulate social practices. That is, the selective appropriation, relocation, and refocusing of key semiotic elements in relation to other discourses results in the creation of new abstract orders and orderings which are enacted as social practices (Bernstein, 1990; Van Leeuwen, 2008).

In this chapter, we present the findings from a pilot study which builds on and expands Van Leeuwen's (2008) recontextualisation principles to analyse violent extremist propaganda materials and the multimodal contextualisation and recontextualisation of images from these sources. More specifically, the aim is to develop a mixed-methods approach (see O'Halloran, Tan, Pham, Bateman, & Vande Moere, 2016) to analyse how violent extremist groups use language and images to propagate and legitimise their views, incite violence and influence recruits in online propaganda materials, and how the images from these materials are re-used in different media platforms to support and resist violent extremism. In doing so, the overall aim is to develop empirical approaches for the analysis of large datasets of multimodal texts (e.g., Bateman, 2014; O'Halloran, Chua, & Podlasov, 2014; O'Halloran, Tan, Pham, Bateman, & Vande Moere, 2016) and to develop the theory and practice of Multimodal Discourse Analysis.

One of the major problems with large datasets is that texts and images need to be interpreted in relation to context. For this reason, the proposed

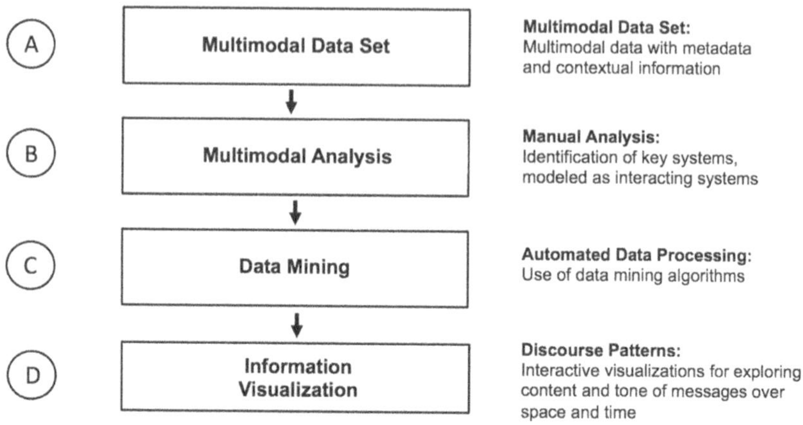

Figure 12.1 A mixed-methods approach to the multimodal analysis of big data (O'Halloran, Tan, Pham, Bateman, & Vande Moere, 2016)

approach (see O'Halloran, Tan, Pham, Bateman, & Vande Moere, 2016; O'Halloran et al., 2016) involves compiling multimodal datasets with accompanying metadata (e.g., date, location, source, URL) and contextual information (e.g., higher-order semantic classifications of keywords and objects derived from Wikipedia classifications). From there, the results derived from manual analysis using software applications (e.g., Multimodal Analysis Image) are used to identify key patterns of interacting system choices. Machine learning techniques are then applied to these results in order to develop automated data mining techniques for analysis of large datasets, using the contextual information provided by the metadata and Wikipedia. The resulting discourse patterns are then explored qualitatively using interactive visualisation applications. The proposed research framework is displayed in Figure 12.1.

In what follows, we discuss the initial results of a pilot project which is the first step towards the development of the mixed-methods approach described above. The online magazine *Dabiq*,[1] produced by Islamic State (henceforth referred to as ISIS, also known as ISIL), is chosen for this purpose. In this study, we developed a framework for categorising the images and article types in *Dabiq*. Following this, we developed and used an interactive visualisation application to (a) investigate how the images, article types and their combinations in *Dabiq* change over time, and (b) trace recontextualised images imported into *Dabiq* and recontextualisations of images from *Dabiq* across different media platforms. In what follows, we describe the multimodal dataset under consideration, the background of ISIS, and some preliminary findings from this pilot project.

2. The Multimodal Dataset

The multimodal dataset which forms the basis of investigations in this pilot study comes from the English language edition of ISIS's official online magazine *Dabiq*. ISIS is chosen for this study because of their notoriety as a violent extremist group and their prolific media output (Zelin, 2015). *Dabiq* is chosen because it is "one of the few original sources of data that directly comes from ISIS" (Vergani & Bliuc, 2015, p. 8). In what follows, the background of ISIS and their beliefs about Islam are briefly reviewed.

2.1 *ISIS Background*

ISIS has, since June 2014, referred to itself as 'Al Dawla al-Islamiyya'. The Arabic name is most often translated into English as 'Islamic State'. Translations into English imply that the kind of 'state' envisaged is akin to a modern nation state. However, the Arabic name is as much religious as it is political. The 'state' imagined by ISIS is a totalitarian theocracy characterised by a strict implementation of Shari'a. It is an attempt to re-imagine and re-create a caliphate, the type of government that originated during the expansion of Islam in the time of the Prophet Muhammad and his successors.

The leader of a caliphate, the caliph, is an absolute, autocratic ruler considered to be the religious, political, and military successor to the Prophet Muhammad and the leader of the entire Muslim community (Bowering et al., 2012, p. 81–86). On 29 June 2014, ISIS declared a caliphate covering territory it controlled in Iraq and Syria. One major platform in the ISIS agenda is to consolidate and expand its caliphate.

2.2 *ISIS's Interpretation of Islam*

The rationale behind the interpretation of Islam adopted by ISIS is an extreme reading of the doctrines of an Islamic movement known as Salafism. Salafism is a socially and religiously conservative, fundamentalist faction of Sunni Islam which is followed by around "3% of the world's Muslim population" (Rashid, 2015, p. 23). The name refers to the generation of Muslims who were contemporaries of the Prophet Muhammad and the two subsequent generations (Olidort, 2015). Salafists consider this earliest form of Islam to be the pure form and reject any subsequent innovations. Salafists have a highly literal, 'black and white' approach to interpreting Islamic scripture and see no separation between religion and state, as Allah alone is seen as having the right to make laws, which were revealed through the Prophet Muhammad.

Salafism itself is not a unified movement (Blanchard, 2007). Salafists can be broadly divided into three groups: The purists, who are the largest group and who avoid politics; the second largest group are the activists, who are politically active but work through existing political institutions; and the smallest group, the jihadists, who form a small minority but have the largest public profile. It is this latter faction, Jihadist Salafism (Kepel, 2002), that provides the theological, ideological, and practical bases for movements like ISIS. Jihadist Salafists operate under an extreme, militaristic definition of 'jihad', which they regard as an obligation to conduct a military campaign against everyone who they perceive to be threats to and enemies of Islam. Islam's enemies are regarded as either consisting of or being orchestrated by "an insidious alliance of Crusaders and Jews" (Tabarani, 2011, p. 11).

2.3 Dabiq Magazine

ISIS puts forward an explicit and unequivocal agenda and an integral instrument for disseminating that agenda is its online magazine *Dabiq*. *Dabiq* is published in a number of languages, including English, and is one place where ISIS makes its agenda accessible to the non-Arabic speaking world. Fifteen issues of *Dabiq* have been published between 5 July 2015 and 31 July 2016, making it a rich source of data on ISIS. As the material from the latest issue had yet to be extracted at the time of writing, the material from Issue 15 is not included in the discussion below.

3. Theoretical Approach: Van Leeuwen's Social Semiotics

The analytical approach adopted here is multimodal social semiotic theory, which studies human signifying processes as social practices and which is concerned with different sign systems and their integration in texts and social activities, interpreted within the context of the situation and culture (e.g., Halliday, 1978; Van Leeuwen, 2005). One of the key tenets of social semiotic theory is the premise that language and other semiotic resources are structured according to the functions which the resources have evolved to serve in society: (a) experiential and logical meaning to structure our experience of the world; (b) interpersonal meaning to enact social relations and create a stance towards happenings and entities in the world; and (c) textual meaning to organise experiential, logical and interpersonal meanings into coherent messages (e.g., Halliday & Matthiessen, 2014). Although initially applied to language, the metafunctional principle has since been adapted and expanded to the study of visual images and other semiotic artefacts and phenomena to account for the ways in which linguistic and non-linguistic resources combine in the communication of meaning (e.g., Kress & Van Leeuwen, 2006; Van Leeuwen, 2005). According to Van Leeuwen (2005, p. 1) "social semiotics is a form of enquiry. It does not offer ready-made answers. It offers ideas for formulating questions and ways of searching for answers". It is this broad view of social semiotics that provides the theoretical foundations for interpreting the text and image combinations in *Dabiq* in the first phase of this study. A more systemically oriented approach in which semiotic resources are conceptualised as systems of meaning with networks of options from which choices are made in the communication of meaning in multimodal texts will be undertaken in the next phase of the project. In this case, choices in the metafunctionally organised systems of lower-level features such as Participant Type, Dress, Gaze, Gesture, Shot Distance, Camera Angle, Colour Contrast, Camera Focus, and Compositional Vectors will be used to inform machine learning techniques to develop data mining algorithms for the automated analysis of the larger dataset. These will then be combined with the higher order semantic classifications of keywords derived from Wikipedia (see O'Halloran et al., 2016) in an attempt to build on and expand Van Leeuwen's social semiotic frameworks to the analysis of large multimodal datasets.

4. Exploring (Re)Contextualisations of Social Practices Through Text-Image Combinations in *Dabiq*

As Kress and Van Leeuwen (2006, p. 177) explain, when analysing composite multimodal texts comprising text-image combinations, the question arises "whether the meanings of the whole should be treated as the sum of the meanings of the parts or whether the parts should be looked upon as interacting with and affecting one another". Rather than looking at the contributions of individual semiotic resources, this pilot study looks the overall meaning that arises from the text-image combinations in *Dabiq*.

In the first phase of the study, 14 issues of *Dabiq* were downloaded. Each image, as well as the page it appeared on, was extracted and image files were catalogued according to (a) which issue the image was from; and (b) what page of the issue it was from. In total 1,012 images were classified into 11 superordinate categories and 75 sub-categories according to distinguishing features, their subject matter (i.e. experiential meaning) and their context. Table 12.1 shows the superordinate image categories and defines key terms used in the classification.

The articles in *Dabiq* were classified according to article titles and matched with issues to determine their distribution across issues (see Table 12.2). The labels we assign to *Dabiq* article types, although different in wording, more or less match the content of those used by Colas (2016, p. 3–5).

The images were then matched to the article types, which provide contextual information for identifying and classifying the different image types. The resulting text-image combinations reflect ISIS's motivations and interests and thus form the basis for understanding the worldview adopted by ISIS in its online magazine (e.g., see Colas, 2016; Wignell, Tan, & O'Halloran, 2017). This is in line with Van Leeuwen's (2008) conceptualisation of discourse as recontextualised social practice.

Before exploring the larger patterns of text-image connections and their recontextualisations in *Dabiq* and other media in Section 5, we first discuss the typical text-image combinations that are found in *Dabiq*, and make some initial observations about (a) how these serve to contextualise ISIS's

Table 12.1 Image classifications and explanations of key terms

	Image Category	*Description (Experiential Meaning)*
1.	FAR ENEMY	The term Far Enemy is used by Jihadist Salafists to refer to Western sponsors of Arab regimes: the United States, its Western allies and Israel (Burke, 2004, p. 19).
2.	NEAR ENEMY	The term Near Enemy was initially applied to secular Arab regimes considered apostate by jihadis (Byman, 2003, p. 146). It is also used to refer to other secular Muslim regimes (Gerges, 2009, p. 1).
3.	ISIS HEROES	Heroes are people, living and dead, regarded by ISIS as worthy of emulation. Hero images are sub-classified according to whether the hero is alive—mostly mujahideen, or dead—martyrs.
4.	ISIS ICONS	The concept of 'icons' is derived from SFL work on iconisation (Martin & Stenglin, 2007; Martin & Zappavigna, 2013; Tann, 2013). Three prominent ISIS icons are identified: the ISIS flag, the AK47 assault rifle, and what we refer to as the Tawheed gesture. These icons are often used in combination with other image categories.
5.	HISTORICAL RECREATIONS	Historical re-creations are usually staged or photoshopped, representations of apocalyptic events and historical events.
6.	ISIS LAW ENFORCEMENT	These are typically in situ documentary shots showing ISIS involved in aspects of Shari'a law enforcement.
7.	ISIS SOCIAL WELFARE	These are a combination of in situ documentary shots and in situ posed shots showing ISIS engaged in social welfare activities.
8.	OTHER ISIS OBJECTS, PLACES, EVENTS	Assorted ISIS-related imagery.
9.	OTHER OBJECTS, PLACES, EVENTS	Assorted non-ISIS-related imagery.
10.	PLEDGES OF ALLEGIANCE	Images of actions signifying allegiance to ISIS.
11.	SCRIPTURE	Includes images of scripture in Arabic. Also includes enacted creed, depicting mujahideen reading scripture, or showing them in prayer after 'victory'.

beliefs, values, and social practices, and (b) how these multimodal propaganda materials may appeal to audiences. Examples of typical image-article type combinations in *Dabiq* are shown in Figure 12.2.

Foreword: The Foreword (called the Introduction in Issue 1) features in every issue of *Dabiq*. The articles are akin to editorials and reflect ISIS

Table 12.2 Article types in *Dabiq*

	Article Type / *Issue*	*1*	*2*	*3*	*4*	*5*	*6*	*7*	*8*	*9*	*10*	*11*	*12*	*13*	*14*
1.	Cover	■	■	■	■	■	■	■	■	■	■	■	■	■	■
2.	Table of Contents	■	■	■	■	■	■	■	■	■	■	■	■	■	■
3.	Last Page Message	■	■	■	■	■	■	■	■	■	■	■	■	■	■
4.	Foreword	■	■	■	■	■	■	■	■	■	■	■	■	■	■
5.	Hikmah (Wisdom)	■	■	■	■	■	■	■	■	■	■	■	■	■	■
6.	In the Words of the Enemy	■	■	■	■	■	■	■	■	■	■	■	■	■	■
7.	Feature Articles	■	■	■	■	■	■	■	■	■	■	■	■	■	■
8.	ISIS Reports		■	■	■	■	■	■	■	■		■	■	■	■
9.	Advertisements		■	■				■	■	■	■	■	■	■	■
10.	Far Enemy Captives			■	■			■				■	■		
11.	John Cantlie (Captive British Journalist)				■	■	■	■	■	■			■		■
12.	Near Enemy Issues						■		■	■	■	■	■	■	
13.	Amongst the Believers are Men							■	■	■	■	■	■	■	■
14.	From the Pages of History							■	■	■	■	■	■	■	■
15.	From/To Our Sisters							■	■	■	■	■	■	■	
16.	Interviews								■	■	■	■	■	■	■

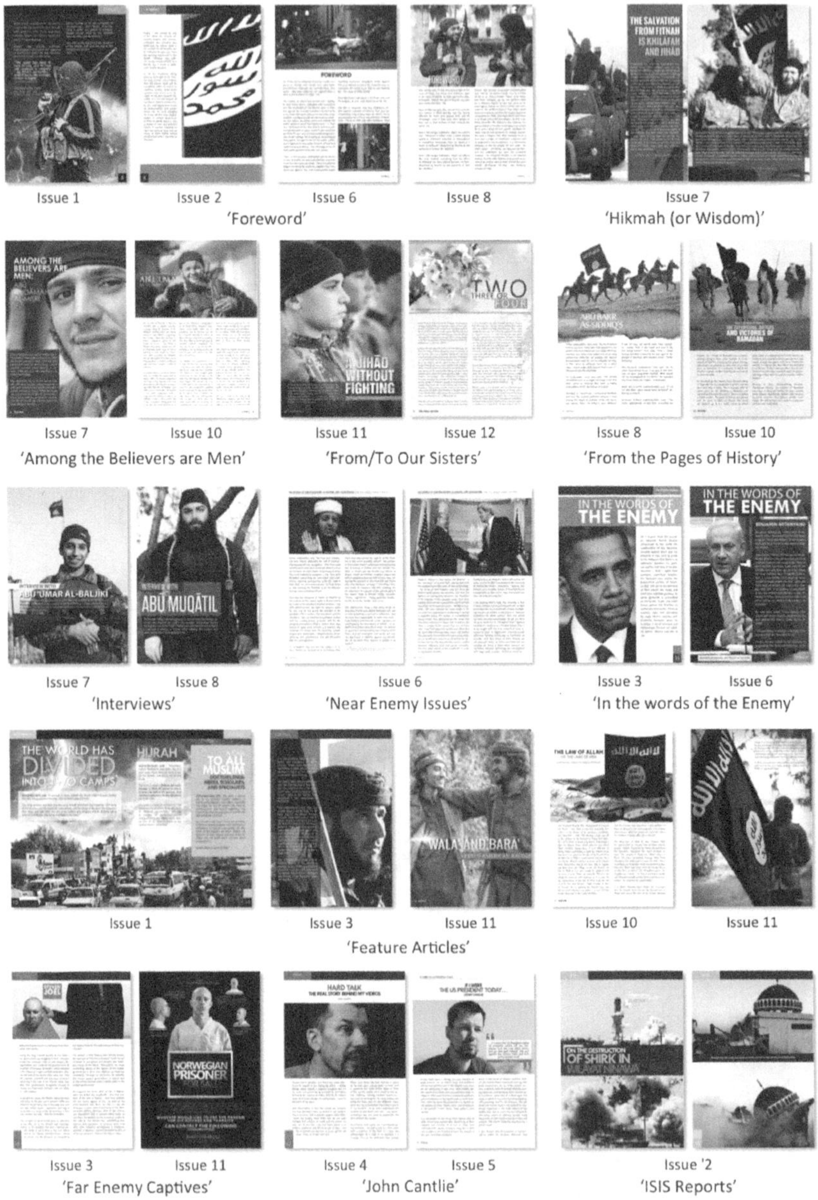

Figure 12.2 Examples of image-article type combinations in *Dabiq*, Issues 1–14

values. Topics are varied and include migration to ISIS territory, encouragement of lone-wolf attacks, gloating reports on attacks on Western countries, denunciations of the Far Enemy, promises of ISIS victory, and gloating reports about attacks on the Near Enemy (especially Shi'a Muslims), which are all legitimised by ISIS through references to selected Islamic scripture that pervade the articles. The images included with this type of article (48) range over 18 different categories and sub-categories. By far the most commonly featured images (15 out of 48) depict Attacks by ISIS on the Far Enemy (e.g. Issues 6, 8, 10, 12–14). However, in terms of their interpersonal appeal, these images, which tend to be imported from mainstream news media, are not necessarily salient. As Colas (2016, p. 3) aptly points out, a 'page count', or in this case, an image count, "does not equate to a reader's emotional response". Kress and Van Leeuwen (2006) and Van Leeuwen (2005) refer to salience as the way which visual elements attract the viewer's attention because of their size, colour, contrast, etc. In this sense, the images of an ISIS Hero and an ISIS Flag in Issues 1 and 2, which set out ISIS's agenda and values, are far more prominent and eye-catching.

Hikmah (or Wisdom) and Among the Believers Are Men: 'Hikmah (or Wisdom)' is a series of religiously inspired feature articles which appear in every issue of *Dabiq*, Hikmah articles usually contain large, striking images (25 in total, from 19 different categories and sub-categories), often occupying the whole page. The most frequently featured images are, again, of ISIS Heroes (seven images), specifically mujahideen engaged in the act of celebration (e.g. Issue 7) and pre and post martyrdom images of martyrs. In Issues 7 to 14, Hikmah articles are usually followed by the article type 'Among the Believers are Men', mostly stories of ISIS Heroes, particularly of exemplary martyrs. The image sub-category martyrs-in-narrative, which depicts the life and exploits of the martyr, features prominently in the majority of images (17 out of 20). These image-article type combinations reflect ISIS's ideology and social practices as embodied through emblems, logos, flags, rituals, and ceremonies (for a more detailed discussion of ISIS's worldview and values as represented through 'bonding icons' in *Dabiq*, see Wignell, Tan, & O'Halloran, 2017).

From/To Our Sisters: In the later issues of *Dabiq* (7–13), articles paying homage to martyrs are frequently followed by the article type 'From/To Our Sisters', which deals with a range of topics on what ISIS considers women's issues. Topics include: migration to ISIS lands, slave girls or prostitutes, advice to wives of Muslims fighting against ISIS, the role of women in jihad, how many wives a man can have, how widows should behave, and an interview with the widow of a martyr. The most frequently appearing images are of ISIS children dressed in military fatigues (e.g., Issues 10 and 11), perhaps with the intent to appeal to female ISIS sympathisers. They also contain images of a martyred husband (Issue 7), or a series of innocuous background images likely sourced from image banks (e.g., Issues 8, 9, and 12). Although these articles have a woman's name as the by-line, and appear to be written by a woman, they do not contain any images of women at all. In other words, although women are included as social actors in the linguistic text, all women are visually excluded from the discourse[2] (e.g., see Van Leeuwen, 2008 for a discussion on the representation of social actors).

From the Pages of History: Another article type that appears only in the later issues of *Dabiq* (7–14) is 'From the Pages of History'. A common topic in these articles is the placing of blame on the Near and Far Enemies. However, images depicting the Near and Far Enemies, although frequent (13 out of 30 images, Issues 7, 9, 11, and 13), are not necessarily salient in terms of their size and compositional placement within the page. Instead, the dynamicity portrayed by men on horseback with swords in staged images of historical conquests, which are paired with articles about the reconstruction of past Islamic 'glory days' (Issues 8, 10, and 14), makes them interpersonally more engaging.

Interviews: Interviews, usually with leaders of other organisations that have pledged allegiance to ISIS, are likewise found only in the later issues of *Dabiq* (7–14). The articles contain a variety of diverse images (49), ranging over 23 categories and sub-categories. The most frequently occurring images are depictions of the Near Enemy (23 images), with Near Enemy Leaders and Public Figures being the most common (14 images). However, like in articles 'From the Pages of History', these images are usually non-salient and embedded within the article. Generally, large, ISIS-related images are only placed at the beginning of the article. Many of those images feature ISIS Heroes (e.g., Issues 7, 8, 12, and 13), although they may not always be the subject of the interview. Often staged or posed, these 'heroes' occupy the whole page and address the reader directly through their gaze, which possibly makes them interpersonally appealing to both ISIS supporters and those that resist terrorist discourses (see discussion in Section 5.4 on the results of the reverse image search).

Near Enemy Issues and In the Words of the Enemy: Near Enemy Issues are articles that criticise the Near Enemy. They are found in Issue 6 and Issues 8–13. Not surprisingly, images depicting the Near Enemy (44 out of 74 images from 26 categories and sub-categories) are most frequently featured in this type of article. The article type 'In the words of the Enemy' appears in every issue of *Dabiq*. These articles are mostly concerned with highlighting the strength of ISIS, and showing enemies as disunited, or showing Far Enemy Leaders, Jews, and Near Enemy leaders as being in collusion, which is also reflected in the images. Most images (46 over 12 different categories and sub-categories) appear to be imported and are usually large, unflattering close shots of grim or pensive looking Far Enemy Leaders and Public Figures (25 images in total).

Feature Articles: Feature articles (40) appear in every issue of *Dabiq* (often more than one article per issue) and are the most varied article type. They cover a wide variety of different topics, including, why ISIS is the legitimate ruler of all Muslims, advice to mujahideen on their obligations, jihad, denunciation of Jews, Shi'a Muslims and Crusaders, conspiracies between the Far and Near Enemy and why ISIS is right and other jihadist and nationalist groups are wrong. Feature articles usually contain a plethora of citations from Islamic scripture to support the points they are making. The images (255) included with feature articles are similarly diverse, ranging over 78 categories and sub-categories. While the most frequently occurring images are from the Far and Near Enemy categories (74 images), few of these images are very salient. Instead, the most prominent images with the power to engage readers at an interpersonal level are those that directly reflect ISIS's values (e.g., see Wignell, Tan, & O'Halloran, 2017), depicting a variety of ISIS Heroes (57 images), and ISIS Icons (18 images), such as ISIS flags and Tawheed gestures (one arm raised with the index finger pointing skywards, which is meant to signify the indivisible oneness of Allah (Zelinsky, 2014)). The most salient and interpersonally engaging images (in terms of compositional arrangement, framing, colour, and size) are perhaps found in Issue 1.

Far Enemy Captives: Another type of feature article is concerned explicitly with the fate of Far Enemy captives. The articles, found in Issues 3, 4, 7, 11, and 12, are about the punishment of captives for 'crimes' against ISIS by the country the captive is from. The majority of images (15 out of 22 images) show Far Enemy Captives wearing a 'Guantanamo jumpsuit', often posed as if about to be executed (all captives depicted in these images were subsequently killed). Some images display the body of the captive(s) after death (e.g., Issue 4 and 12). Images of this kind serve a dual purpose: attracting ISIS sympathisers to their cause, and shocking and intimidating mainstream audiences who may find these images distasteful and offensive.

John Cantlie: John Cantlie is a British journalist who was captured by ISIS in 2012 and who writes commentaries in support of ISIS (under duress). These articles, which appear in Issues 4–9, 12, and 14, stand out from the rest of the articles in *Dabiq*, as they follow typical Western journalistic editorial or op-ed style, written mostly in the first person. The articles are usually positioned towards the end of the magazine, and include a total of 28 images from 12 categories and sub-categories. In some issues, the articles include large, prominent images of the author, often on the first and last page of the article (Issues 4–6). Two of the articles depict the author as a Far Enemy Captive wearing a 'Guantanamo jumpsuit' (Issue 4 and 12), while other issues show him dressed in civilian clothes, perhaps in an attempt to show that Cantlie has accepted or even embraced ISIS's way of life, and to legitimise the views expressed as his own.

ISIS Reports: These articles, which can be found in Issues 1–9, 11, 13, and 14, are mostly local and district reports of ISIS military activity and successes. The reports are news-like, matter of fact, and often composed almost entirely of images with captions, particularly in the early issues of *Dabiq*. Although the images themselves (321, ranging over 81 categories and sub-categories) are mainly shot in documentary style, their compositional arrangement, size, framing, and large headlines and captions render them interpersonally salient. The most frequently featured images are concerned with the Near Enemy (124 images), specifically Actions by ISIS against the Near Enemy (94 images), blowing things up and destroying 'shirk' (objects related to polytheism and idol-worship) (37 and 22 images respectively). Explicit images of Near Enemy battle casualties (10 images) also feature frequently. Documentary images of this kind serve to create authenticity and provide evidence of ISIS's successes in expanding the caliphate.

In the above section, we discussed some of the social practices (re)contextualised in the text-image combinations typically found in *Dabiq*. These serve as a basis for exploring larger patterns of distribution, which are discussed in the following section.

5. Exploring Text-Image Connections and Recontextualisations Through Interactive Visualisations

Information visualisation permits exploration of patterns in large, multidimensional datasets through a range of tasks, such as overviewing the whole dataset, zooming into items of interest, filtering out items, selecting details-on-demand, and extracting sub-collections (Shneiderman, 1996). In this case, the prototype Multimodal Analysis Visualisation application (MMA Visualisation app) has several different visualisations for displaying *Dabiq* image categories and text types, combinations of images and texts in *Dabiq* and the results of reverse image searches, which show where images in *Dabiq* are located across different online media sites over time. In what follows, we illustrate some of the initial findings of text-image connections in *Dabiq* and the reserve image search.

5.1 Image-Article Type Distribution

Image-article type distributions can be visualised by means of simple pie charts. Our analysis revealed that the distribution of images and articles types in *Dabiq* is not constant but shifts in tandem with the state of affairs and evolving agenda of ISIS over time. Figure 12.3a (top), for example, shows that, in the first issue of *Dabiq*, greater emphasis is placed on ISIS Heroes (29% of all images). Figure 12.3a (bottom) reveals that the emphasis on ISIS Heroes diminishes in the later issues of *Dabiq*, such as in Issue 12, which was released more than a year later on 18 November 2015 (almost immediately after the Paris attacks on 13 November 2015), where images of ISIS Heroes account for only 15%. Here, emphasis is placed on the Near and Far Enemy, which together make up more than half of all images (52%), reflecting ISIS's concern with attacks on Near and Far Enemy countries. At the same time, while there were only seven article types in the first issue, the diversity of article types also increased in the later issues of *Dabiq*.

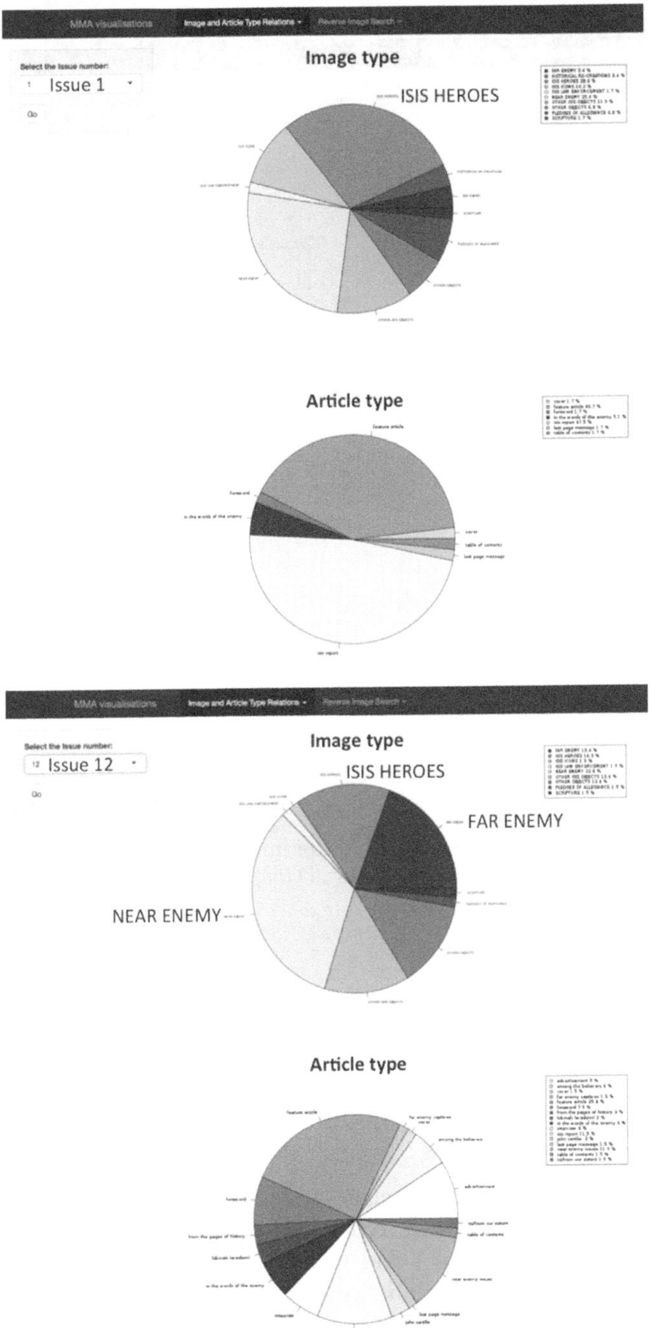

Figure 12.3a Comparison of image-article type distribution in *Dabiq* Issue 1 (top) and Issue 12 (bottom)

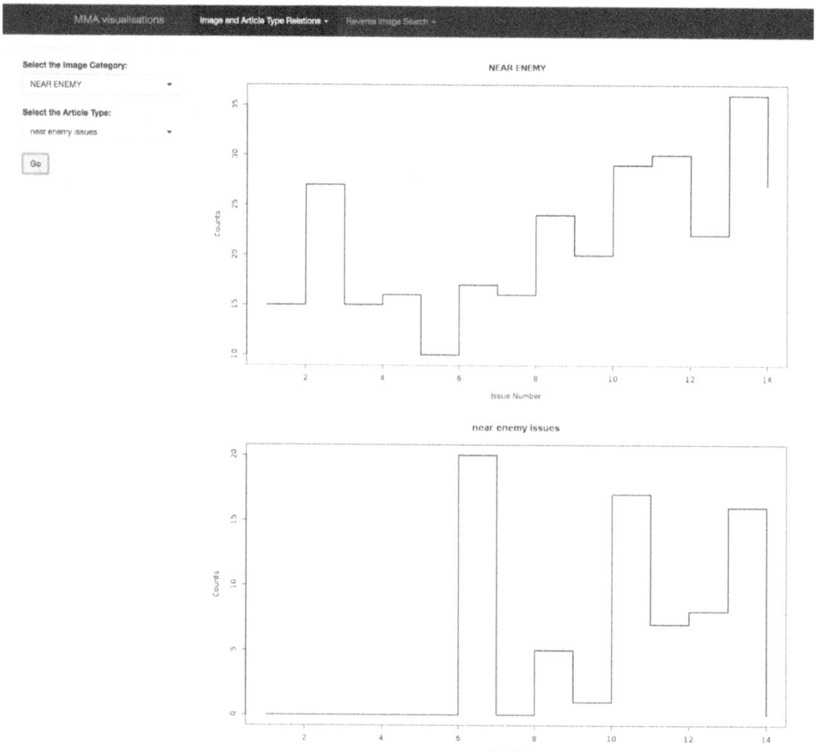

Figure 12.3b Image-article type frequency analysis for image category 'Near Enemy' and article type 'Near Enemy Issues', *Dabiq* Issues 1–14

5.2 Image-Article Type Frequency Analysis

The increasing concern with Near Enemy issues over time can also be visualised in terms of an image-article type frequency analysis (see Figure 12.3b).

5.3 Image-Article Type Connections

The change in emphasis over time of image and article types can also be investigated by means of image-article type connections using arc graphs and interactive tables. Taking Issues 1 and 12 as examples, there are fewer and different image/article type combinations in Issue 1 than in Issue 12. This can be attributed to the greater variety of articles types in Issue 12 compared to Issue 1 (16 versus seven). An interrogation of image-article type connections for the categories (and subcategories) of Far and Near Enemies, for example, reveals a concentration of Near Enemy image categories and

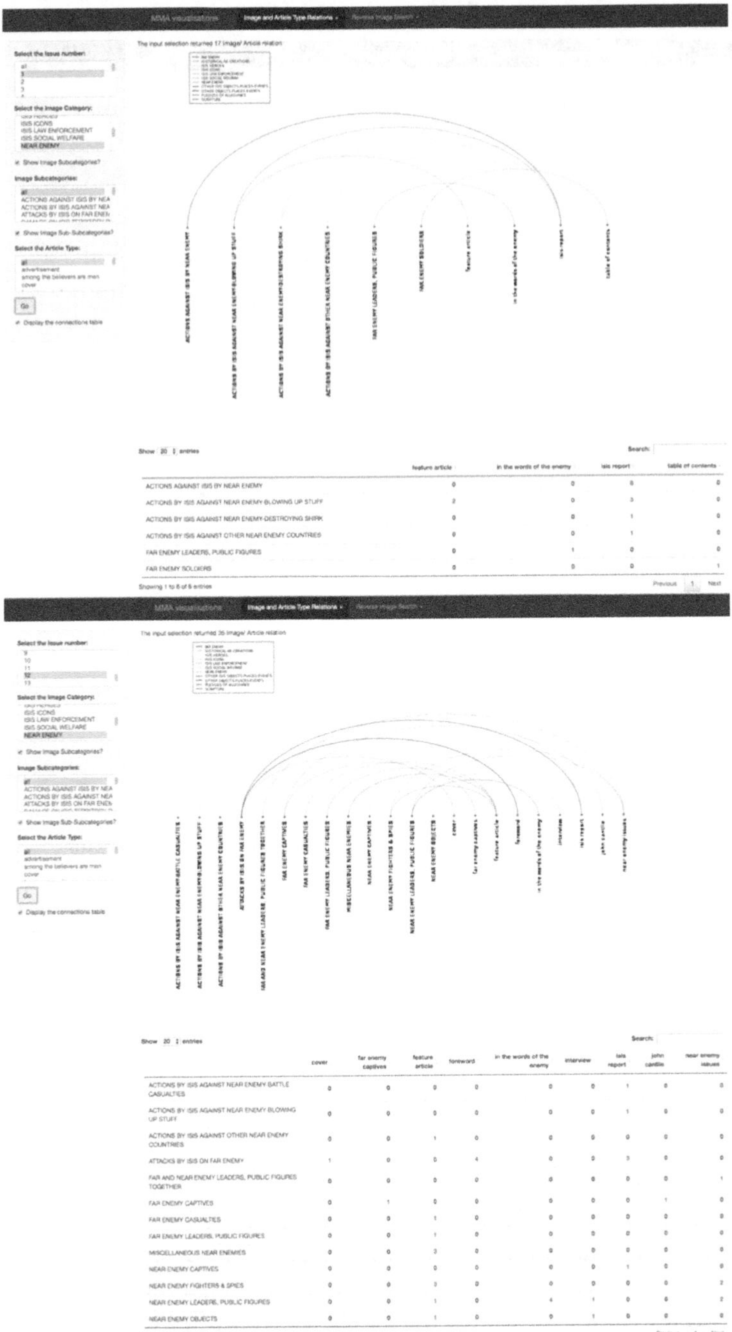

	feature article	in the words of the enemy	isis report	table of contents
ACTIONS AGAINST ISIS BY NEAR ENEMY	0	0	0	0
ACTIONS BY ISIS AGAINST NEAR ENEMY-BLOWING UP STUFF	2	0	3	0
ACTIONS BY ISIS AGAINST NEAR ENEMY-DESTROYING SHIRK	0	0	1	0
ACTIONS BY ISIS AGAINST OTHER NEAR ENEMY COUNTRIES	0	0	1	0
FAR ENEMY LEADERS, PUBLIC FIGURES	0	1	0	0
FAR ENEMY SOLDIERS	0	0	0	1

	cover	far enemy captives	feature article	foreword	in the words of the enemy	interview	isis report	john cantlie	near enemy issues
ACTIONS BY ISIS AGAINST NEAR ENEMY BATTLE CASUALTIES	0	0	0	0	0	0	1	0	0
ACTIONS BY ISIS AGAINST NEAR ENEMY BLOWING UP STUFF	0	0	0	0	0	0	1	0	0
ACTIONS BY ISIS AGAINST OTHER NEAR ENEMY COUNTRIES	0	0	1	0	0	0	0	0	0
ATTACKS BY ISIS ON FAR ENEMY	1	0	0	4	0	0	3	0	0
FAR AND NEAR ENEMY LEADERS, PUBLIC FIGURES TOGETHER	0	0	0	0	0	0	0	0	1
FAR ENEMY CAPTIVES	0	1	0	0	0	0	0	1	0
FAR ENEMY CASUALTIES	0	0	1	0	0	0	0	0	0
FAR ENEMY LEADERS, PUBLIC FIGURES	0	0	1	0	0	0	0	0	0
MISCELLANEOUS NEAR ENEMIES	0	0	3	0	0	0	0	0	0
NEAR ENEMY CAPTIVES	0	0	0	0	0	0	1	0	0
NEAR ENEMY FIGHTERS & SPIES	0	0	3	0	0	0	0	0	2
NEAR ENEMY LEADERS, PUBLIC FIGURES	0	0	1	0	4	1	0	0	2
NEAR ENEMY OBJECTS	0	0	1	0	0	1	0	0	0

Figure 12.3c Comparison of image-article type connections for the image categories and sub-categories of Far and Near Enemies in *Dabiq* Issue 1 (top) and 12 (bottom) (Note: Near Enemy sub-categories are represented by blue arcs, Far Enemy sub-categories by red arcs.)

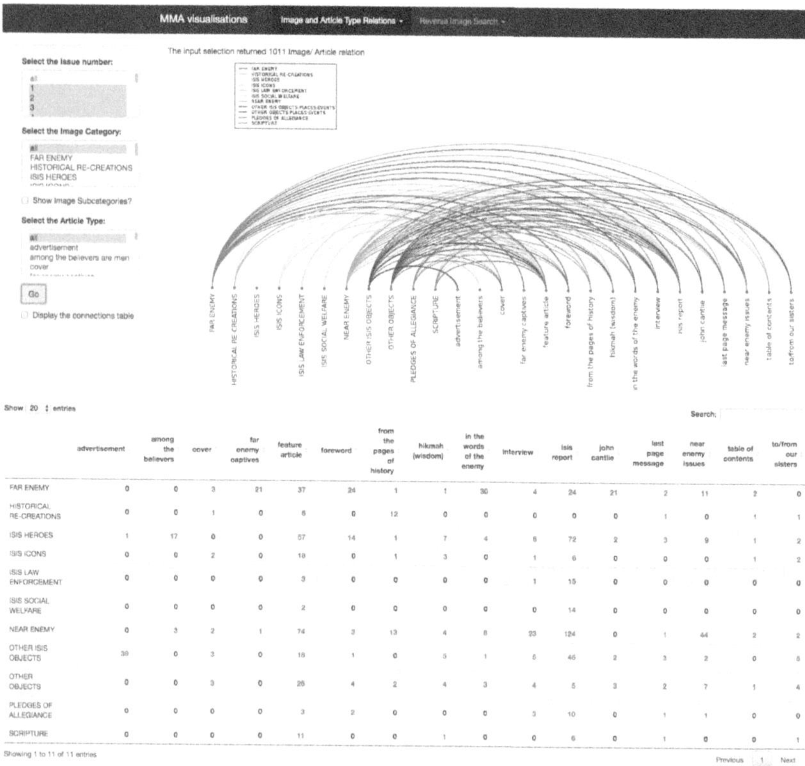

	advertisement	among the believers	cover	far enemy captives	feature article	foreword	from the pages of history	hikmah (wisdom)	in the words of the enemy	interview	isis report	john cantlie	last page message	near enemy issues	table of contents	to/from our sisters
FAR ENEMY	0	0	3	21	37	24	1	1	30	4	24	21	2	11	2	0
HISTORICAL RE-CREATIONS	0	0	1	0	6	0	12	0	0	0	0	0	1	0	1	1
ISIS HEROES	1	17	0	0	57	14	1	7	4	6	72	2	3	9	1	2
ISIS ICONS	0	0	2	0	18	0	1	3	0	1	6	0	0	0	1	2
ISIS LAW ENFORCEMENT	0	0	0	0	3	0	0	0	0	1	15	0	0	0	0	0
ISIS SOCIAL WELFARE	0	0	0	0	2	0	0	0	0	0	14	0	0	0	0	0
NEAR ENEMY	0	3	2	1	74	3	13	4	8	23	124	0	1	44	2	2
OTHER ISIS OBJECTS	39	0	3	0	18	1	0	5	1	6	46	2	3	2	0	8
OTHER OBJECTS	0	0	3	0	26	4	2	4	3	4	5	3	2	7	1	4
PLEDGES OF ALLEGIANCE	0	0	0	0	3	2	0	0	0	3	10	0	1	1	0	0
SCRIPTURE	0	0	0	0	11	0	0	1	0	0	6	0	1	0	0	1

Figure 12.3d Total number of image-article type connections in *Dabiq* Issues 1–14

subcategories in ISIS Reports in Issue 1. Both the graph and table in Figure 12.3c (top) show a total of four Near Enemy sub-categories distributed over two article types. In contrast, Figure 12.3c (bottom) reflects a much wider spread and diversity of image/article type connections in Issue 12.

The overall pattern of all image-article type combinations in the 14 issues of *Dabiq* is displayed in Figure 12.3d.

5.4 Reverse Image Search

The MMA Visualisation app has facilities for showing the results of the reverse image search which is used to trace the online locations of images found in *Dabiq*. The reverse image search was undertaken using TinEye,[3] which functions in a similar fashion to Google image search. That is, TinEye uses image identification technology rather than keywords, metadata, or watermarks, so searches are based on images. Upon submitting an image, TinEye creates a digital signature of the image and matches it with other indexed images. This procedure is able to match even heavily edited versions

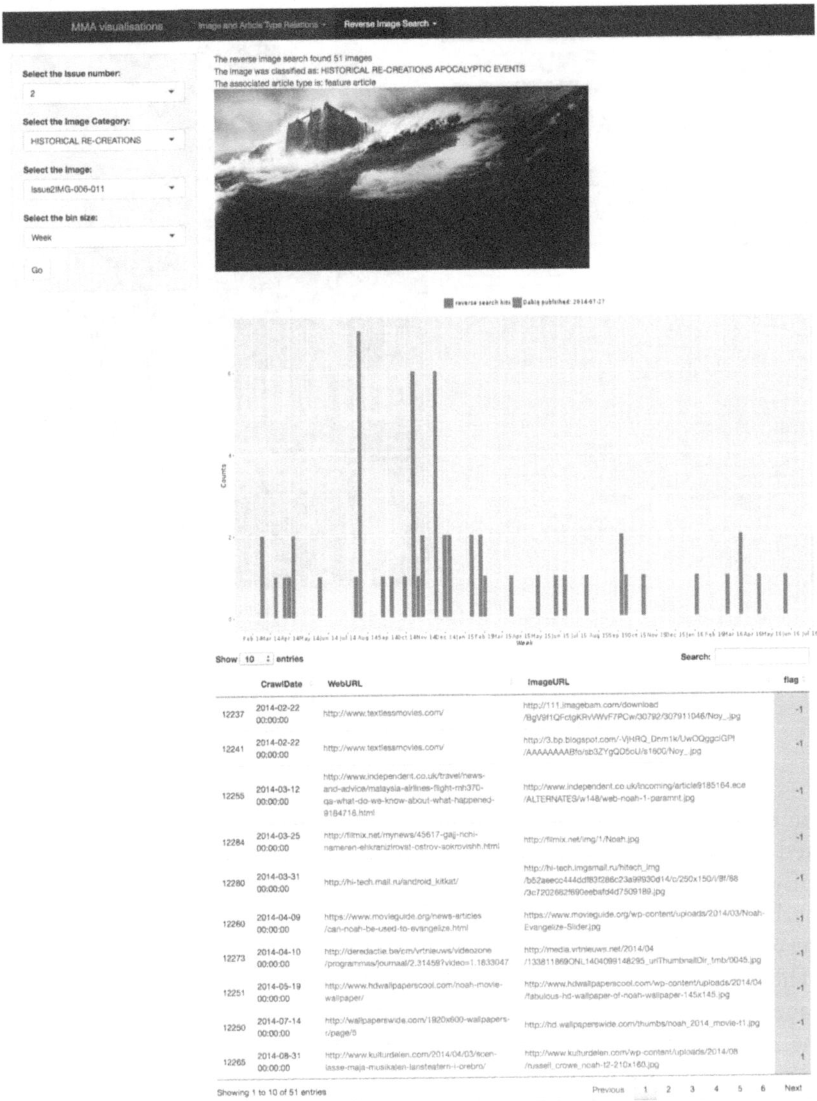

Figure 12.3e Reserve image search results for 'The Flood' in *Dabiq* Issue 2

of the submitted image. The results of the reverse image search include the URLs where the image is located and the date in which the site was indexed.

For example, the results of the reverse image search for the image of 'The Flood', which is featured in Issue 2 of *Dabiq* and categorised as an Apocalyptic Event, is displayed in Figure 12.3e. In the bar graph, the red bar is a marker of the publication date when the image appeared in *Dabiq*, and the grey bars indicate the frequency of appearances in other

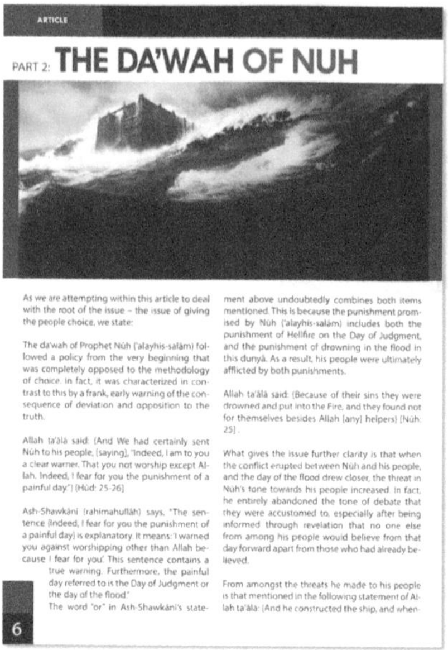

ARTICLE

PART 2: THE DA'WAH OF NUH

As we are attempting within this article to deal with the root of the issue – the issue of giving the people choice, we state:

The da'wah of Prophet Nûh ('alayhis-salâm) followed a policy from the very beginning that was completely opposed to the methodology of choice. In fact, it was characterized in contrast to this by a frank, early warning of the consequence of deviation and opposition to the truth.

Allah ta'âlâ said: {And We had certainly sent Nûh to his people, [saying], "Indeed, I am to you a clear warner. That you not worship except Allah. Indeed, I fear for you the punishment of a painful day."} [Hûd: 25-26]

Ash-Shawkânî (rahimahullâh) says, "The sentence {Indeed, I fear for you the punishment of a painful day} is explanatory. It means: 'I warned you against worshipping other than Allah because I fear for you.' This sentence contains a true warning. Furthermore, the painful day referred to is the Day of Judgment or the day of the flood."

The word "or" in Ash-Shawkânî's statement above undoubtedly combines both items mentioned. This is because the punishment promised by Nûh ('alayhis-salâm) includes both the punishment of Hellfire on the Day of Judgment, and the punishment of drowning in the flood in this dunyâ. As a result, his people were ultimately afflicted by both punishments.

Allah ta'âlâ said: {Because of their sins they were drowned and put into the Fire, and they found not for themselves besides Allah [any] helpers} [Nûh: 25].

What gives the issue further clarity is that when the conflict erupted between Nûh and his people, and the day of the flood drew closer, the threat in Nûh's tone towards his people increased. In fact, he entirely abandoned the tone of debate that they were accustomed to, especially after being informed through revelation that no one else from among his people would believe from that day forward apart from those who had already believed.

From amongst the threats he made to his people is that mentioned in the following statement of Allah ta'âlâ: {And he constructed the ship, and when-

6

Issue 2

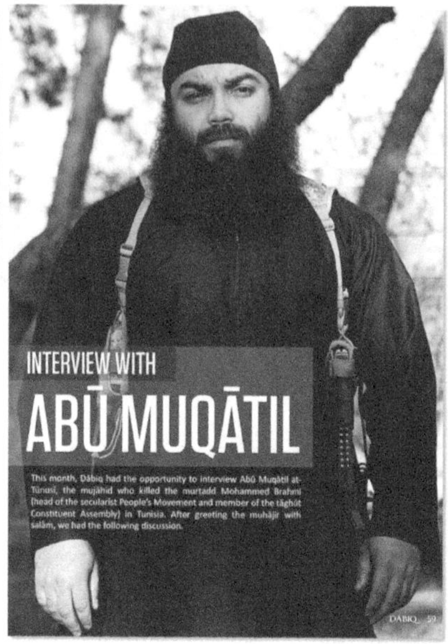
INTERVIEW WITH
ABŪ MUQĀTIL
This month, Dâbiq had the opportunity to interview Abû Muqâtil at-Tûnusi, the mujâhid who killed the murtadd Mohammed Brahmi (head of the secularist People's Movement and member of the tâghût Constituent Assembly) in Tunisia. After greeting the muhâjir with salâm, we had the following discussion.

Issue 8

Figure 12.3f Images which have been recontextualised in *Dabiq*, e.g., Apocalyptic Event (Issue 2, left), and images which have been recontextualised elsewhere after appearing in *Dabiq*, e.g., ISIS Hero (Issue 8, right).

online sites according to date. The various appearances of the image are listed below the graph according to an ID number, the crawl date of the TinEye search, the web URL, the image URL, and a flag which indicates whether the image appeared before it was published in *Dabiq* (-1) or afterwards (+1).

The reverse image search tool thus allows us to explore which type of images in *Dabiq* appeared or reappeared across different online sites over time. The reverse image search tool is particularly useful for investigating the recontextualised use of images either imported into or originating in *Dabiq*. For example, the results of the reverse image search for the image of 'The Flood' displayed in Figure 12.3e (reproduced in Figure 12.3f, left) reveals that the image appears to be cropped from a movie poster for the feature film *Noah* starring Russell Crowe, which was used by movieguide.org[4] in the context of evangelisation. An image identical to the one used in *Dabiq* also appeared on a wallpaper repository site, WallpapersWide.com,[5] before it was recontextualised by *Dabiq* as a warning to those who resist ISIS. There are other early records of the appearance of the image (as can be seen from the grey bars, which appear to the left of the red bar in Figure 12.3e), but in some cases, these websites are no longer accessible (e.g., the server cannot be found or access is prohibited).

A reverse image search can also yield insights about the recontextualised uses of images from *Dabiq* in discourses that function to resist terrorism. The recontextualised use of some images in counter-discourses is more evident in some cases than in others. For example, the reverse image search of an image that features an ISIS Hero 'Abū Muqātil', which appeared in *Dabiq* Issue 8 (Figure 12.3f, right), found images of the same person, renamed 'Abu Muquack' and with the face of a rubber duck in place of his own face in the magazine MAXIM (maxim.com).[6] This image, which originated as part of a campaign called 'Allahu Quackbar' by the hacker group Anonymous, has found its way on to a number of social media, entertainment news and magazine websites and reveals that the same image was recontextualised explicitly for the purpose of resisting violent extremist discourse, as shown by the case of MAXIM magazine. As such, MMA Visualisation app has the potential to permit widespread investigation of exactly how violent extremist images are re-used across different media sites for different purposes.

The MMA Visualisation app also provides an overview of the websites in which images from *Dabiq* are found by means of an integrated word-cloud tool. For example, the word cloud in Figure 12.3g (top) reveals that images from the Far Enemy category in Issue 1 appeared mainly on news websites, such as bbc.com, heraldsun.com, merdeka.com, but also

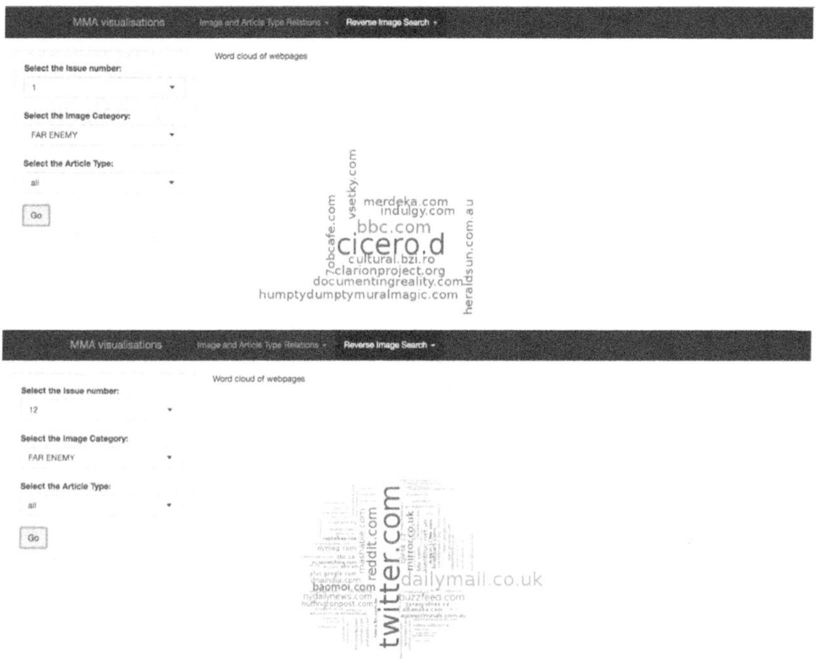

Figure 12.3g Word cloud of URLs of websites with the same or similar images categorised as 'Far Enemy' in *Dabiq* Issue 1

on some more sinister websites, such as documentingrealtiy.com, which is a source for death pictures and death videos. In contrast, images from the same category in Issue 12 (Figure 12.3g, bottom) also circulated on social media, social news, and entertainment networking sites, such as twitter.com, reddit.com, mashable.com, buzzfeed.com, etc. In this way, it is possible to explore trends in relation to the appearance of different images over different media sites over time.

6. Conclusion and Future Directions

While the pilot project has yielded some interesting patterns and results, the next stage involves applying these insights to the analysis of large datasets. The contextualisation of images in *Dabiq* provides a baseline and reference point for analysing recontextualisations both before and after publication in *Dabiq*. Going forward, we are faced with some fundamental questions which have yet to be resolved. For instance, machine learning techniques can be applied to the text and images which have been manually analysed for big data analytics, but what about the new materials (i.e. textual and visual) found on websites where the re-used images appear? A mixed-methods approach (O'Halloran, Tan, Pham, Bateman, & Vande Moere, 2016) proposes to overcome the problems associated with analysing large datasets by using contextual information derived from metadata and Wikipedia's categorisation system which provides higher order semantic classifications of key words and objects to assist with the interpretative process. Together with natural language processing algorithms (e.g., keyword identification, sentiment analysis), we hope to automatically ascertain information about the nature of the multimodal recontextualisations of the images across different media sites. This process will not be straightforward, however, given the large number of different media platforms in which the images are found and the wide range of texts which are involved.

With this in mind, our next step is to apply image-processing techniques to the *Dabiq* images in order to identify the key characteristics of the images (e.g., icons, objects, faces, focus, perspective) which are associated with the different image categories. From here, we can build up a picture of the visual systems which are at play in these images and how choices from these systems are exploited in order to support and resist violent extremism. Following this, we aim to explore the use of natural language processing algorithms and Wikipedia categorisation trees for automatic classifications of the texts in which these images appear, with a view to developing interactive visualisations for exploring the patterns thus established. In this way, we aim to investigate the potential of multimodal semiotics for understanding how multimodal recontextualisations reconfigure social practices, building upon the theoretical principles developed by Van Leeuwen (2005, 2008).

Notes

1 www.clarionproject.org/news/islamic-state-isis-isil-propaganda-magazine-dabiq
2 Even in cases where women are present in the images, they are categorically pixelated in *Dabiq*.
3 www.tineye.com/
4 www.movieguide.org/news-articles/can-noah-be-used-to-evangelize.html
5 http://wallpaperswide.com/1920x600-wallpapers-r/page/5
6 www.maxim.com/maxim-man/article/isis-fighters-duck-photoshop-2015-12

References

Bateman, J. (2014). Using multimodal corpora for empirical research. In C. Jewitt (Ed.), *The Routledge handbook of mutimodal analysis* (pp. 238–252). London/New York: Routedge.

Bernstein, B. (1990). *Class, codes and control, Volume IV: The structuring of pedagogic discourse*. London: Routledge.

Blanchard, C. (2007). *The Islamic traditions of Wahhabism and Salafiyya*. Washington, DC: Congressional Research Service.

Bowering, G., Crone, P., Kadi, W., Stewart, D. J., Zaman, M. Q., & Mirza, M. (2012). *The Princeton encyclopedia of Islamic political thought*. Princeton, NJ: Princeton University Press.

Burke, J. (2004, May–June). Al Qaeda. *Foreign Policy, 142*. Washington, DC: Washington Post Newsweek.

Byman, D. L. (2003). Al-Qaeda as an adversary: Do we understand our enemy? *World Politics, 56/1*, 139–163. doi:10.1353/wp.2004.0002.

Colas, B. (2016). What does *Dabiq* do? ISIS hermeneutics and organizational fractures within *Dabiq* Magazine. *Studies in Conflict & Terrorism, 40*(3), 173–190. doi:10.1080/1057610X.2016.1184062

Gerges, F. (2009). *The far enemy: Why Jihad went global*. New York: Cambridge University Press.

Halliday, M. A. K. (1978). *Language as social semiotic: The social interpretation of language and meaning*. London: Edward Arnold.

Halliday, M. A. K., & Matthiessen, C. M. I. M. (2014). *Halliday's introduction to functional grammar* (4th ed., revised by C. M. I. M. Matthiessen, Ed.). London/New York: Routledge.

Kepel, G. (2002). *The trail of political Islam*. Cambridge: Harvard University Press.

Kress, G., & Van Leeuwen, T. (2006). *Reading images: The grammar of visual design* (2nd ed.). London: Routledge.

Martin, J., & Stenglin, M. (2007). Materialising reconciliation: Negotiating difference in a transcolonial exhibition. In T. Royce & W. Bowcher (Eds.), *New directions in the analysis of multimodal discourse* (pp. 215–238). Mahwah, NJ: Lawrence Erlbaum Associates, Publishers.

Martin, J. R., & Zappavigna, M. (2013). Youth justice conferencing: Ceremonial redress. *International Journal of Law, Language & Discourse, 3/2*, 103–142.

O'Halloran, K. L., Chua, A., & Podlasov, A. (2014). The role of images in social media analytics: A multimodal digital humanities approach. In D. Machin (Ed.), *Visual communication* (pp. 565–588). Berlin: Gruyter.

O'Halloran, K. L., Tan, S., Pham, D.-S., Bateman, J., & Vande Moere, A. (2016). A digital mixed methods research design: Integrating multimodal analysis with data mining and information visualization for big data analytics. *Journal of Mixed Methods Research*. doi:10.1177/1558689816651015

O'Halloran, K. L., Tan, S., Wignell, P., Bateman, J. A., Pham, D.-S., Grossman, M., & Moere, A. V. (2016). Interpreting text and image relations in violent extremist discourse: A mixed methods approach for big data analytics. *Terrorism and Political Violence*, 1–21. doi:10.1080/09546553.2016.1233871.

Olidort, J. (2015, November 24). What is Salafism? *Foreign Affairs*. Retrieved from www.foreignaffairs.com/articles/syria/2015-11-24/what-salafism

Rashid, A. (2015). *ISIS: Race to Armageddon*. New Delhi: Vij Books.

Shneiderman, B. (1996). The eyes have it: A task by data type taxonomy for information visualisations. In *Proceedings of IEEE Symposium on Visual Languages* (pp. 336–343). Boulder, CO: IEEE.

Tabarani, G. (2011). *Jihad's new Heartlands: Why the West has failed to contain Islamic Fundamentalism*. Milton Keynes: Author House.

Tann, K. (2013). The language of identity discourse: Introducing a framework for functional iconography. *Linguistics and the Human Sciences*, *8*(3), 361–391.

Van Leeuwen, T. (2005). *Introducing social semiotics*. London: Routledge.

Van Leeuwen, T. (2008). *Discourse and practice: New tools for critical discourse analysis*. Oxford: Oxford Univerity Press.

Vergani, M., & Bliuc, A.-M. (2015). The evolution of the ISIS' language: A quantitative analysis of the language of the first year of *Dabiq* Magazine. *Sicurezza, Terrorismo e Società*, *1*(2), 7–20.

Wignell, P., Tan, S., & O'Halloran, K. L. (2017). Violent extremism and iconisation: Commanding good and forbidding evil? *Critical Discourse Studies*, *14*(1), 1–22. doi:10.1080/17405904.2016.1250652

Zelin, A. Y. (2015). Picture or it didn't happen: A snapshot of the Islamic State's official media output. *Perspectives on Terrorism*, *9*(4), 85–96.

Zelinsky, N. (2014, September 3). ISIS sends a message: What gestures say about today's middle east. *Foreign Affairs*. Retrieved from www.foreignaffairs.com/articles/middle-east/2014-09-03/isis-sends-message

Revisiting the Family Silver: A Visual Essay on the Grammar of Visual Design

Morten Boeriis

In this visual essay, a number of the key grammatical notions in visual social semiotics are treated from a multimodal perspective. The aim is to discuss and develop the theory by conducting visual commutations, i.e. displaying the consequences of various available choices and thereby attempting to isolate the parameters, their interplay, and their semiotic consequences in visual meaning-making. As much as the article is a visual discussion of theoretical and descriptive issues, it is also an implicit meta-discussion about what can be discussed visually and how, exploring ways to shed light on theoretical issues.

Topics are:

Process fusion: Material processes (facial muscular action) at the Component level fuse into expressing cognitive, affective, and expressive processes at the Figure level. Several processes at the Figure level fuse into one Group-level process.

Frontal planes: Rhetor positions the perceiver at a specific viewpoint, but objects in visual texts can have several frontal planes.

The human body: Five frontal planes (face, shoulder, pelvis, knee and feet) + gaze. But what about Components such as arms, legs, fingers?

Groups: Parallel lines but also combined frontal planes of the Figures that make up the Group.

Vertical viewpoint: Dominant vs. subservient; exerting power vs. negating power; complaisant vs. unaccommodating.

Horizontal viewpoint: Partial or complete involvement; material or mental involvement.

Viewpoint distance: At a certain level the motif changes (dynamic rank scale).

Grids as meaning: Systems; segregation; separation.

Aspect ratio: The meaning of frame proportions.

Empty space: In front or behind participants; circumstantial setting; mental activity; elided participant; tension; cohesive-logical setup.

Ideational information value: Perceived processual variance between mirrored images; information value constrains the transitivity; more vs. less smiling; determination vs. melancholy, more vs. less leaning back or forth; more vs. less squinting of eyes; more vs. less lifted eyebrows; determined visionary gaze vs. melancholic dreaming gaze.

Process fusion

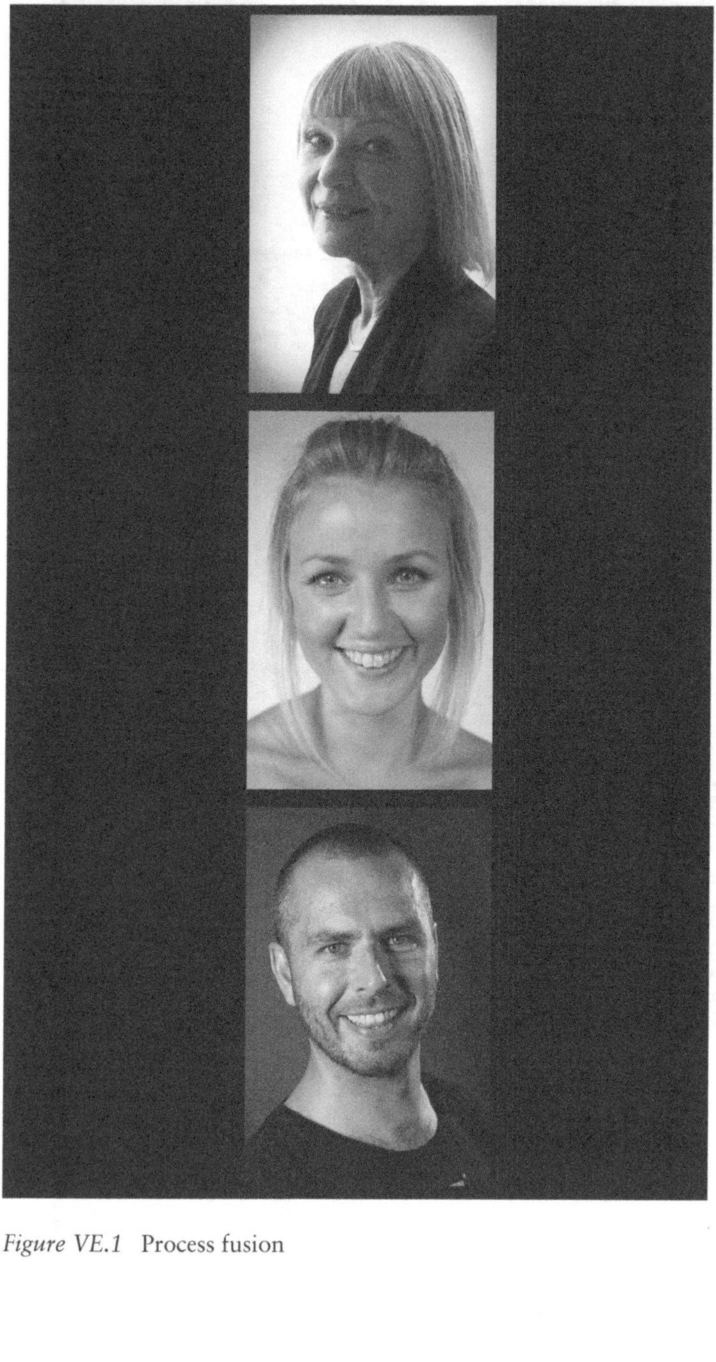

Figure VE.1 Process fusion

Frontal planes

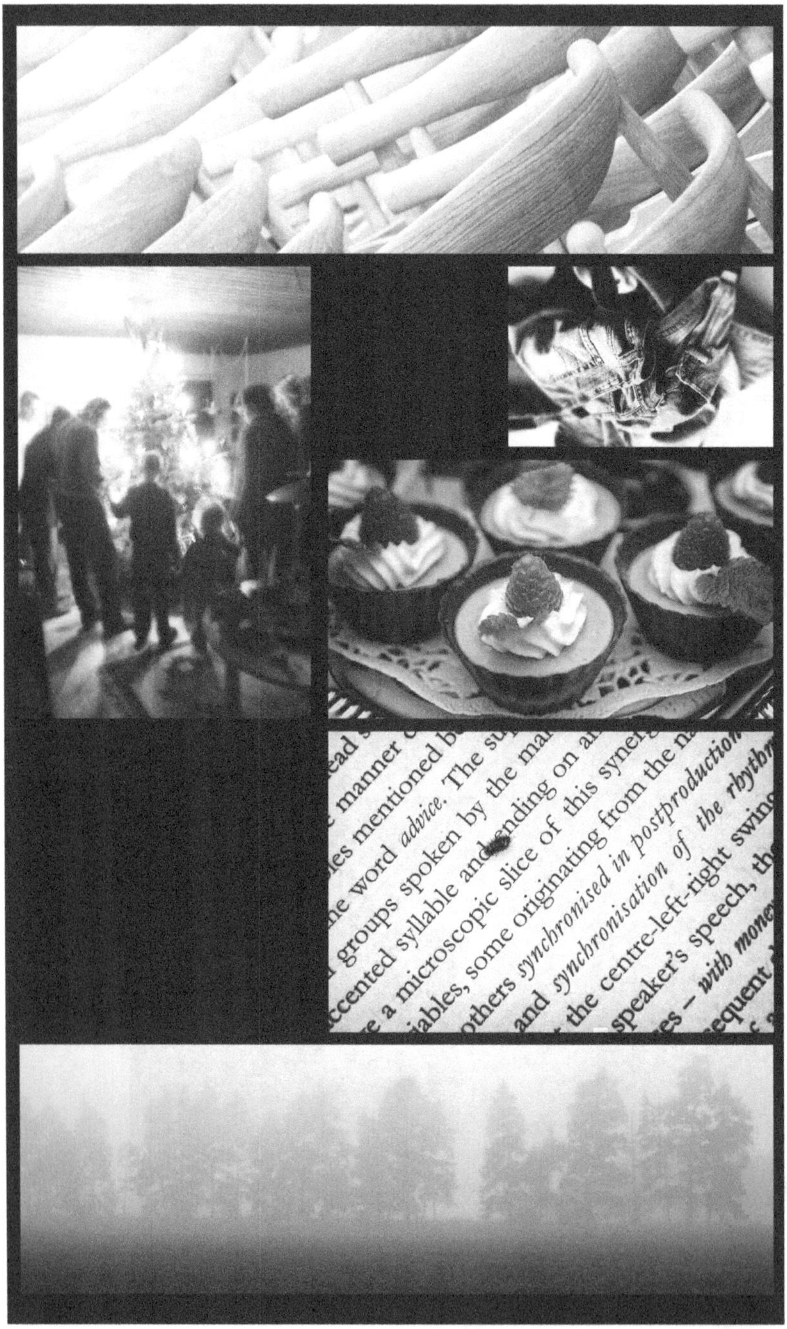

Figure VE.2 Frontal planes

Vertical viewpoint

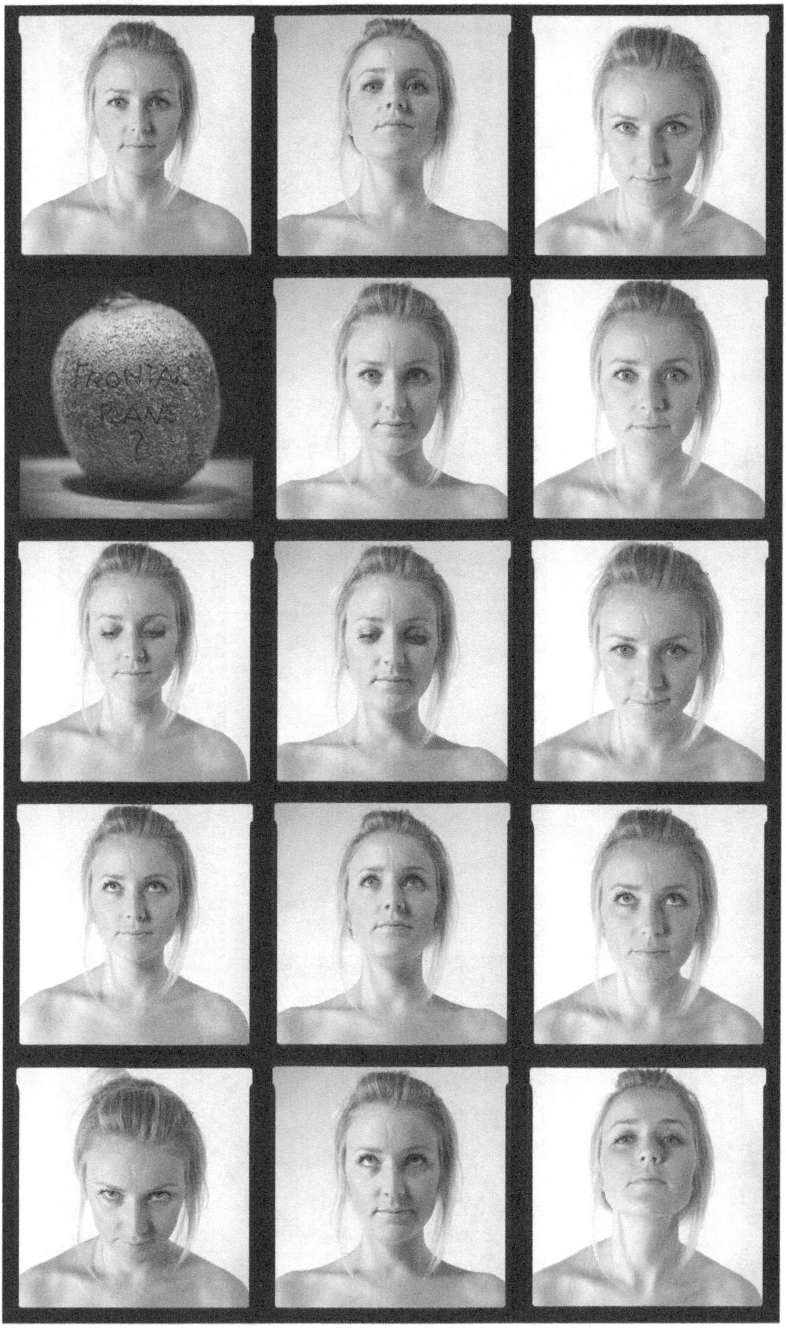

Figure VE.3 Vertical viewpoint

Horizontal viewpoint

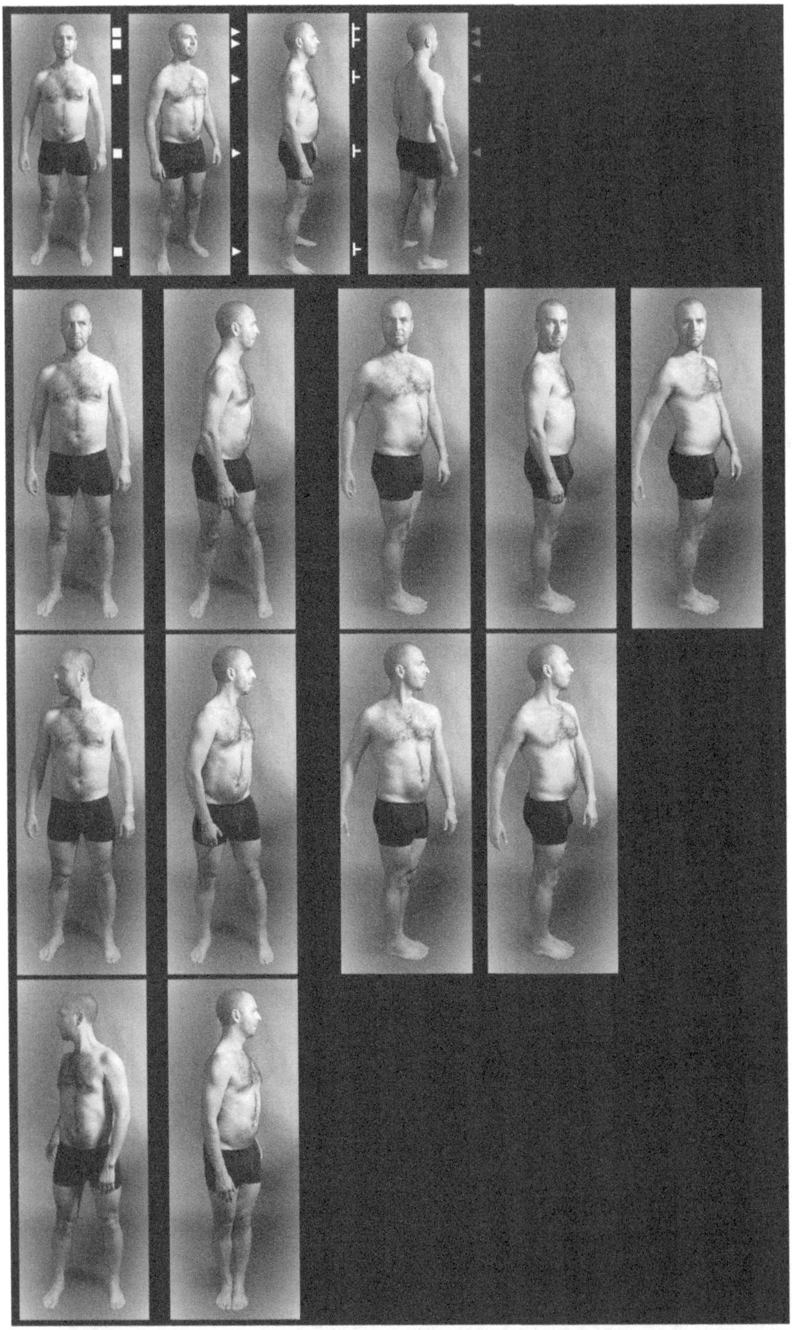

Figure VE.4 Horizontal viewpoint

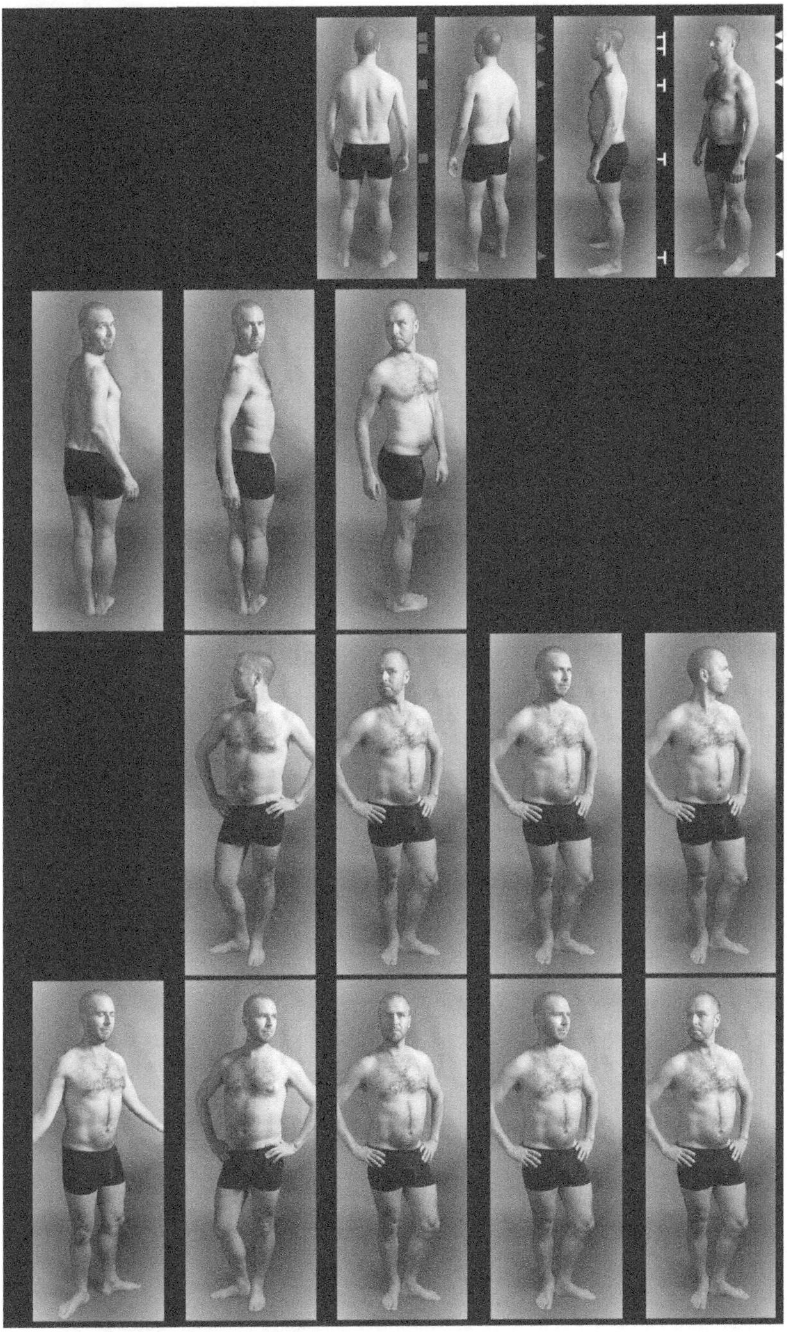

Figure VE.5 Horizontal viewpoint 2

Viewpoint distance

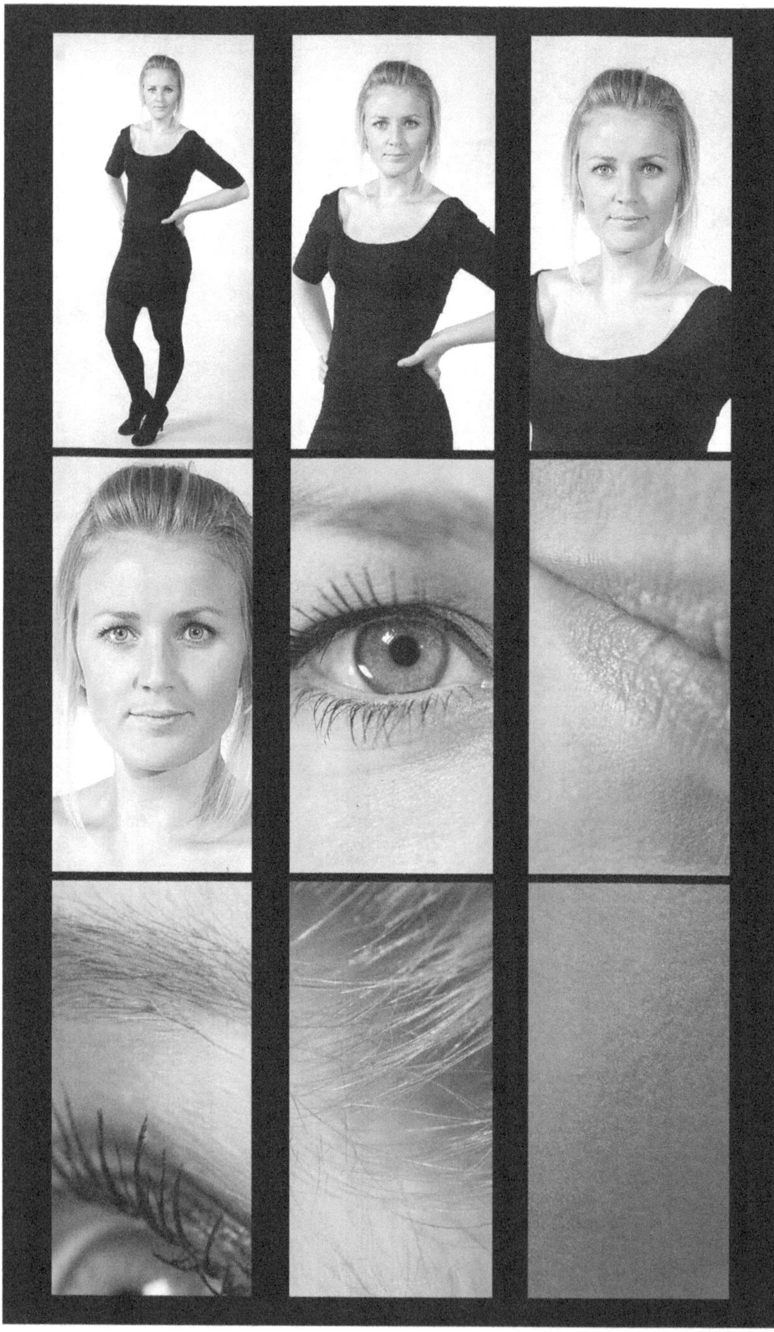

Figure VE.6 Viewpoint distance

Grids as meaning

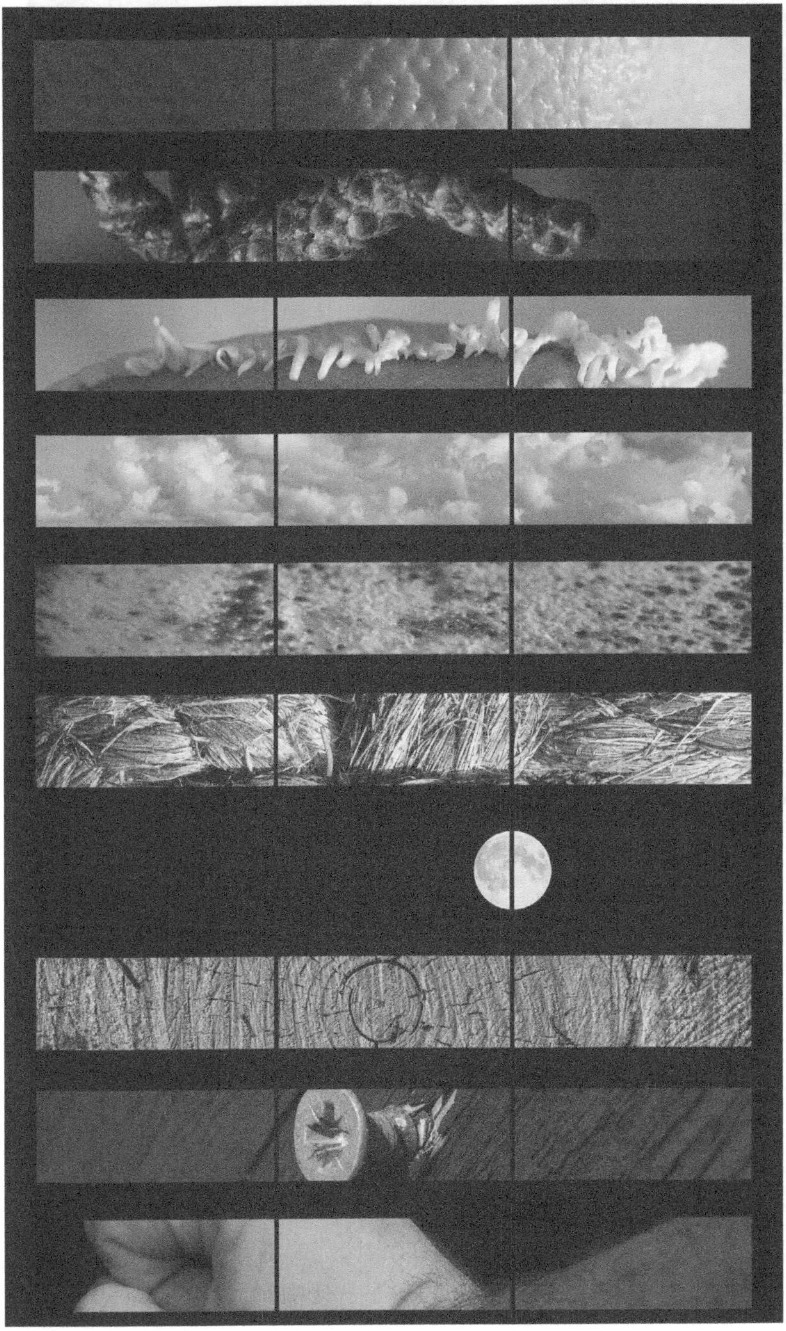

Figure VE.7 Grids as meaning

Framing

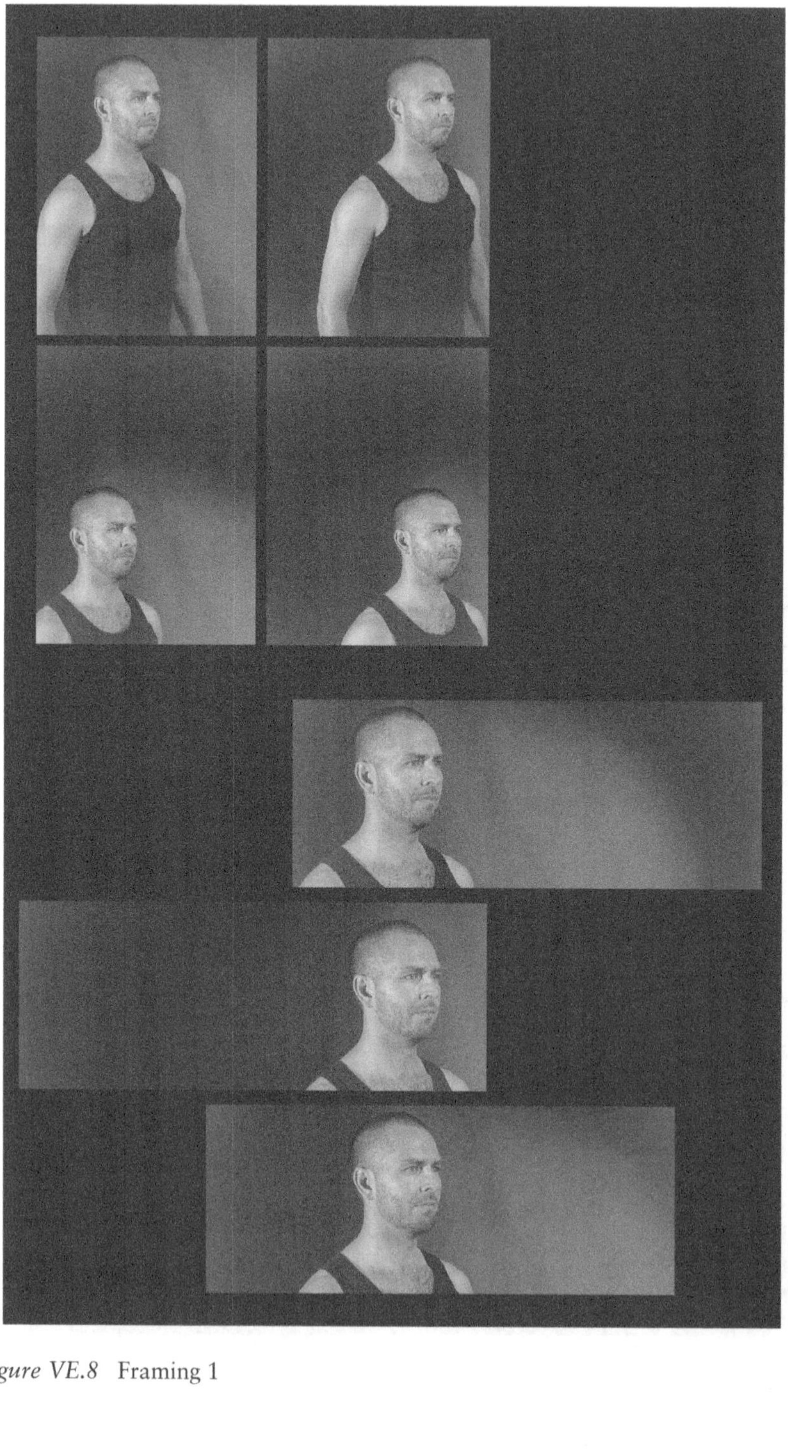

Figure VE.8 Framing 1

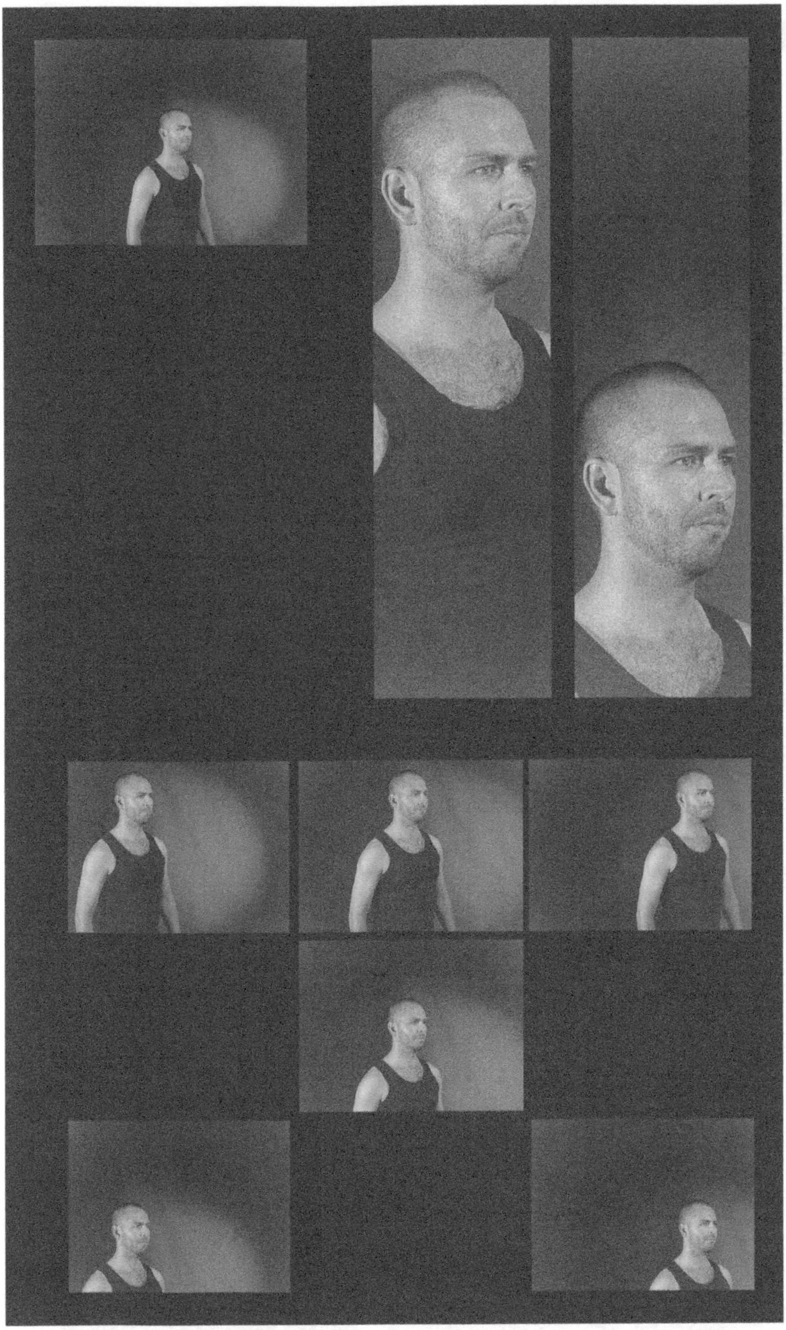

Figure VE.9 Framing 2

Ideational information value

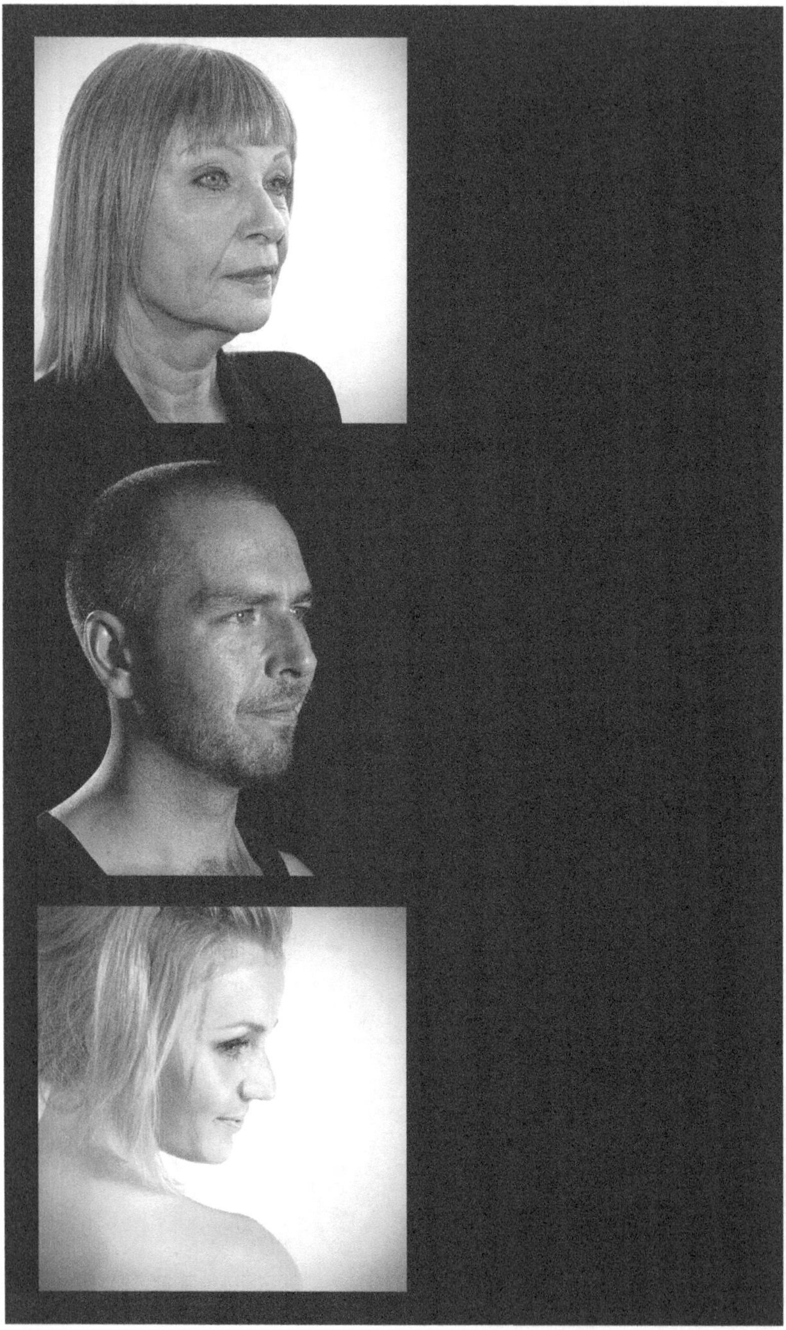

Figure VE.10 Ideational information value 1

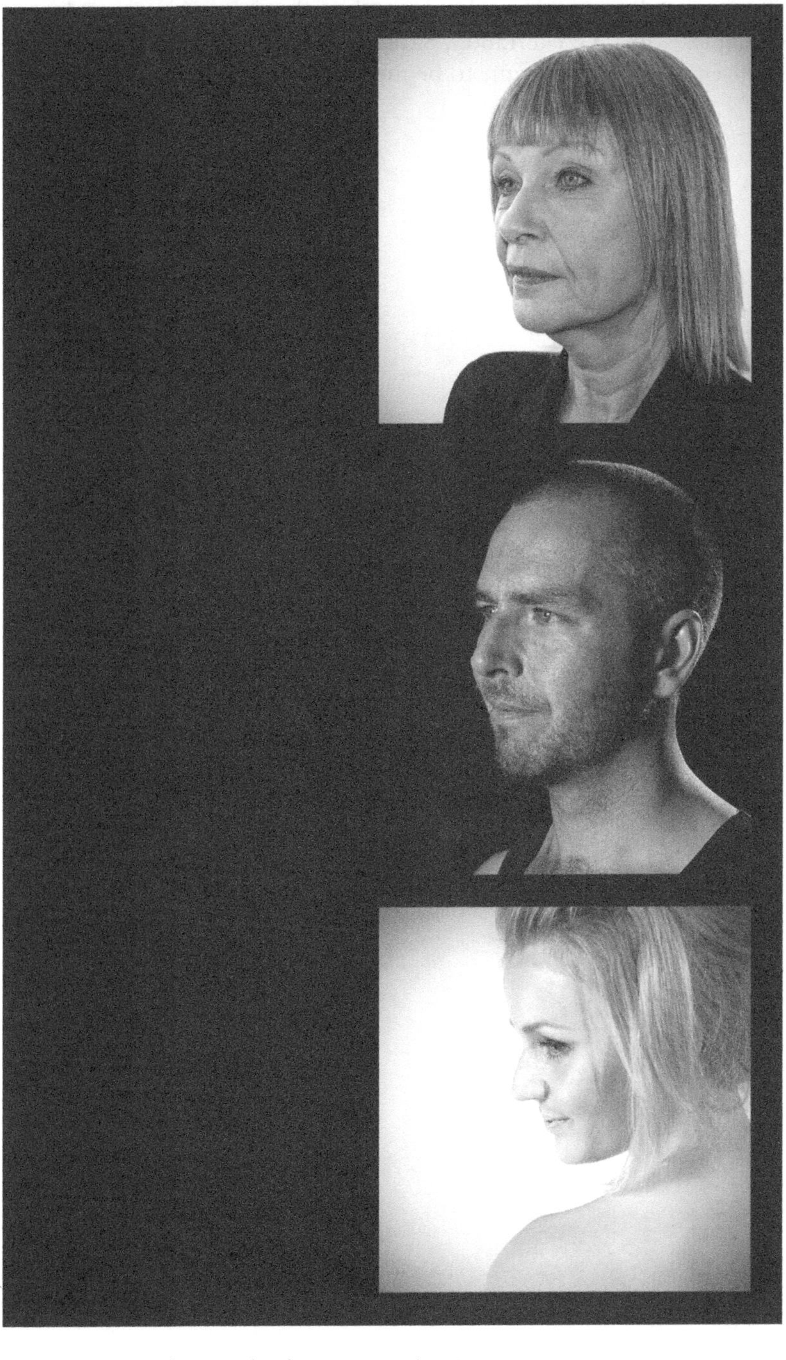

Figure VE.11 Ideational information value 2

Acknowledgement

All photos are taken and edited by the author. Special thanks to my beautiful colleagues Anna Vibeke Lindø, Sarah Bro Pedersen, and Kasper Østerholdt Jensen for taking the time to be motifs.

Index

abstraction 23, 40, 42, 53, 56–7, 110, 147, 162
aesthetic(s) 8, 54, 56, 63, 118, 150, 165, 168, 171, 176
aestheticisation 173
affordance 2, 4, 6, 13, 84, 86, 92
agency 74–5, 83, 87, 147, 148, 162, 168
analysis: discourse-historical 46; discourse (*see* Critical Discourse Analysis; Multimodal (Discourse) Analysis); lexical 40; methods and principles of 8, 10, 24, 27, 36, 47, 50, 52, 68, 73, 90, 131, 137, 142, 150–1, 169, 182; semiotic 2, 52–3, 57, 62–5, 68–9, 95, 169; sentiment 200; social semiotic 84, 90–1, 119, 132, 137
anti-consumerism 167–168
artefacts 81, 88–9, 165; semiotic 10, 184; upcycled 166–9, 171, 173, 178–9; value of 170
artificial intelligence 117–18, 125, 128
aural mode 83, 86, 154
aural realism 119
aural parameters 115, 119
authenticity 7, 154, 156, 172, 192

Bakhtin, Mikhail Mikhailovich 70, 168
Barthes, Roland 1, 55–6, 176, 178
body 80, 83, 89, 91, 124, 147–8, 158, 160–1; as metaphor (*see* body-border politics under politics)
border *see* moralisation; *see also* body-border politics
brand(ing) 8, 160, 166, 168, 173, 176–8
Bernstein, Basil 8, 181
codification 148, 157, 162
coding orientation 52–4, 62–3, 64, 119
coherence 11, 13, 23, 27, 28, 132, 135, 144, 147, 152, 153, 162
cohesion 11, 23, 27, 136, 139, 141, 143, 149
colour 1, 4, 7, 70, 83, 95, 109–10, 152, 169, 176, 178, 185, 189
commodification 148–9, 162
community currency 95–7, 101, 103, 105–7, 109, 110–11
connotative provenance 171–2, 173, 176, 177
consumerism 9, 148, 165, 168; *see also* anti-consumerism
context 3, 6, 8, 10, 11, 35–7, 38, 51–2, 62, 65, 67–8, 69–70, 75, 85–6, 87, 89, 91, 132, 151, 184; of culture 2, 66; epistemic 68, 71, 73; of situation 2, 66; social 2, 68, 73, 82, 115
contextualisation 63; *see also* recontextualisation
choice 3–4, 7, 10, 14, 24, 55, 95, 102, 106, 108, 110–11, 135, 151, 185, 200, 203
Critical Discourse Analysis/Studies (CDA) 8, 24, 181
common sense 32, 35–6, 46, 52, 55

data 21, 158; big 181–2; meta- (*see* metadata); mining 185; visualisation (*see* visualisation)
dataset, large 181–2, 185, 200
discourse: critical (*see* critical discourse analysis/studies); of immigration 33, 38; legitimation (*see* legitimation); multimodal (*see* multimodal discourse); racist

58, 65; technologisation of 148; terrorism/terrorist 41, 46, 190, 199
design 5, 11, 24, 26–8, 89, 96–7, 103, 106, 148, 150, 166, 169; learning 74; software 10–11; sound 120, 128; visual 4, 11, 21, 149
distribution 5, 8, 26, 28
dynamic *see* sound

Eco, Umberto 51, 56
epistemic context 68, 71, 73–4, 75

film techniques: character development 136, 142–3; intercut 138, 140–1; multiple endings 131–2, 134–5, 143; score 116–17, 124–25; soundtrack (*see* soundtrack)
framing 7, 36, 69, 75, 151–2, 153–4, 158, 191, 212

genre 7, 9, 23, 26–7, 52, 71, 131–2; structure 133–4, 136–7
gesture 23, 80–1, 191
grammar 4, 21–2, 25–6, 50, 86; *see also* sound grammar; visual grammar

Halliday, M. A. K. 4, 9, 20–1, 22–3, 51, 66, 75, 82, 86–7
Hasan, Ruquaia 51

identity 8, 106–8, 110, 118, 141, 148; politics (*see* politics)
image: analytical 107–8; analytical methods 20–4, 27–8, 52, 55–6, 61, 65, 181–2, 185–6, 196–7, 200 (*see also* reverse image search); conceptual 52; -text (article) relation 52, 54, 185, 188, 192–4
immigration *see* immigration discourse in discourse
institution 42, 148
institutional context 2–3, 73
institutional domain 71, 74
institutional framing 69, 75
interactive fiction 135
intertextual(ity) 6, 67–8, 125, 176, 178–9

Language as Ideology (1978) 19–20
legitimation 35–6, 46; strategies 31–4, 41–2, 45; *see also* rationalisation
lexical analysis *see* analysis
Lexis 4, 22
learning 68–9, 73–5, 89; *see also* machine learning
logical relations 133, 142, 144

marketisation 149, 162
materiality 2, 5–6, 22–3, 79, 81–2, 83–4, 86, 150–1, 169–170
material resources *see* resources
meaning potential 2, 4, 6, 74, 84, 88–9
media 10, 27–8, 46, 132, 149, 164–5, 199
metadata 182, 196, 200
metafunctions 4, 75, 82, 87, 184; ideational/experiential 4, 6–7, 20, 80, 82, 85, 86–7, 115, 125, 171–2, 185–6, 204, 214; interpersonal 4, 6, 20–1, 79–80, 82, 86–7, 184, 191; textual 4, 6, 20, 86–7
modality 4, 5, 22, 24, 53, 109–10; in sound 115, 119
mode 4–5, 10, 20, 22–3, 25–7, 79, 80–1, 82–4, 86, 87–8, 90–1
money 95–7, 106, 109–11
moralisation 42; of borders 34–5, 44, 46
Multimodal Discourse (2001) 3–4, 5, 24, 26–8
multimodal (discourse) analysis (MDA) 5, 9, 28, 81, 83, 181, 182
multimodality 3, 4–5, 25, 28, 83–4, 91
multiple endings *see* film techniques
music 6, 20, 23, 83, 115, 116–17, 120, 124–5

narrative 73, 117, 120, 131, 134–5, 136, 142
narrative strands 138–40, 143
narrative structure 134, 137, 138
neoliberal(ism) 26, 148, 150–1, 154
new writing 11, 147, 148–50, 152–4, 156, 158, 160
noise 115–16
norm/normative/normativity 10, 34, 36, 83, 90–1

objects 2, 4, 5, 25, 80, 85, 88, 90, 151, 170, 176, 179; responsive 88–9; upcycled 167, 168, 173

parametric system 6–7
performance management 158, 161
photograph(ic) 52, 55, 56–7, 58, 63, 65

politics 32, 46, 183; border-and-body 31, 34; of fear 47
popular culture 9
post-truth society 28
power 19, 22, 68, 70, 81, 83, 90, 91, 151, 162, 203
practitioners 115, 128
production 5–6, 8, 26, 28, 89
provenance 6–7, 85, 115, 124, 151, 156, 161, 171–3, 176–7, 178–9; *see also* connotative provenance

rationalisation 31–2, 35, 42–43, 44–7
Reading Images (1996/2006) 3–4, 6, 21, 24–5, 26–7
realism 24; *see also* aural realism
recontextualisation 8, 47, 165, 167–9, 170–1, 178–9, 181, 192, 200
recycling 165, 178
reification 57–8, 65
resources: material 5, 6, 7, 10, 20, 84, 167; semiotic (*see* semiotic resources)
responsive objects *see* objects
reverse image search 196–7, 198–9
Rhetorical Structure Theory 132
rhyming 152–3, 154

salience 7, 189; science fiction 116–17, 128, 138, 139
self-management 162
semantic classification 182, 185
semiotic artefact *see* artefact
semiotic change 3, 27, 165
semiotic mode *see* mode
semiotic potential 7, 82, 168–9, 170–1, 173, 177
semiotic regimes 3, 171
semiotic resources 2–3, 5–6, 10–11, 23, 53, 74, 79, 81–2, 83–5, 86, 91–2, 147, 149, 151, 169, 171–2, 176, 178–9, 184–5
semiotic technology/software technologies 9, 10–11, 14
senses/sensory 81–2, 83–6, 91, 92, 176
sensory coding 4, 119–20
social, the 23, 26, 27, 28, 75, 88
social actor 8, 9, 43, 88, 190
social context 2, 12, 68, 74, 82
social norms 83, 90; *see also* norms
social practices 1, 2, 5, 7, 8–9, 31, 147, 149–50, 154, 162, 165, 169–70, 181, 185, 189, 200
social semiotics 2, 7, 8, 10, 11, 24, 27, 28, 68, 73, 81, 82–3, 88, 90, 91, 128, 151, 168, 170, 184, 203
Sontag, Susan 52
sound 5–6, 20, 81–2, 86–7, 115–16, 117, 119–20, 125–6, 128
sound resources: pitch 82, 115, 119, 120, 126, 128; timbre 6, 7, 81, 115, 119, 120, 126; voice quality 115, 120, 126
soundtrack 115, 117, 118, 119–20, 126, 139
space 11, 150–1, 154, 156
speech 19–20, 22–3, 24–5, 116
stratification 133
stratum/strata 5, 28, 132–3, 139
subjective experience 115, 120
synaesthesia 7
synthesizer 117, 122, 128
Systemic Functional Linguistics (SFL)/ Semiotics (SFS) 4, 6, 9, 31, 51

tactile 7, 82, 84–5, 86–7, 89, 90, 106, 110
taste 7
text 10, 23, 24, 27, 51, 52, 56–7, 62–63, 64, 65–6, 67–8, 69–70, 132–3, 144, 149, 162
texture 7, 82, 85–6, 88, 95, 105–06, 110, 150, 151–2, 154, 172–3, 177
Topos/Topoi 33, 36–7, 41–2, 43, 44–6
touch: materiality of 83–4; as mode 86–87, 89; properties of 90–1; types of 88
touch communication 79–80, 89
typography 5, 7

upcycled artefacts *see* artefact
upcycling 165–7, 169–70, 171, 173, 178–9

value 97, 101, 110, 165–6, 168–9, 170–1, 173, 178–9
visual design *see* design
visualisation 182, 192, 196, 199